American
Diabetes
Association®

LIFE *with* DIABETES

A Series of Teaching Outlines
by the Michigan Diabetes Research
and Training Center

— 4th Edition —

Director, Book Publishing, Robert Anthony; Managing Editor, Book Publishing, Abe Ogden; Editor, Rebekah Renshaw; Production Manager, Melissa Sprott; Composition, ADA; Cover Design, Koncept, Inc.; Illustrations, Duckwell Productions; Printer, R.R. Donnelley

Printed in the United States of America
1 3 5 7 9 10 8 6 4 2

The suggestions and information contained in this publication are generally consistent with the *Clinical Practice Recommendations* and other policies of the American Diabetes Association, but they do not represent the policy or position of the Association or any of its boards or committees. Reasonable steps have been taken to ensure the accuracy of the information presented. However, the American Diabetes Association cannot ensure the safety or efficacy of any product or service described in this publication. Individuals are advised to consult a physician or other appropriate health care professional before undertaking any diet or exercise program or taking any medication referred to in this publication. Professionals must use and apply their own professional judgment, experience, and training and should not rely solely on the information contained in this publication before prescribing any diet, exercise, or medication. The American Diabetes Association—its officers, directors, employees, volunteers, and members—assumes no responsibility or liability for personal or other injury, loss, or damage that may result from the suggestions or information in this publication.

♾ The paper in this publication meets the requirements of the ANSI Standard Z39.48-1992 (permanence of paper).

ADA titles may be purchased for business or promotional use or for special sales. To purchase more than 50 copies of this book at a discount, or for custom editions of this book with your logo, contact the American Diabetes Association at the address below, at booksales@diabetes.org, or by calling 703-299-2046.

American Diabetes Association
1701 North Beauregard Street
Alexandria, Virginia 22311

DOI: 10.2337/9781580403320

Library of Congress Cataloging-in-Publication Data

Funnell, Martha Mitchell.
Life with diabetes / Martha M. Funnell. — 4th ed.
    p. cm.
Includes bibliographical references and index.
ISBN 978-1-58040-332-0 (alk. paper)
1. Diabetes—Outlines, syllabi, etc. 2. Diabetes—Study and teaching. 3. Patient education. I. Title.
RC660.L54 2009
616.4'62–dc22
                        2009027385

Contents

➡ SUPPLEMENTARY OUTLINES

➡ SUPPORT MATERIALS

▶ ▶ ▶ ▶ ▶

These materials were originally developed under the direction of the Patient Education Committee of the Michigan Diabetes Research and Training Center. They were designed for use in teaching patients on the Diabetes Center Unit and were edited for their first publication in 1984 by Linda K. Strodtman, MS, RN; Patricia A. Barr, BS; John C. Floyd, Jr., MD; and me.

The second and third editions of these outlines were published in 1987 and 1991 by the Michigan DRTC after revisions to reflect both technological advances and changes in care and education. The American Diabetes Association took over publication of *Life with Diabetes* in 1997. This fourth edition of *Life with Diabetes* was revised to include current content areas necessary for meeting the National Standards for Diabetes Self-Management Education and for achieving recognition from the American Diabetes Association Education Recognition Program. It also incorporates new therapies and new information about the prevention and treatment of diabetes.

In the 25 years since the first publication of this resource, the advances in diabetes care and education continue to occur. The advances that have been made in the care and treatment of this devastating disease and its complications offer great benefit and hope. Equally impressive changes have been made in how we provide education and on-going support for people with diabetes and their families.

Beginning as early as 1984, and with each revision, we have made these materials more patient-centered, reflecting the empowerment philosophy which has been studied and promulgated by our Center, including Bob Anderson, EdD, and our colleagues around the country and the world. The importance of the psychosocial aspects of diabetes and the impact of emotions on behavior and the critical need to provide on-going support for diabetes self-management has been increasingly recognized in recent years. As a result, we have incorporated psychosocial and behavioral issues and strategies into each of the content areas so that the instructor can better help participants integrate diabetes into their lives. Diabetes education has clearly evolved from didactic content presentations to more theoretically-based empowerment models. We have moved beyond knowledge and behavior into a more holistic and realistic view of diabetes education. The purpose of education is not just to provide knowledge about diabetes, but to help participants better understand themselves and to make informed choices about how they will live with diabetes, and then to sustain those decisions and changes.

I continue to believe that being a diabetes educator is the best job in the world because we have the opportunity to bring help and hope, and help our patients live with this burdensome disease more effectively and peacefully. I hope that you will find these materials helpful in your practice and in your work as you bring caring, compassion, and competence to people with diabetes and pre-diabetes.

Martha M. Funnell, MS, RN, CDE
Michigan Diabetes Research and Training Center
Ann Arbor, Michigan

Acknowledgments

▶ ▶ ▶ ▶ ▶

Many have contributed to the outlines in the past two decades. They have been the joint effort of many staff members of the Michigan Diabetes Research and Training Center Education Committee, the Clinical Implementation Core, the Educational Development and Evaluation Core, and the Continuing Education and Outreach Core. Martha M. Funnell, MS, RN, CDE; Marilynn S. Arnold, MS, RD, CDE; and Patricia A. Barr, BS, served as lead authors and editors of the first edition published by the American Diabetes Association, and Andrea J. Lasichak, MS, RD, CDE, joined them on the 2nd and 3rd editions. Martha Funnell and Andrea Lasichak updated the text for this 4th edition.

Additional contributors are listed as completely as memory permits:

Marilyn Allard, BSN
Diana Barlage, RN, CDE
Carol Barnett, MS, RN
Lucy Bauman, MS, RN
Marilyn Bowbeer, BA
Nugget Burkhart, MA, RN, CDE
Catherine Eichel, MS, RN
John Floyd, Jr., MD
Mary Frey, MS, RN
Margaret Howard, BSN
Patricia Johnson, MSN, RN, CDE
Ralph Knopf, MD
Catherine Martin, MS, RN, CDE
Patricia McNitt, BSN

Sandra Merkle, MS, RN
Mara Mesa, RN, MA, MSW
Lisa Root Parker, BSN
Patricia Rahe, BSN
Cecilia Sauter, MS, RD, CDE
Margaret Smith, RN, BA
Irene Soble, MS, RN
Martha Spencer, MD
Renate Starr, BSN
Linda Strodtman, MS, RN
Carolyn Templeton, MS, RD
Neil White, MD
Linda Zucker, BSN

Graphic Artists

Linda A. Alvira
Nancy Fortino Bates
Michele Dansereau
Holly Harrington
Christine Lux
Kathryn E. Simpson

Reviewers of Current and Previous Editions

Samuel L. Abbate, MD, CDE
Barbara Anderson, PhD
Connie Crawley, RD, BS, MS
John T. Devlin, MD
Paulina Duker, MPH, APRN-BC, CDE
Margie Fox, CDE
Charlotte Hayes, MS, RD, CDE
Lois Jovanovic, MD
Joseph B. Nelson, MA
Clara Schneider, MS, RD, RN, LD, CDE
Jacqueline Siegel, RN
Neil White, MD
Gretchen A. Youssef, MS, RD, CDE

▶ ▶ ▶ ▶ ▶

PURPOSE

The primary purpose of *Life with Diabetes: A Series of Teaching Outlines by the Michigan Diabetes Research and Training Center* is to guide health professionals in the education of patients with diabetes mellitus. The outlines provide information on many diabetes-related topics. Although the content is generally for adults with either type 1 or type 2 diabetes, the information can easily be adapted for use with younger people, pregnant women, or those with special learning needs. The detail portions of the outlines are purposely worded to be brief so that the instructor can quickly scan the outline before teaching a session. The information included in the outlines comes from many sources and has been reviewed by content experts. In some cases, what has been included, and the way it has been stated or drawn, reflects our best compromise.

These outlines are only one component of an educational program and educational process. They are not a substitute for staff development and education nor are they intended to teach the instructor diabetes content or teaching methods. Health care professionals need to be educated in diabetes content and diabetes care as well as in the process of behavior change, teaching, counseling, and the impact of psychosocial and cultural concerns before they engage in diabetes education activities, if they are to be effective teachers.

A great deal has been learned in recent years about the effectiveness of diabetes education and about particular programatic and teaching strategies. As examples, multiple meta-analyses have shown that diabetes education is effective in producing positive outcomes, at least in the short term. These studies have also shown that group education is effective and that patient participation and collaboration appear to produce more favorable results than didactic presentations. We have also learned that while no one education program is more effective than others, programs that incorporate the behavioral and affective aspects of diabetes produce better outcomes. We also have greater appreciation for the impact of psychosocial and emotional concerns on self-management behaviors and the need for on-going diabetes self-management support to sustain the gains made during the education program and process. We encourage you to use this information as you prepare your program and work with participants. An approach that we have found to be effective is "ask the experts." In this format, session topics are generated by questions asked by participants. The instructor then builds on content generated by these questions to present related topics. Over the course of a program, a comprehensive curriculum can be presented. Keeping track of topics will help ensure that this occurs and that all content areas are addressed. Programs that need to provide specific clinical content during planned sessions can also use this approach by reminding participants of the topic area and asking if there are any questions or concerns. In addition, suggesting that participants try "behavioral experiments" between sessions gives them valuable experiences with behavior change. Beginning the following session with a discussion of what was learned from their experiment (regardless of its outcome) can be used to generate topics and content areas for the group to address at that session and helps to keep participants actively involved. This approach is effective in both diabetes self-management education and diabetes self-management support programs.

FORMAT AND TIPS FOR USE

These outlines are bound into a book that allows you to more easily make copies of the pages. In addition, the book is accompanied by a full-content CD-ROM. Some educators find they use sections of these outlines exactly as they appear, but most prefer to use specific outlines, portions, or combinations, to develop curricula appropriate for their patients and population. With the content on the CD, you can copy and combine the text, handouts, and graphics you specifically need for an education session. You are invited to use any of the materials in this book that are helpful to you in delivering self-management education and support and to make any changes necessary to adapt the materials to meet specific needs. The American Diabetes Association requests that any use of these materials be credited with a notification reading:

"These materials were adapted from *Life with Diabetes: A Series of Teaching Outlines by the Michigan Diabetes Research and Training Center,* 4th Edition. American Diabetes Association, 2009."

Publication of these materials is not allowed without written permission from the American Diabetes Association. Duplication of patient handouts is allowed for classroom use.

The first section consists of core outlines that include the basic information generally taught to people with diabetes. The second section includes supplementary information that is useful for particular situations. It is not the intent nor is it necessary to teach the sessions in the order that they are arranged in this book or to include all of the content from each outline or a session.

Each outline includes a statement of purpose; prerequisites that should be known by participants before attending a particular session; materials needed for teaching the session; a content outline that includes the general concepts to be covered, specific details, and instructor's notes or teaching tips with potential questions to help patients reflect on the management of diabetes in relation to their lives, experiences, and concerns; an evaluation and documentation plan; and suggested readings related to each topic. The content areas in the National Standards for Diabetes Self-Management Education were specifically written to allow for maximum flexibility and creativity in presentation style and method. Key behavioral and psychosocial aspects of each content area were incorporated to help participants to better integrate these aspects into their lives and self-management activities.

The material in each outline includes basic information about diabetes, diabetes self-care, and general health care practices. It does not include specific information for particular ethnic, cultural, or age-related groups, but it does make distinctions as to type 1 and type 2 diabetes. It is important to assess the individual and group needs of the participants because the effectiveness of education is enhanced by personalizing the education program to the specific needs of the audience. Information may need to be added or deleted, depending on your patients and their assessed needs. Again, the content on the CD-ROM will facilitate just that.

It is particularly important to consider the literacy skills of your participants. Fully 25% of adults in the United States have difficulty reading even simple text, and their ability to understand complex information presented orally is also limited. Simplify concepts; use plain, straightforward language; close the loop to ensure comprehension; and explain any unfamiliar words you use when teaching.

OVERVIEW OF NUTRITION OUTLINES

A significant portion of this curriculum addresses nutrition, often the most difficult aspect of diabetes self-care. Many different approaches to meal planning have been developed in recent years. Some are less rigid than earlier plans and may be less difficult for patients to use; however, the increase in meal-planning options presents an even greater challenge for educators, who need the information and skill to explain the choices to their participants and to further collaborate with them in developing individual plans that help them to reach personal goals.

The nutrition outlines are based on the understanding that dietary changes are difficult to initiate and sustain and that the fewer the changes, the more likely they will be attempted and maintained. Fewer but more effective and reasonable changes can be developed when the participant and health care professional are aware of usual, cultural, and preferred eating patterns. The outlines provide activities intended to help class members become aware of when, how much, and what they are eating, before information about meal planning is given. People are often frustrated by changing dietary recommendations. Inform class members that the information provided is based on current interpretation of scientific findings—which do change.

Although there are many potential benefits that can occur as a result of food choices, blood glucose management is the benefit unique to diabetes. It contributes to reducing acute and long-term complications and allows many people to feel better on a day-to-day basis. Therefore, the primary focus of the core nutrition outlines is blood glucose management. Although this is presented in the context of overall healthy food choices, it is important for the educator to distinguish between changes that benefit overall health and those that contribute directly to blood glucose management.

The sequence of topics has been chosen intentionally to help participants focus on one or two aspects of their diet at once and to encourage behavioral steps toward long-term goals. Blood glucose monitoring is encouraged to provide participants with information about the effects of different food choices on their blood glucose levels. The nutrition information to support blood glucose management is found in the Core Outlines section.

Additional content outlines are found in the Supplementary Outlines section. These include special issues and more intensive meal-planning approaches.

EVALUATION

The educational process is not complete without the evaluation of the outcomes achieved. This can be done in several ways. In terms of diabetes self-management skills and content, a conventional method is to assess the participant's preprogram knowledge, develop learning objectives based on the needs assessment, and then help participants determine whether they met their learning objectives at the conclusion of the program. Diabetes self-care skills need to be evaluated by observation.

Application of knowledge is more difficult to evaluate than content learned. One method for evaluating behavior change is through personal goals, the development and implementation of a plan to achieve those goals, and progress toward goal attainment. In this approach, participants define and articulate meaningful and personal goals relevant to their diabetes care. It is generally most effective for participants to begin by choosing an overall or long-term goal related to their diabetes: for example, to lose 10 pounds over the next four months. They then experiment with short-term behaviors to reach that goal and learn from their experiences. The opportunity to reflect on lessons they learned during this trial is used as a basis for decision-making for additional short-term behavioral goal-setting or problem-solving. It can also be used to monitor the educational progress over time, i.e., over several encounters with the health care system.

In addition to achievement of individual learning objectives and behavioral goals, other outcome measures can be used to evaluate the program's effectiveness. Participant outcomes that can be measured include levels of metabolic control, acute complications, process measures for monitoring complications, hospitalizations related to diabetes, lost work or school days, and psychosocial indicators, such as diabetes distress, quality of life, self-efficacy, and empowerment using standardized, reliable, and valid instruments. The outcome measures selected depend on the program design, target population, resources, and program goals.

RESOURCE MATERIALS

Additional information has been included to help you in using these teaching guides, including a participant assessment, education record forms, a curriculum review guide, sample objectives, supplemental readings, and resources for patients and health care professionals.

DIABETES EDUCATION RECOGNITION PROCESS

The American Diabetes Association's Education Recognition Program is a national voluntary process that formally identifies diabetes self-management education programs that meet the National Standards for Diabetes Self-Management Education. For more information, visit http://www.diabetes.org/recognition/education or call 1-800-DIABETES.

Core
Outlines

| #1 | **What Is Diabetes?** |

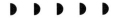

STATEMENT OF PURPOSE

This session is intended to provide basic information about the definition, pathophysiology, and treatment of diabetes.

PREREQUISITES

None.

OBJECTIVES

At the end of this session, participants will be able to:

1. identify diabetes as a chronic disorder of metabolism in which the body is unable to use food properly for energy, resulting in hyperglycemia;
2. state the importance of their role in decision-making;
3. identify the pancreas as the organ that makes the hormone, insulin;
4. state that the normal range for fasting plasma glucose is 70–100 mg/dl;
5. define *hyperglycemia* and list the symptoms;
6. state which of the two types of diabetes they have: type 1 or type 2;
7. list several factors that may contribute to the development of diabetes;
8. state that diabetes is a lifelong condition;
9. state that learning about diabetes and self-care is an important factor in the management of diabetes and prevention of complications;
10. list 3 components of the treatment of diabetes.

CONTENT

Describe the diabetes disease process and treatment options.

MATERIALS NEEDED

VISUALS PROVIDED	ADDITIONAL
1. Pancreas	■ Body model
2. Normal Glucose Metabolism	■ Video programs that provide an overview of the
3. How Insulin Works	pathophysiology and treatment of diabetes

MATERIALS NEEDED *continued*

VISUALS PROVIDED	ADDITIONAL

4. Normal Blood Glucose and Insulin Levels
5. Glucose Metabolism in Diabetes
6. Oral Glucose Tolerance Test
7. Natural History of Type 2 Diabetes
8. Insulin Resistance Due to Excess Weight

METHOD OF PRESENTATION

Start by introducing yourself and telling what you do. Ask participants to introduce themselves, say how long they have had diabetes, and how their diabetes is currently treated. Explain that the purpose of this session is to provide a basic overview of diabetes. Ask participants to identify what would be useful areas for discussion.

Show one of the videotapes, if desired. Present material in a question/discussion format, using the first question as a starting point. Provide appropriate content outlined below in response. Ask if there are additional questions, and respond, repeating the process for the entire session. Use the questions in the Instructor's Notes section to generate discussion if no questions are forthcoming after a period of silence. Keeping track of the content discussed in each session, using the Diabetes Self-Management Record, the Participant Follow-up Record, or another form, helps you to evaluate if all needed content has been discussed.

Because participants are more interested in their own diabetes than in a general discussion of diabetes, you can also use their laboratory results as a starting point for this session if available. One option is to use the Diabetes Complications Risk Profile tool available at http://www.med.umich.edu/mdrtc/profs/index.htm#risk, or a similar form to present their results. After giving participants time to review, ask if there are questions related to the results. Provide the content outlined below in response to their questions.

CONTENT OUTLINE

CONCEPT	DETAIL	INSTRUCTOR'S NOTES
1. Definition of diabetes mellitus	1.1 Define *diabetes mellitus*.	*Diabetes* = running through *Mellitus* = sweet
	1.2 Diabetes is a disorder of metabolism.	Ask, "What questions or concerns do you have about your diabetes? How would you explain what living with diabetes is like to another person?" Point out the difference between textbook knowledge of diabetes and their experiences.

CONTENT OUTLINE

CONCEPT	DETAIL	INSTRUCTOR'S NOTES
2. Self-care	2.1 Caring for diabetes is different than caring for other illnesses. You provide most of your own daily care. The choices and decisions you make each day affect both how you feel today and your long-term health.	Ask, "How is caring for diabetes different? What are some choices you make that affect your diabetes?"
	2.2 Caring for diabetes is not easy. It is a lot of work and can be frustrating when your efforts do not seem to pay off.	
	2.3 Diabetes causes many feelings that can affect your quality of life and how you care for yourself.	Ask, "What feelings have you experienced as a result of your diabetes?" Common feelings are anger, fear, frustration, and guilt. Avoid making judgments or trying to change or minimize the feelings identified.
	2.4 Although your health professionals are experts on diabetes, you are the expert on yourself and what will work best for you.	
3. Pancreas and liver	3.1 In diabetes, there is insufficient insulin activity. Insulin is needed to use the food we eat for energy. Insulin is made by the pancreas.	Ask, "What is diabetes?"
	3.2 The pancreas is a large, elongated gland located behind the stomach.	Show pancreas on the body model or Visual #1, Pancreas.
	3.3 The pancreas has two functions:	
	a. Secretion of pancreatic juice that aids in digestion (exocrine function).	This is done by 99% of the pancreas.
	b. Secretion of hormones that control various body processes (endocrine function). Insulin is a hormone made by beta cells in the pancreas. Insulin regulates carbohydrate metabolism.	Only 1% of the pancreas—the islets of Langerhans—performs this job.

5

CONTENT OUTLINE

CONCEPT	DETAIL	INSTRUCTOR'S NOTES
	3.4 Amylin is a hormone produced by the alpha cells of the pancreas that helps insulin work better.	Amylin production is reduced among people with diabetes.
	3.5 Glucagon is a hormone produced by the alpha cells of the pancreas. It is released when the blood glucose level is low.	Point out that while this is complex, it will help them better understand their glucose levels and diabetes therapy. Glucagon causes the liver to convert stored glycogen into glucose.
	3.6 Among its many other functions, the liver helps the body digest the food you eat. It helps break down and store glucose and the other sugars your body needs for energy.	One of the many functions of the liver is to stabilize blood glucose levels.
4. Normal metabolism	4.1 To understand and manage diabetes, you need to know what happens when you eat. Food is broken into simple forms by enzymes (chemicals) in the digestive system.	Some of these enzymes are produced by the pancreas.
	4.2 Most of the food you eat is broken down into glucose and other simple sugars.	
	4.3 Glucose is absorbed into the bloodstream to be used by cells for energy. Cells need glucose to work.	Use Visual #2, Normal Glucose Metabolism. Some of the non-glucose simple sugar is converted to glucose by the liver.
	4.4 Blood glucose rises promptly after food is eaten. Insulin is released from the pancreas as blood glucose levels go up.	
	4.5 Cells have receptor sites on the outside. When insulin attaches to the receptor sites, a passageway is made and glucose goes into the cell. Insulin "opens" the cells, like a key.	Most cells need insulin for glucose to enter. Brain, liver, and kidney cells do not; these cells receive glucose even though there is little insulin activity. Use Visual #3, How Insulin Works.
	4.6 Because glucose goes out of the blood and into the cells, plasma blood glucose levels stay in the normal range.	Ask, "What are normal blood glucose levels?" Use Visual #4, Normal Blood Glucose and Insulin Levels.
	4.7 Excess calories are generally converted into fat and stored.	Usually blood glucose rises (to <140 mg/dl) and returns to

CONTENT OUTLINE

CONCEPT	DETAIL	INSTRUCTOR'S NOTES
	Excess glucose is stored in the liver for future use.	normal 2 hours after beginning to eat.
	4.8 When your blood glucose starts to go down, your pancreas slows down how quickly and how much insulin it makes. When insulin levels drop, the liver releases some of the glucose it has stored. This keeps the blood glucose from dropping too low. Your liver also puts out extra glucose when your blood glucose drops too low.	This role of the liver is especially important during times of fasting, such as overnight, or when you need energy quickly, such as during exercise. Ask, "Have you ever had your blood glucose go up overnight? After exercise?" Point out that bedtime and morning fasting glucose levels should be in the same range.
5. Food metabolism in diabetes	5.1 Food is broken down in the normal way.	
	5.2 Digestive enzymes act in the normal way.	The digestive enzymes produced by the pancreas are not affected by diabetes.
	5.3 Glucose is absorbed into the bloodstream in the normal way.	
	5.4 But, there is not enough insulin action.	The key to the cells (insulin) is missing.
	5.5 Because insulin action is affected by diabetes, your liver may put out extra sugar even when the blood glucose is high. This can further raise the blood glucose level.	Point out that this does not mean that the liver is damaged, just that the signals are not interpreted correctly.
	5.6 Hormones made in the gut stimulate the production of insulin when glucose levels are elevated after meals, inhibit glucagon production, and slow emptying of the stomach. This effect is blunted or delayed among people with diabetes.	These are the incretin hormones (GLP1 and GIP).
	5.7 Without insulin action, glucose can't get into most cells to be used for energy.	Use Visual #5, Glucose Metabolism in Diabetes.
	5.8 Glucose stays in the blood. There is not enough insulin action to maintain a normal blood glucose level.	

CONTENT OUTLINE

CONCEPT	DETAIL	INSTRUCTOR'S NOTES
	5.9 Blood glucose level rises, leading to *hyperglycemia.*	Insulin maintains euglycemia by allowing glucose to move into the cells.
	5.10 Most cells are drowning in glucose on the outside and starving for it on the inside.	
6. Signs and symptoms of hyperglycemia	6.1 The symptoms are caused by high glucose levels and by your body's efforts to get rid of the extra sugar.	Ask, "What symptoms did you have before you found out you had diabetes?" *hyper* = high *glyc* = sugar *emia* = blood
	6.2 The kidneys work as filters to remove waste products from the blood, including excess glucose. The higher the glucose levels in the blood, the more glucose will appear in the urine, and the harder the kidneys have to work.	Glucose leaving the body in the urine is called *glycosuria.* In some patients, hyperglycemia must be extreme before glycosuria develops. The renal threshold is the level at which glycosuria develops.
	6.3 This leads to extra urine production. Your body must make more urine to get rid of the extra glucose. This is called *polyuria.*	High levels of glucose in the urine increase urination correspondingly, as your body dilutes the sugar.
	6.4 When you urinate a lot, your body needs more water. This increases your thirst. Increased thirst is called *polydipsia* and is due to polyuria.	Getting up too often during the night to urinate is common.
	6.5 *Polyphagia* (increased hunger) is due to starvation of the cells because glucose stays in the blood and is not available to the cells.	Loss of glucose through the urine means loss of calories.
	6.6 Dehydration, weight loss, weakness, and fatigue also happen.	Other factors, such as anorexia, may contribute to weight loss.
	6.7 Blurred vision results from hyperglycemia. Sugar accumulates in the lens of the eye, causing the lens to swell and distort vision. As blood glucose returns to normal, the lens usually recovers its shape and vision changes again.	Participants need to wait 6–8 weeks after blood glucose levels are regulated before undergoing vision testing for glasses. Reassure participants that these changes are not related to blindness (retinopathy) from diabetes.

CONTENT OUTLINE

CONCEPT	DETAIL	INSTRUCTOR'S NOTES
	6.8 Another symptom of high blood glucose is itching, especially in the genital area.	Itching can be caused by dry skin from dehydration, or an overgrowth of microorganisms.
	6.9 Slow or confused thinking can occur if hyperglycemia and dehydration are marked; coma and cerebrovascular accident can result.	The brain cannot function well if fluids are unbalanced.
	6.10 Delayed healing and an increased number of infections can also occur.	Vaginal and bladder infections are common examples.
	6.11 These symptoms come on acutely in type 1 diabetes, but more slowly in type 2 diabetes. Many people attribute these symptoms to aging and ignore them.	Point out that people have type 2 diabetes for 7 years on average before diagnosis. It is sadly not uncommon to be diagnosed when a complication develops.
7. Tests used to diagnose diabetes	7.1 One test to diagnose diabetes is called the fasting plasma glucose test. A blood sample is taken after a 10–12 hour-fast, usually before breakfast. A normal result is 70–99 mg/dl. Values above 126 mg/dl more than once are diagnostic of diabetes.	Ask, "How was your diabetes diagnosed? Were you ever told you had pre-diabetes?"
	7.2 Another test is called the random plasma glucose test. A nonfasting plasma glucose level of >200 mg/dl along with classic symptoms is diagnostic.	In the absence of unequivocal hyperglycemia with any of the diagnostic methods, the results must be confirmed on a subsequent day.
	7.3 A1C levels may be used to diagnose diabetes. Diabetes is diagnosed when the A1C level is >6.5%.	Those with an A1C >6% and <6.5% need appropriate preventative counseling.
	7.4 Another test is the oral glucose tolerance test (OGTT). After a 10- to 12-hour fast, a blood sample is taken. A glucose dose is then given and blood samples are taken every half hour for 2–5 hours. This test is done if there is a question of pre-diabetes or diabetes. A two-hour level of more than 200 mg/dl is diagnostic.	Use Visual #6, Oral Glucose Tolerance Test, if patients have had this test and are interested. A 75-gram glucose load or its equivalent is recommended.

CONTENT OUTLINE

CONCEPT	DETAIL	INSTRUCTOR'S NOTES
	7.5 A 2-hour postprandial plasma glucose test may be used for diagnostic purposes. A high-carbohydrate meal may be given before the test, especially to children.	
	7.6 Pre-diabetes is defined as a fasting plasma glucose value of more than 100 and less than 126, or/and a 2-hour plasma glucose value more than 140 and less than 200.	Contrast this with the old designation of borderline diabetes. Review the results of the Diabetes Prevention Program (DPP), which indicated that modest weight loss (5–7%) and moderate exercise (e.g., walking 150 minutes per week) were shown to significantly reduce the risk for and potentially delay the onset of type 2. Additional educational materials and curricula based on the DPP are available at: www.yourdiabetesinfo.org.
8. Type 1 diabetes	8.1 There are several types of diabetes. The two most common types are type 1 and type 2.	
	8.2 In type 1, the pancreas makes little or no insulin.	Old names for type 1 are insulin-dependent, juvenile-onset, ketosis-prone, unstable, or brittle diabetes.
	8.3 People with type 1 are prone to develop ketosis.	Ketosis will be explained later.
	8.4 People with type 1 need insulin in order to stay alive.	
	8.5 Type 1 can begin at any age, but it usually occurs in children and young adults.	The incidence of type 2 diabetes among children and adolescents is increasing.
9. Type 2 diabetes	9.1 The pancreas is producing insulin, but the amount is not adequate, or the insulin is not effective in lowering blood glucose because the cells are resistant.	Old names for type 2 are maturity-onset, adult-onset, and insulin-resistant diabetes. Use Visual #7, Natural History of Type 2 Diabetes.

CONTENT OUTLINE

CONCEPT	DETAIL	INSTRUCTOR'S NOTES

9.2 With insulin resistance, the pancreas produces more insulin than usual, but the cells are unable to use the insulin because there are fewer receptors.

The insulin also remains in the bloodstream.

9.3 People with type 2 are unlikely to develop ketosis.

9.4 Onset is possible at any age, but type 2 is more commonly diagnosed after age 30.

Type 2 diabetes may occur at younger ages in high-risk populations.

9.5 The treatment for type 2 diabetes is done in phases or stages: nutrition therapy and exercise, and oral medications and/or other non-insulin injectables and/or insulin.

Exercise and weight loss may help decrease insulin resistance. Meal planning and exercise are important during all phases.

9.6 Although diabetes is often thought of as a "sugar problem," in reality it is an "insulin problem." Because pancreatic function declines over time, insulin is often needed to achieve blood glucose targets. Insulin is a natural and the most effective therapy for diabetes.

Emphasize that people with type 2 often progress to insulin and that it is not a failure or a sign that their diabetes is worse. Clarify the difference between type 1 and type 2 diabetes.

10. Factors contributing to the development of diabetes

10.1 The exact cause of diabetes is unknown. Heredity is a factor in both types of diabetes, but is more often associated with type 2. If one parent has type 2, the risk is 10–15% that children will get it as adults. If one parent has type 1, the risk is 2–5%.

You don't catch diabetes or get it from eating sweets. Studies show that if one identical twin gets type 1, the other doesn't always (25–50%). This indicates that something in the environment has brought out the diabetes in one twin. If one twin gets type 2, the other usually does too (60–75%). Stress the importance of preventing type 2 diabetes among their children and grandchildren.

10.2 Being overweight is a factor in developing type 2 diabetes. More and larger body cells require energy. Also, cells are more resistant to insulin than normal because, as cells get larger, receptor sites are

More than 80% of people are obese at the time of diagnosis. Use Visual #8, Insulin Resistance Due to Excess Weight. Note the large body cell with fewer receptor sites. The insulin

11

CONTENT OUTLINE

CONCEPT	DETAIL	INSTRUCTOR'S NOTES
	lost. Thus, more insulin is needed for both reasons.	molecule cannot attach to the cell; therefore, the glucose molecule cannot attach to the insulin molecule.
	10.3 Stresses, both emotional and physical, may precipitate or aggravate type 1 and type 2: ■ pregnancy (gestational diabetes) ■ illness or surgery ■ medications such as glucosteroids (e.g., prednisone).	Gestational diabetes may go away after the pregnancy, but may reappear as type 2 diabetes later in life. There is increasing evidence that depression may precede diabetes.
	10.4 Age is a factor (incidence of diabetes increases with age).	
	10.5 Injury to the pancreas (infection, surgery, tumor, or trauma) may lead to diabetes, even in low-hereditary-risk groups.	People with diabetes as a result of pancreatectomy are considered to have type 1 diabetes.
	10.6 Ethnic background can contribute (Native Americans, Hispanic Americans, and Asian Americans have a higher incidence of type 2 diabetes).	
	10.7 In combination with hereditary factors predisposing one to the development of type 1 are the following: ■ immunologic factors (antibodies against the islet cells that produce insulin) ■ viral factors (post-mumps, rubella, or coxsackie).	
11. Treatment of diabetes mellitus	11.1 Diabetes is a serious, lifelong condition. It is not curable, but it is treatable.	Stress the seriousness of both types of diabetes.

CONTENT OUTLINE

CONCEPT	DETAIL	INSTRUCTOR'S NOTES
	11.2 Most (95–99%) of the daily care of diabetes is self-care. You make many decisions each day that affect your blood glucose levels and long-term outcomes.	Stress the importance of the role of the person with diabetes as a care provider. Recent evidence demonstrates that 98% of outcomes are patient-related.
	11.3 Most problems in diabetes are linked to blood glucose levels that are too high or too low. One of the most important things you can do is to learn about diabetes and how to manage blood glucose levels.	
	11.4 The first step is to decide your personal blood glucose targets. Treatment, including self-care, is then based on working toward this target.	Keeping blood glucose levels near normal helps decrease symptoms and reduces the risks for the acute and long-term complications of diabetes.
	11.5 The treatment of type 1 diabetes always includes insulin. The intensity (number of shots each day, meal plan, and exercise) of the treatment is based on your personal blood glucose targets and other goals.	Ask, "How is your diabetes treated? How has your treatment changed since you were diagnosed?"
	11.6 The treatment of type 2 diabetes is usually done in stages or phases— starting with meal planning and exercise, then oral medicines (if needed), and then injectables and/or insulin, alone or with oral medications. Each stage will be tried for 3–6 months. Effectiveness is evaluated based on blood glucose goals. Using oral medications from the time of diagnosis is more and more common. Metformin is often the drug of first choice.	Stress that they may stay in one phase or stage for a while, but that they should not stay with a form of treatment that is not effective. Remind participants that treatment failures are not personal failures and that progression of therapy does not mean that their diabetes has "progressed" or worsened.
	11.7 A meal plan for glucose control distributes carbohydrates throughout the day to smooth out blood glucose levels and balance with insulin or oral medicines, if taken.	They will design their diabetes meal plan in collaboration with a dietitian.

CONTENT OUTLINE

CONCEPT	DETAIL	INSTRUCTOR'S NOTES
	11.8 A meal plan for weight control reduces calorie intake within the framework of glucose control.	Even a small amount of weight loss (5–10%) can lower blood glucose significantly for two reasons: 1) receptor sites return, making the patient more sensitive to his/her own available insulin; 2) there is less metabolic demand on the body.
	11.9 Exercise usually lowers blood glucose because exercise increases the rate of burning blood glucose (metabolism). It also provides a sense of well-being, aids the vascular system, and helps in weight reduction and maintenance.	Ask, "What are your personal reasons for meal planning? Exercise?"
	11.10 Medication involves oral agents (which are not insulin) and/or other injectibles and/or insulin.	Emphasize the need to use meal plans and exercise along with medications.
	11.11 Caring for diabetes often involves making changes in your lifestyle and other health behaviors.	Ask, "What changes have you made to care for your diabetes? What helped or hindered your efforts?"
	11.12 It is unrealistic to think that you can make all the changes at one time. Many people find choosing long-term blood glucose and other goals and then choosing and reaching short-term goals is helpful.	Ask participants to select a long-term goal related to diabetes and an appropriate short-term goal that can be achieved by the next class. Examples: If the long-term goal is to lose 30 lb, the short-term goal could be to eat 1 1/2 sandwiches for lunch instead of 2. If the long-term goal is a lower A1C level, then the short-term goal may be to walk three times a week for 20 minutes. The purpose of this is to give participants a chance to experiment and learn by trying to make a behavior change.

CONTENT OUTLINE

CONCEPT	DETAIL	INSTRUCTOR'S NOTES
	11.13 Reward yourself when you accomplish your short-term goals.	
	11.14 These classes will also offer tips to carry out needed care.	
	11.15 Choose one thing you will do this week to care for your diabetes.	Close the session by asking participants to identify one action step they will take this week.

SKILLS CHECKLIST

None.

EVALUATION PLAN

Knowledge will be evaluated by achievement of learning objectives and by responses to questions during the session. The ability to apply knowledge will be evaluated by the recognition of feelings about diabetes, the development of personal self-care goals, the development and implementation of a plan to achieve those goals, and through program outcome measures.

DOCUMENTATION PLAN

Record class attendance and achieved objectives as appropriate.

SUGGESTED READINGS

AADE White Paper: White paper on the prevention of type 2 diabetes and the role of the diabetes educator. *The Diabetes Educator* 28:964–970, 2002

American College of Physicians: *ACP Diabetes Care Guide*. Philadelphia, PA: American College of Physicians, 2007

American Diabetes Association and National Institute of Diabetes and Digestive and Kidney Diseases: The prevention or delay of type 2 diabetes. *Diabetes Care* 25:742–749, 2002

American Diabetes Association: *Annual Review of Diabetes*. Alexandria, VA: American Diabetes Association, 2008

American Diabetes Association: Clinical practice recommendations. *Diabetes Care* 32(Suppl 1):S1–S104, 2009

American Diabetes Association: *The Complete Guide to Diabetes*, 3rd Edition. Alexandria, VA: American Diabetes Association, 2003

SUGGESTED READINGS *continued*

American Diabetes Association: Consensus Statement. Type 2 diabetes in children. *Diabetes Care* 23:281–338, 2000

American Diabetes Association: *Diabetes A to Z,* 5th Edition. Alexandria, VA: American Diabetes Association, 2003

American Diabetes Association: *Diabetes 411.* Alexandria, VA: American Diabetes Association, 2008

American Diabetes Association: *Diabetes Ready-Reference Guide for Health Care Professionals,* 2nd Edition. Alexandria, VA: American Diabetes Association, 2004

American Diabetes Association: Diagnosis and classification of diabetes mellitus. *Diabetes Care* 32(Suppl 1):S55–S60, 2009

American Diabetes Association: *Medical Management of Type 1 Diabetes*, 5th Edition. Alexandria, VA: American Diabetes Association, 2008

American Diabetes Association: *Medical Management of Type 2 Diabetes*, 6th Edition. Alexandria, VA: American Diabetes Association, 2008

American Diabetes Association: Screening for type 2 diabetes. *Diabetes Care* 27(Suppl 1):S11–S14, 2004

American Diabetes Association: Standards for medical care in diabetes. *Diabetes Care.* 31(Suppl. 1):S12–S54, 2008

American Diabetes Association: *Therapy for Diabetes Mellitus and Related Disorders*, 5th Edition. Alexandria, VA: American Diabetes Association, 2009

Appel SJ: Sizing up patients for metabolic syndrome. *Nursing* 35(12):20–21, 2005

Aronoff SL, Kerokwitz K, Shreiner B, Want L: Glucose metabolism and regulation: beyond insulin and glucagon. *Diabetes Spectrum* 17:73–77, 2004

Bloomgarden Z: Achieving glycemic goals in type 2 diabetes. *Diabetes Care* 30:174–180, 2007

Bloomgarden ZT: Glycemic treatment in type 1 and type 2 diabetes. *Diabetes Care* 29:2549–2555, 2006

Bloomgarden ZT: Insulin resistance, concepts. *Diabetes Care* 30:1320–1326, 2007

Brophy S, Brunt H, Davies H, Mannan S, Williams R: Interventions for latent autoimmune diabetes (LADA) in adults. *Cochrane Database of Systematic Reviews* no. CD006165, 2007

Bunker K: 30 things you should know about managing diabetes. *Diabetes Forecast* 61(4):54–55, 2008

Childs, B, Cypress M, Spollett S: *Complete Nurses Guide to Diabetes Care,* 2nd edition Alexandria, VA: American Diabetes Association, 2009

Clark NG, Fox KM, Grandy S, for the SHIELD study group: Symptoms of diabetes and their association with the risk and presence of diabetes. *Diabetes Care* 20:2868–2873, 2007

Cramer JS, Sibley RF, Bartlett DP, Kahn LS, Loffredo L: An adaptation of the Diabetes Prevention Program for use with high-risk minority patients with type 2 diabetes. *The Diabetes Educator* 33:503–508, 2007

D'Arrigo T: The inflammation factor. *Diabetes Forecast* 60(11):48–50, 2007

De Simone G, Devereaux RB, Chinali M, Best LG, et al.: Prognostic impact of metabolic syndrome by different definitions in a population with high prevalence of obesity and diabetes. *Diabetes Care* 30:1851–1856, 2007

Fowler MJ: Classification of diabetes: not all hyperglycemia is the same. *Clinical Diabetes* 25:74–76, 2007

Ford ES, Li C, Little RR, Mokdad AH: Trends in A1C concentrations among U.S. adults with diagnosed diabetes from 1999–2004. *Diabetes Care* 31:102–107, 2008

Ford ES, Giles WH, Mokdad AH: Increasing prevalence of the metabolic syndrome among U.S. adults. *Diabetes Care* 27:2444–2449, 2004

Funnell MM: Standards of care for diabetes. *Nursing* 38(10):47–49, 2008

Gaede P, Lund-Andersen H, Parving H-H, Pedersen O: Effect of a multifactoral intervention on mortality in type 2 diabetes. *The New England Journal of Medicine* 258:580–591, 2008

SUGGESTED READINGS *continued*

Gebel E, Neithercott T: Back to basics. *Diabetes Forecast* 62(4):31–55, 2009

Gebel E. Keeping trouble at bay. *Diabetes Forecast* 61(12):45–46, 2008

Gebel E: What is diabetes? *Diabetes Forecast* 61(4):49–50, 2008

Gilles CL, Abrams KR, Lambert PC, Cooper NJ, et al.: Pharmacological and lifestyle interventions to prevent or delay type 2 diabetes in people with impaired glucose tolerance: systematic review and meta-analysis. *BMJ* 334:209–302, 2007

International Expert Committee report on the role of the A1C assay in the diagnosis of diabetes. *Diabetes Care* 32:1327–1334, 2009

Jackson L: Translating the diabetes prevention program into practice: a review of community interventions. *The Diabetes Educator* 35:309–318, 2009

Kruger DF, Martin CE, Sadler CE: New insights into glucose regulation. *The Diabetes Educator* 32:221–228, 2006

Lee D-H, Lee I-K, Jim S-H, Steffes M, Jacobs DR, Jr: Association between serum concentrations of persistent organic pollutants and insulin resistance among nondiabetic adults. *Diabetes Care* 30:622–628, 2007

Lipscombe LL, Jamal SA, Booth GL, Hawker GA: The risk of hip fractures in older individuals with diabetes. *Diabetes Care* 30:835–841, 2007

Mensing C, Cypress M, Halstenson C, McLaughlin S, Walker EA: *The Art and Science of Diabetes Self-management Education.* Chicago, IL: American Association of Diabetes Educators, 2006

Narayan KMV, Boyle JP, Geiss LS, Saaddine JB, Thompson TJ: Impact of recent increase in incidence on future diabetes burden. *Diabetes Care* 29:2114–2116, 2006

Nathan DM, Buse JB, Davidson MB, Ferrannini E, et al.: Medical management of hyperglycemia in type 2 diabetes: a consensus statement of the American Diabetes Association and the European Association for the Study of Diabetes. *Diabetes Care* 32:193–203, 2009

Nichols GA, Hiller TA, Brown JB: Progression from newly acquired impaired fasting glucose to type 2 diabetes. *Diabetes Care* 30:228–233, 2007

Padwal R, Majumdar SR, Johnson JA, Varney J, McAlister FA: A systematic review of drug therapy to delay or prevent type 2 diabetes. *Diabetes Care* 28:736–744, 2005

Piette JD, Kerr EA: The impact of comorbid chronic conditions on diabetic care. *Diabetes Care* 29:725–731, 2006

Roberts SS: Ties that bind: the pancreas piece of the diabetes puzzle. *Diabetes Forecast* 59(11):25–28, 2006

Seidel MC, Powerell RO, Zgibor JC, Siminerio LM, Piatt GA: Translating the diabetes prevention program into an urban medically underserved community. *Diabetes Care* 31:684–689, 2008

Statten P, Bjor O, Ferrari P, et al.: Prospective study of hyperglycemia and cancer risk. *Diabetes Care* 30:561–567, 2007

The DPP Research Group: Impact of intensive lifestyle and metformin therapy on cardiovascular disease risk factors in the diabetes prevention program. *Diabetes Care* 28:888–894, 2005

The DPP Research Group: Strategies to identify adults at high risk for type 2 diabetes. *Diabetes Care* 28:138–144, 2005

Tuncell K, Bradley CJ, Lafata JE, Pladevall M, Divine GW, Goodman AC, Vijan S: Glycemic control and absenteeism among individuals with diabetes. *Diabetes Care* 30:1282–1285, 2007

Vinik A: Advancing therapy in type 2 diabetes mellitus with early, comprehensive progression from oral agents to insulin therapy. *Clinical Therapeutics* 29:1236–1252, 2007

Pancreas

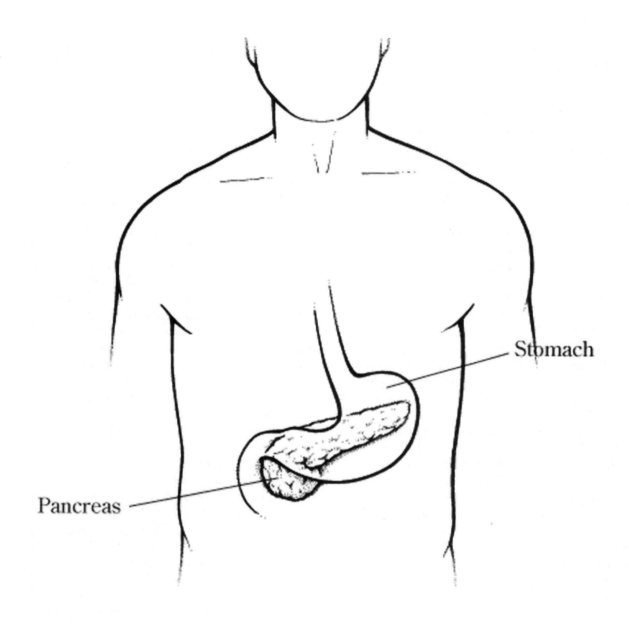

Stomach

Pancreas

◑ Normal Glucose Metabolism

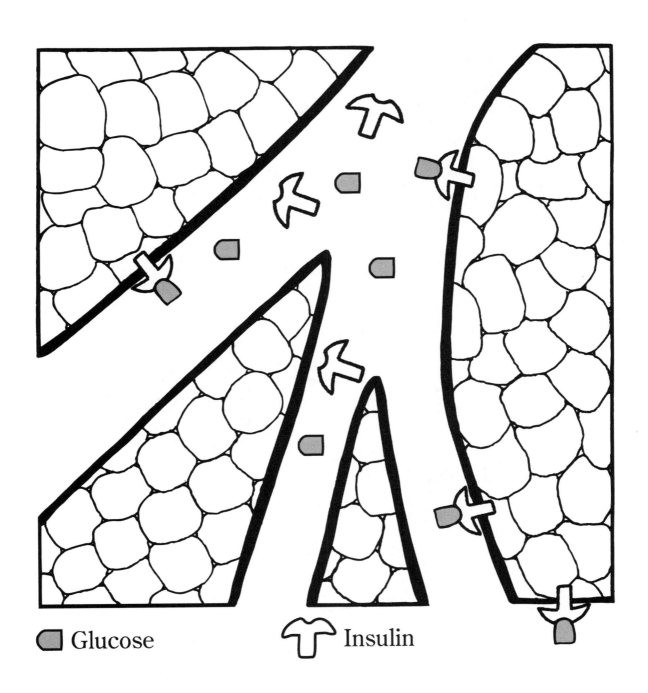

⬤ Glucose   ⬆ Insulin

➲ How Insulin Works

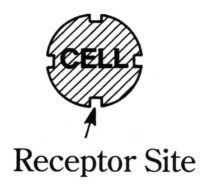

Receptor Site

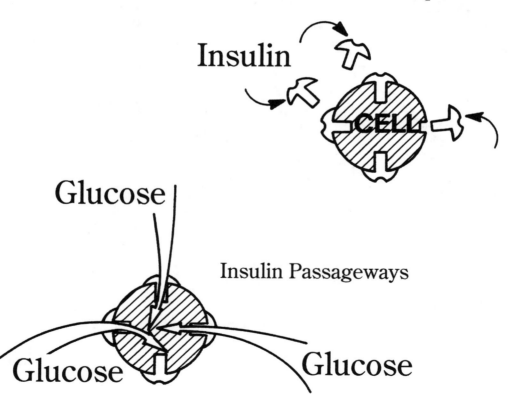

Insulin Fills Receptor Sites

Insulin

Glucose

Insulin Passageways

Glucose

Glucose

Normal Blood Glucose and Insulin Levels

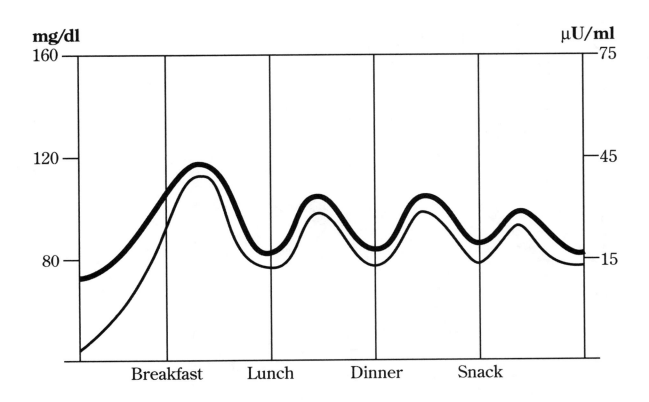

Legend:
- **Blood Glucose Level**
- Plasma Insulin Level

⮕ Glucose Metabolism in Diabetes

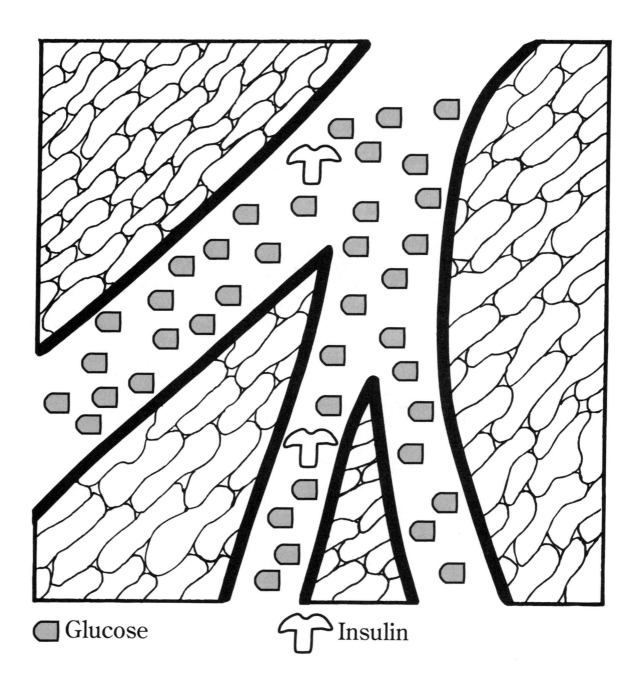

⬡ Glucose   ⬦ Insulin

➔ Oral Glucose Tolerance Test

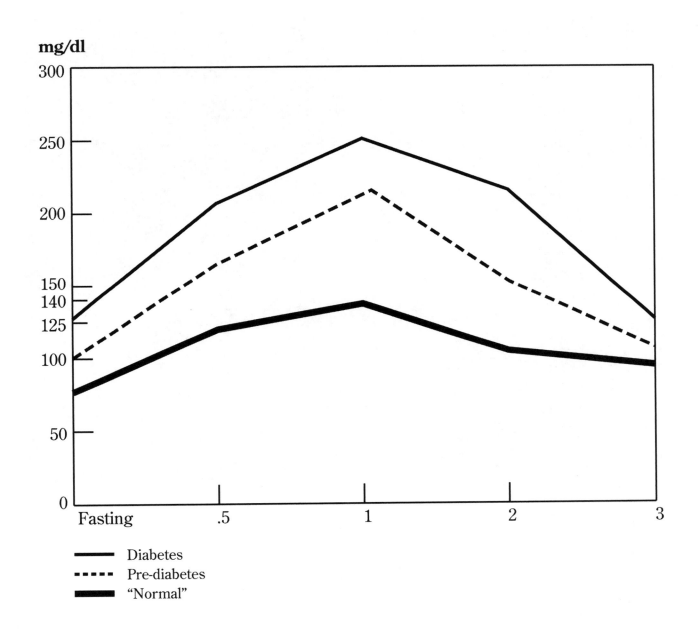

mg/dl

Diabetes

Pre-diabetes

"Normal"

➡ Natural History of Type 2 Diabetes

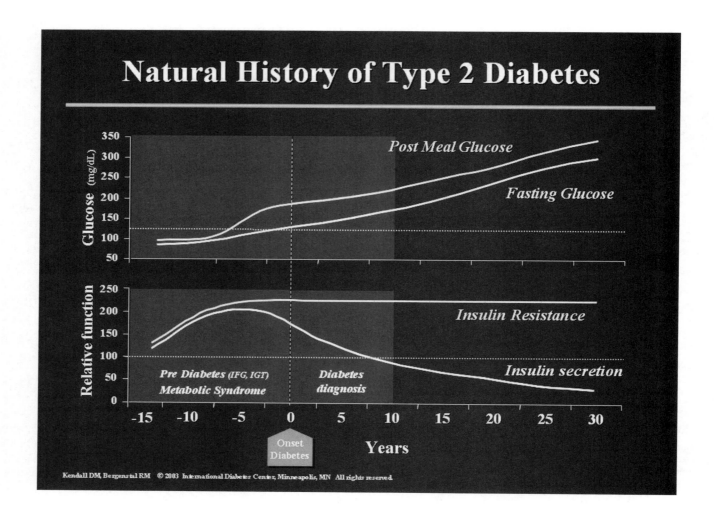

Insulin Resistance Due to Excess Weight

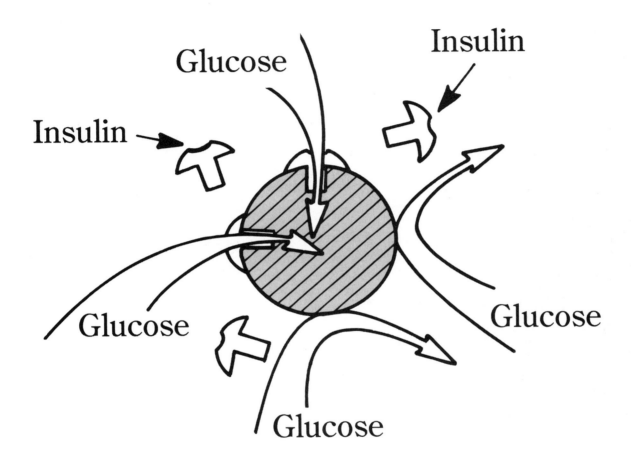

#2   Learning to Live with Diabetes

▶ ▶ ▶ ▶ ▶

STATEMENT OF PURPOSE

This session is intended to encourage people with diabetes and their significant others to recognize and express feelings about having diabetes and how it affects their lives.

PREREQUISITES

None.

OBJECTIVES

At the end of this session, participants will be able to:

1. express the effects diabetes has had or may have on their way of life and the lives of their families;

2. state who they have told about their diabetes, and state who needs to be told and why;

3. express feelings about having diabetes;

4. share experiences, personal successes, and problems in coping with diabetes;

5. identify a source of emotional support, or state one way to increase support.

CONTENT

Developing personal strategies to address psychosocial issues and concerns.

MATERIALS NEEDED

VISUALS PROVIDED	ADDITIONAL
None.	■ Information about local diabetes support groups and other local resources
	■ "Trigger" videotapes to initiate discussion of these issues

METHOD OF PRESENTATION

Start by introducing yourself and telling what you do. Ask participants to introduce themselves. Explain that the purpose of this session is not only to give information, but to provide a time for participants to express their thoughts about living with diabetes. You may wish to use a videotape as an introduction to the topic, and then facilitate a group discussion.

It is important to acknowledge and validate any feelings expressed by participants. If your spouse, parents, or other family members are present, you can draw them into the discussion by asking about their thoughts and concerns. You may wish to combine this with Outline #12, *Stress and Coping* (p. 255), or Outline #15, *Changing Behavior* (p. 315). Another option is to close with an exercise from Outline #16, *Putting the Pieces Together* (p. 331), such as situation two, three, and/or ten.

Show one of the videotapes, if desired. Begin by asking how they did with their short-term goal and what they learned from it. Present material in a question/discussion format, using the first question as a starting point. Provide appropriate content outlined below in response. Ask if there are additional questions, and respond, repeating the process for the entire session. Use the questions in the Instructor's Notes section to generate discussion if no questions are forthcoming after a period of silence. Keeping track of the content discussed in each session, using the Diabetes Self-Management Record, the Participant Follow-up Record, or another form, helps you to evaluate if all needed content has been discussed.

CONTENT OUTLINE

CONCEPT	DETAIL	INSTRUCTOR'S NOTES
1. Diabetes as a chronic illness	1.1 Diabetes is a lifelong condition.	Feelings are a critical component of diabetes self-management and need to be acknowledged and incorporated throughout the educational program.
	1.2 As such, it affects many aspects of a person's life.	Ask, "What are your thoughts/ feelings about diabetes? What is the hardest thing about living with diabetes for you?"
2. Possible effects on the way one lives	2.1 Some of the effects diabetes may have on your life are: ■ the need for a more regular schedule ■ a change in eating habits ■ daily medication and monitoring	Ask, "What effect has diabetes had on your life?" Acknowledge the difficulties of living with diabetes every day. If family members are present, acknowledge their struggles as well.

CONTENT OUTLINE

CONCEPT	DETAIL	INSTRUCTOR'S NOTES
	■ possible changes in recreational or occupational pursuits ■ possible changes in relationships with people ■ fear of future effects on life and health ■ anger about having to deal with a chronic illness ■ frustration when efforts are not reflected in outcomes ■ guilt for having developed diabetes.	
3. Identification of self as a person with diabetes	3.1 Who have you told?	Ask, "Who have you told? Why? How have others reacted when you've told them you have diabetes? How would you like them to respond?"
	3.2 Who needs to know and why (family, employer, co-workers, school, or responsible adult)?	School personnel need preparation to accommodate the child with diabetes. Other classmates need reassurance that diabetes isn't contagious. Co-workers may be helpful in emergencies.
4. Feelings about having diabetes	4.1 Everyone has feelings or thoughts about having diabetes. Diabetes is burdensome and distressing and it is common for negative feelings to persist or reoccur many years after diagnosis.	Ask, "What were your feelings (thoughts) when you first found out you had diabetes? What are your feelings (thoughts) now about diabetes?"
	4.2 Feelings may vary from day to day and change over time.	It is important for the instructor to realize that feelings are not problems to be solved. The instructor's role is to assist participants to acknowledge and clarify feelings with questions such as, "You felt *(feeling)* because of *(reason)*?" It is unlikely that participants will resolve their feelings by the end of this class session.

Property of
Baker College
of Allen Park

CONTENT OUTLINE

CONCEPT	DETAIL	INSTRUCTOR'S NOTES
	4.3 Fear or worry about long-term effects of diabetes is also common.	
	4.4 Your feelings and stress levels affect your blood glucose levels, and your blood glucose levels affect your mood and your ability to cope with stress.	
	4.5 Family members, especially parents, may feel guilty. Adult children may worry about getting diabetes, and siblings may feel jealous of the attention paid to the family member with diabetes. Spouses may worry about the effects of diabetes on their future or feel responsible for your self-management decisions.	Ask, "Have any of you ever felt 'nagged' by your family or that you live with the 'diabetes police'? Is that helpful for you? What would you prefer?"
	4.6 It is common to go through stages of the grieving process: denial, anger, depression, and adaptation.	
	4.7 **Denial.** People may find it hard to believe they have diabetes, that they really have to take care of it, or that certain aspects of their treatment are needed.	Learning may be difficult at this stage. When a participant is experiencing denial, it is important to support the person without supporting his/her denial. An appropriate response might be, "I can see you are _____, but can I tell you why I'm concerned about you."
	4.8 **Anger.** People may wonder, "Why me?" or act angrily to family and friends. They are really angry about having diabetes.	Ask, "Do you find that you get angry more easily?" Anger about an illness can be expressed as anger toward other people. Again, it is essential to continue accepting the participants as they are.

CONTENT OUTLINE

CONCEPT	DETAIL	INSTRUCTOR'S NOTES
	4.9 **Depression.** Anger, bottled up inside over time, can lead to feeling very sad and blue— even hopeless.	Ask, "What are signs of depression?" Accepting the participant and actively listening can be positive interventions. Statements such as, "It sounds as if you're sad about _____" can help the participant talk about the issue.
	4.10 People with diabetes are twice as likely to suffer from depression. While everyone feels sad now and then, clinical depression is a serious medical problem. Feeling sad most of the time for more than 2 weeks may indicate clinical depression. This type of depression can be successfully treated with a combination of medication and counseling.	Screening questions for clinical depression are: "Over the past 2 weeks, have you felt down, depressed, and hopeless?" and "Over the past 2 weeks, have you felt little interest or pleasure in doing things?" A variety of screening instruments are available online. Cognitive behavioral therapy has been shown to be an effective treatment approach for people with diabetes.
	4.11 The direct effects of depression on glycemic control are not known, but many people find it hard to care for themselves when they are depressed.	Point out the similarity of symptoms of high blood glucose and diabetes. There is some evidence that depression can lead to diabetes.
	4.12 **Acceptance.** Gradually, most people adjust or adapt. They still wish they did not have diabetes, but they are better able to live with it.	Ask, "Have you ever had any of these feelings? How did they affect you? How did they affect your relationships with family and friends?" This adjustment process can take time. If participants are "stuck" at a particular stage, it may be a sign that additional help is needed. Remember that this process may be repeated if other diabetes-related changes occur (e.g., starting insulin, complications).

CONTENT OUTLINE

CONCEPT	DETAIL	INSTRUCTOR'S NOTES
5. Coping with feelings	5.1 Feelings do not happen in a particular order. They come and go, and you may have two or more of these feelings at once.	Feelings change from day to day—it's normal to have more than one feeling at a time.
	5.2 These are common responses to problems. The way you have handled your feelings in the past can help you deal with your feelings now.	Point out that this process is the same as for other problems or losses. Ask, "How have you handled difficulties in the past?" Ask participants what they believe will be helpful, based on these past coping strategies. Ask participants to identify coping strategies. Write these on the board and discuss. Coping strategies are more likely to be meaningful and implemented if identified by the person with the problem.
	5.3 Feelings also affect behavior because thoughts influence feelings, which influence motivation.	Point out that although they didn't choose to have diabetes, they can choose how they respond to and care for it.
	5.4 For example, people who think of diabetes as a disaster or burden feel and behave differently from those who view it as a challenge or opportunity.	Ask, "How do you view diabetes?" Point out that to change their emotional response, motivation, or behavior, they first need to understand the influence of their thoughts. Reframing is a strategy for modifying thoughts.
	5.5 The role of the health care team is to provide information and inspiration to help you change behavior, and support to ensure success with your diabetes plan.	
6. Getting the support you want and need	6.1 Most people find a support person helpful when living with diabetes.	Ask, "What have you found helpful in living with diabetes? Who do you turn to when you have a problem? Could he or she help you with your diabetes?"

CONTENT OUTLINE

CONCEPT	DETAIL	INSTRUCTOR'S NOTES
	6.2 Support can come from family, friends, your health care team, and/or others with diabetes.	Support groups may be particularly helpful for those with limited family support.
	6.3 Families and friends generally want to be supportive, but may not know how.	Ask, "How have your family and friends responded to your diabetes? How do you feel about their responses?"
	6.4 Family and friends need to know about diabetes and what you want them to do to help you.	Ask the group to brainstorm ideas for ways others can be supportive. Write these on the board. (Examples: exercise or eat healthy, notice positives rather than negatives, go to a support group with you, listen to your concerns, etc.)
	6.5 Also, family and friends may have feelings about your having diabetes. You need to recognize these feelings and their impact on support.	You need to understand their feelings just as you want them to understand yours. Honest communication is critical to avoid conflict.
	6.6 Studies have shown that people with diabetes do better when they get support for managing diabetes after this type of education program.	Ask, "What type of on-going support do you feel would be helpful for you?"
	6.7 Some find it helpful to join a diabetes support group, or to talk with a counselor or another person with diabetes.	Ask, "Has anyone been in a support group? What was your experience?" Provide information about local support groups or other resources. Ideas for resources include the American Diabetes Association, Community Mental Health Centers, Crisis Counseling Centers, Catholic Social Services, Jewish Family Services, and Pastoral Counseling Services.

CONTENT OUTLINE

CONCEPT	DETAIL	INSTRUCTOR'S NOTES
	6.8 Living with diabetes is difficult, but help and support are available.	You may want to close by discussing situations two, three, and/or ten from Outline #16, *Putting the Pieces Together* (p. 331). Ask participants to share a thought, feeling, or experience that has helped them to live with diabetes.
	6.9 Choose one thing you will do this week to care for your diabetes.	Close the session by asking participants to identify one action step they will take this week.

SKILLS CHECKLIST

None.

EVALUATION PLAN

Knowledge will be evaluated by achievement of learning objectives, by responses to questions during the session, and by the ability to acknowledge thoughts or feelings about diabetes. The ability to apply knowledge will be evaluated by the development of personal self-care goals, by the development and implementation of a plan to achieve those goals, and through program outcome measures.

DOCUMENTATION PLAN

Record class attendance and achieved objectives as appropriate.

SUGGESTED READINGS

American Diabetes Association: *Caring for the Diabetic Soul.* Alexandria, VA: American Diabetes Association, 1997

American Diabetes Association: *Winning with Diabetes.* Alexandria, VA: American Diabetes Association, 1997

Anderson BJ, Rubin RR: *Practical Psychology for Diabetes Clinicians,* 2nd Edition. Alexandria, VA: American Diabetes Association, 2002

Anderson D, Horton C, O'Toole ML, Brownson CA, Fazzone P, Fisher EB: Integrating depression care with diabetes care in real-world settings. *Diabetes Spectrum* 20:10–17, 2007

Anderson RM, Patrias R: Getting out ahead: the diabetes concerns assessment form. *Clinical Diabetes* 25:141–143, 2007

Anderson RM, Fitzgerald JT, Gruppen LD, Funnell MM, Oh MS: The diabetes empowerment scale-short form (DES-SF). *Diabetes Care* 6:1641–1643, 2006

Andrews LW: How to ask for help and get it. *Diabetes Self-Management* 27(3):42–45, 2006

SUGGESTED READINGS *continued*

Beverly E, Wray LA, Miller CK: Practice implications of what couples tell us about type 2 diabetes management. *Diabetes Spectrum* 21:39–45, 2008

D'Arrigo T: Fun in the sun. *Diabetes Forecast* 60(8):54–56, 2007

D'Arrigo T: Emotional eating. *Diabetes Forecast* 60(7):23, 2007

D'Arrigo T: Your biggest fan. *Diabetes Forecast* 60(2):46–49, 2007

Deatcher J: Spiritual self-care and the use of prayer. *Diabetes Self-Management* 19(6):57–59, 2002

DeGroot M, Anderson R, Freedland KE, Clouse RE, Lustman PJ: Association of depression and diabetes complications: a meta-analysis. *Psychosom Med* 63:619–630, 2001

Fisher EB, Thrope CT, DeVellis BM, DeVellis RF: Healthy coping, negative emotions, and diabetes management: a systematic review and appraisal. *The Diabetes Educator* 33:1080–1103, 2007

Fisher K: Assessing psychosocial variables: a tool for diabetes educators. *The Diabetes Educator* 32:51–56, 2006

Fisher L, Skaff MM, Mullen JT, et al.: Clinical depression versus distress among patients with type 2 diabetes. *Diabetes Care* 30:542–548, 2007

Funnell MM: The Diabetes Attitudes, Wishes, and Needs (DAWN) study (review). *Clinical Diabetes* 24:154–155, 2006

Funnell MM: Providing diabetes self-management support. *Practical Diabetology* 26(1): 46–48, 2007

Geil P, Hieronymus L: Maintaining your health during the holidays. *Diabetes Self-Management* 23(6):7–10, 2006

Gendelman N, Snell-Bergeon JK, McFann K, Kinney G, et al.: Prevalence and correlates of depression in individuals with and without type 1 diabetes. *Diabetes Care* 32:575–579 2009

Gilmer TP, Walker C, Johnson ED, Philis-Tsimikas A, Unutzer J: Improving treatment of depression among Latinos with diabetes using project Dulce and IMPACT. *Diabetes Care* 31:1324–1325, 2008

Gonzalez JS, Peyrot M, McCarl LA, Collins EM, et al.: Depression and diabetes treatment nonadherence: a meta-analysis. *Diabetes Care* 31:2398–2403, 2008

Gottlieb SH: Fighting the fear. *Diabetes Forecast* 59(2):28–30, 2006

Katon WJ, Russo JE, Von Korff M, Lin EHB, Ludman E, Ciechanowski PS: Long-term effects on medical costs of improving depression outcomes in patients with depression and diabetes. *Diabetes Care* 31:1155–1159, 2008

Murphey K: Shedding the burden of depression and anxiety. *Nursing* 38(4):34–42, 2008

Perry SJ: My spouse has diabetes. *Diabetes Forecast* 53(6):118–121, 2000

Peyrot M, Rubin RR: Behavioral and psychosocial interventions in diabetes: a conceptual review. *Diabetes Care* 30:2433–2440, 2007

Peyrot M, Rubin RR, Siminerio LM on behalf of the International DAWN Advisory Panel: Physician and nurse use of psychosocial strategies in diabetes care. *Diabetes Care* 29:1256–1262, 2006

Polonsky WH: *Diabetes Burnout*. Alexandria, VA: American Diabetes Association, 1999

Polonsky WH, Fisher L, Earles J, Dudl RJ, Lees J, Mullan J, Jackson RA: Assessing psychosocial distress in diabetes. *Diabetes Care* 28:626–631, 2005

Restinas J: Type 2 diabetes: adjusting to the diagnosis. *Diabetes Self-Management* 20(3):27–30, 2003

Roberts SS: Are you at risk for depression? How to know, what to do. *Diabetes Forecast* 58(7):20–21, 2005

Robertson C: Living alone and living well with diabetes. *Diabetes Self-Management* 22(3):26–31, 2005

Rubin RR, Ma Y, Marrero DG, Peyrot M, Barrett-Connor EL, Kahn SE, et al.: Elevated depression symptoms, antidepressant medicine use, and risk of developing diabetes during the Diabetes Prevention Program. *Diabetes Care* 31:420–426, 2008

Ruder K: Antidepressants: how they affect

SUGGESTED READINGS *continued*

blood glucose control. *Diabetes Forecast* 60(7):30–32, 2007

Ruder K: Driving me crazy. *Diabetes Forecast* 60(8):45, 2007

Ruder K: Finding a therapist. *Diabetes Forecast* 60(7):32, 2007

Siminerio LS, Funnell, MM, Peyrot M, Rubin RR: U.S. nurses' perceptions of their role in diabetes care: results of the cross-national Diabetes Attitudes, Wishes, and Needs (DAWN) study. *The Diabetes Educator* 33:152–162, 2007

Spero D: With a little help from our friends. *Diabetes Self-Management* 20(6):57–63, 2004

Tang TS, Brown MB, Funnell MM, Anderson RM: Social support, quality of life and self-care behaviors among African Americans with type 2 diabetes. *The Diabetes Educator* 34:266–276, 2008

Trif PM: Depression in elderly diabetes patients. *Diabetes Spectrum* 20:71–75, 2007

Unger J: Managing mental illness in patients with diabetes. *Practical Diabetology* 25(2):44–53, 2006

Weiss MA, Funnell MM: Beyond the numbers. *Diabetes Forecast* 57(5):53–54, 2004

Welch GW, Jacobon AM, Polonsky WH: The problem areas in diabetes scale. *Diabetes Care* 20:760–766, 1997

Zhang X, Norris SL, Chowdhury FM, Gregg EW, Zhang P: The effects of interventions on health related quality of life among persons with diabetes: A systematic review. *Medical Care* 45:820–845, 2007

▶ ▶ ▶ ▶ ▶

#3 The Basics of Eating

STATEMENT OF PURPOSE

This session is intended to emphasize the critical role of macronutrient intake in diabetes management. The composition of food groups and their impact on blood glucose are discussed, and participants are asked to consider how they most want to benefit from meal planning. The effects of composition, timing, and amount of food intake on blood glucose are addressed. Practice in measuring food is included. Participants are encouraged to have the person who prepares their food attend the nutrition sessions with them. Participants are asked to assess their own eating by keeping a food diary before the next session.

PREREQUISITES

None.

OBJECTIVES

At the end of this session, participants will be able to:

1. identify three macronutrients and their impact on blood glucose;

2. state the most important personal reason they might use a meal plan;

3. state how the timing of food can help them reach their blood glucose goals;

4. state how the composition of their meal plans can help them reach their blood glucose goals;

5. state how monitoring the amount of food eaten can help them reach their blood glucose or weight goals;

6. demonstrate how to measure liquid and dry ingredients;

7. describe how to keep a food diary;

8. develop an initial understanding of their personal emotional and cultural eating habits and influences.

CONTENT

Incorporating nutritional management into lifestyle.

MATERIALS NEEDED

VISUALS PROVIDED	ADDITIONAL
1. Reasons for Meal Planning	■ Food models
	■ Measuring cups and spoons
Handouts (one per participant)	■ Food scale
1. Food Diary Example	■ Chalkboard and chalk/Board and markers
2. Food Diary	■ Colored water and clear glasses
	■ Cereal and cereal bowls
	■ Other food as desired (see section 6)

METHOD OF PRESENTATION

Start by introducing yourself and telling what you do. Ask participants to introduce themselves. Explain that the purposes of this session are to discuss the role of diet in the treatment of diabetes and provide basic guidelines for eating.

Begin by asking how they did with their short-term goal and what they learned from it. Present material in a question/discussion format, using the first question as a starting point. Provide appropriate content outlined below in response. Ask if there are additional questions, and respond, repeating the process for the entire session. Use the questions in the Instructor's Notes section to generate discussion if no questions are forthcoming after a period of silence. Keeping track of the content discussed in each session, using the Diabetes Self-Management Record, the Participant Follow-up Record, or another form, helps you to evaluate if all needed content has been discussed.

If appropriate, explain that although the information provided is useful for people with type 1 and type 2 diabetes, it is important to realize that their personal meal plan may be different.

CONTENT OUTLINE

CONCEPT	DETAIL	INSTRUCTOR'S NOTES
1. Definition of diabetes mellitus	1.1 Diabetes mellitus is a disorder in which the body either does not produce insulin (type 1) or is unable to use the insulin that it makes (type 2).	Review definition by asking: ■ What is diabetes? ■ What does insulin do? ■ Where does blood glucose come from? ■ What happens if blood glucose cannot enter the cell?
	1.2 Food is composed of protein, fat, carbohydrate, vitamins, minerals, and water.	Ask, "What questions or concerns do you have about diabetes and food?"
	1.3 When food is eaten and digested, it is broken down into simple	

CONTENT OUTLINE

CONCEPT	DETAIL	INSTRUCTOR'S NOTES

substances—one of which is glucose (a form of sugar).

1.4 Glucose is needed by the cells for energy.

1.5 Insulin enables glucose to enter body cells.

1.6 If insulin is not available or effective, the glucose cannot enter the cells.

1.7 If glucose cannot enter the cells, it builds up in the blood, causing hyperglycemia (high blood glucose).

2. Role of diet

2.1 Food raises blood glucose. What, when, and how much food you eat affects how much the blood glucose increases. The more you know about what is in food, the better you'll understand how it affects your blood glucose. This helps you make decisions about what, when, and how much to eat.

Each person's glycemic response to foods varies. Blood glucose monitoring helps people learn about their individual responses. General guidelines are presented here.

2.2 Learning ways to balance food, diabetes medicines, and activity helps to keep blood glucose levels in your target range.

Ask, "What have you noticed about how food, activity, and stress each affect your glucose?"

2.3 Some people with type 2 diabetes can keep their blood glucose in their target range with meal planning alone. However, meal planning is basic for the treatment of all types of diabetes, even when oral agents, other injectibles, or insulin are taken.

3. Reasons for meal planning

3.1 The reasons for meal planning include:

Maintain blood glucose as close to your target range as possible.

Blood glucose management is often the main reason for meal planning.

Ask, "What are your reasons for paying attention to food choices?" Use Visual #1, Reasons for Meal Planning.

See Outline #11, *Managing Blood Glucose* (p. 231).

CONTENT OUTLINE

CONCEPT	DETAIL	INSTRUCTOR'S NOTES

It is also one reason that is different for people with diabetes than for people without diabetes. The closer to normal blood glucose levels can be safely kept, the lower the risk for eye, kidney, nerve, and blood vessel damage for people with diabetes. Most of the other reasons for meal planning apply to everyone.

Point out that nutrition is a growing science, so advice will change from time to time.

3.2 Maintain cholesterol (blood fats) and blood pressure levels as close to your target as possible.

People with diabetes have a greater risk of developing heart and blood vessel disease, especially when blood glucose and blood pressure levels are high for a period of time. High blood pressure levels also increase the risk for microvascular complications.

Diet to normalize cholesterol and other types of fat in the blood may help reduce the risk of heart disease. Information about reducing total fat is provided in Outline #4, *Food and Blood Glucose* (p. 53). More information about this topic is in Outline #18, *Eating for a Healthy Heart* (p. 379).

3.3 Prevent, delay, or treat diabetes-related complications.

Long-term complications with dietary implications include renal disease, gastroparesis, hypertension, and lipid abnormalities. Additional recommendations for protein, fiber, and sodium may be needed. See Outline #14, *Long-Term Complications* (p. 283), and Outline #18, *Eating for a Healthy Heart* (p. 379).

3.4 Improve health through food choices.

As with everyone, eating a variety of foods each day helps provide the many different vitamins and minerals your body needs.

Optimal nutrition helps avoid fatigue and increases resistance to infection. The diet for diabetes is a healthy diet for nearly everyone. Additional vitamins and minerals, specifically for people with diabetes, are not generally recommended at this time. Women who plan to become pregnant need to take folate and should also take

CONTENT OUTLINE

CONCEPT	DETAIL	INSTRUCTOR'S NOTES

calcium to prevent bone loss. It is important to assess vitamin, herbal, and nutritional supplement use by asking, "What vitamins, minerals, other supplements, or alternative therapies do you use?" The American Medical Association recommends that all adults take a multivitamin daily.

Vitamin D (1000 mg/dl) is increasingly being recommended for people with diabetes.

Ask your provider to check your blood to see if you are low in vitamin D.

3.5 **Meet individual nutritional needs.** Food meets both physical and psycho-social needs and is an expression of our cultures and family traditions.

Address individual needs including lifestyle, personal, and cultural preferences and desire to make changes. Point out that psychosocial, lifestyle, cultural, and family needs are critical components of a useful meal plan.

3.6 Calories are needed for:
■ reasonable body weight
■ normal growth and development
■ pregnancy and lactation
■ energy to work/play—physical activity.

3.7 Weight loss in an overweight person with diabetes may help reduce blood glucose, blood fats, and blood pressure. Losing 10–20 lb or 5–10% of body weight can help significantly.

Very high- or low-calorie diets can be disruptive to blood glucose levels. Moderate weight loss of 1–2 lb/week is recommended. Weight loss appears to be most helpful in the early stages of type 2 diabetes.

3.8 A reasonable weight goal is one that:
■ you choose
■ you can achieve and maintain
■ you can stick with over time.

Weight management is covered in Outline #4, *Food and Blood Glucose* (p. 53). Help the group identify the negatives and benefits of weight loss. Write on the board. Ask, "Do the negatives outweigh the positives for you? If not, what would it take to tip the balance?"

CONTENT OUTLINE

CONCEPT	DETAIL	INSTRUCTOR'S NOTES
	3.9 Some reasons may be more important to you than others.	Ask, "What is the most important reason for you to plan meals?"
4. Timing	4.1 Three things that directly affect blood glucose levels are timing of intake, portion sizes, and food composition.	
	4.2 The more you eat at one time, the more insulin you need. If you eat smaller amounts throughout the day, you will need less insulin. Eating a lot of carbohydrate at one time also increases your need for insulin. It takes more insulin to bring down a high blood glucose level than to keep the level in your target range.	Ask, "What have you heard about how often to eat when you have diabetes? Have you noticed differences in your blood glucose based on frequency or timing of meals?"
	4.3 Basic guidelines are:	These guidelines are starting points. The more information participants learn about food and diabetes care, the more flexible they can be and still reach their targets.
	■ Small meals throughout the day help keep glucose levels more even. Try to eat at least three meals a day.	Ask, "How many times do you eat each day?" A minimum of three meals a day is usually encouraged, but two meals and a snack may accomplish the same thing.
	■ Eat each meal and snack at about the same time each day.	Ask, "What times do you usually eat? Do they change from day to day?"
	■ Eat about the same amount of carbohydrate at each meal each day. Each breakfast should have about the same amount of carbs, and each lunch, etc. Day-to-day consistency is especially important for people who take one or two insulin shots per day.	Consistency is less important for those treated with multiple insulin injections who learn to use carbohydrate/insulin ratios.
	■ Skipping a meal after taking insulin or some diabetes medications greatly increases the risk of low blood glucose levels.	Ask, "What happens to you if you skip a meal?" Discuss occasions when a meal might be delayed. Skipping meals early in

CONTENT OUTLINE

CONCEPT	DETAIL	INSTRUCTOR'S NOTES
	It may also mean that you overeat later, which makes it harder to manage both blood glucose and weight.	the day often leads to overeating in the evening. This prevents hunger in the morning, perpetuating the cycle. Carry food with you if a meal will be delayed or you will be more active than usual.
	■ Eat breakfast. Research shows that eating early in the day helps to set an increased metabolic rate, promotes weight loss, and helps you manage overall intake and maintain weight loss.	Some people feel that eating breakfast increases hunger. After a few days, however, the body adjusts and regulates caloric intake so that late-evening hunger is diminished.
	■ Learn to balance the time you take medicine for your diabetes with the time you eat. Insulin and most diabetes medications work better to lower blood glucose if you take them at about the same time each day.	Explain problems associated with not doing this (e.g., taking insulin on rising without eating breakfast or taking short-acting insulin immediately before a meal). Some people find that a nighttime snack helps them maintain blood glucose levels at a safe level overnight and may prevent morning hyperglycemia.
5. Portion size	5.1 Too much food at one time raises blood glucose levels. Too much total food increases body weight.	
	5.2 If your blood glucose is high after some meals or if your weight is going up, eating less may help.	Ask, "What have you learned by monitoring after meals?" Blood glucose monitoring helps you evaluate the effect of different meals on blood glucose levels.
	5.3 Some ways to eat less are: ■ Choose smaller portions (one piece of toast for breakfast or one sandwich for lunch instead of two). ■ Eat only one serving. No seconds. ■ Use a small plate instead of a large plate. ■ Eat more slowly so you are the last one to finish the meal.	Ask, "Can you think of other ways to eat less food?" Brainstorm a list and write it on the board. Discuss and add ideas. Different ideas work for different people. (This section is not appropriate for growing children.)

CONTENT OUTLINE

CONCEPT	DETAIL	INSTRUCTOR'S NOTES

■ Serve plates in the kitchen instead of putting serving dishes on the table.
■ Keep tempting foods out of sight or out of the house.
■ Share dessert.
■ Put your fork down between each bite.
■ Figure out exactly how much you are eating and make a plan to eat a little less the next week. Gradual changes work best and are more likely to be sustained. For example, eat 6 oz of meat instead of 8 oz, or 1 1/2 cups of potatoes instead of 2 cups.
■ Ask someone else to do the tasting when you are cooking.
■ Eat smaller meals with low-calorie snacks to prevent hunger.
■ Identify your cravings to prevent binging.
■ Identify ways to cope with stress other than eating.
■ Ask for the support you need from family and friends.

Ask, "How do you get the support you need from others?"

6. Weighing and measuring food

6.1 Many people do not know how much they eat.

Demonstrate the differences between perceived and actual amounts of food with activities such as the following:
■ Hold up glasses of colored water and ask how much is in each. Pour into a measuring cup to see.
■ Ask three participants to pour a serving of cereal into a bowl (a different size/shape for each) and tell the amount. Measure each.
■ Pass around a piece of bread spread with margarine and jam. Ask participants to estimate the amount of each in teaspoons. Give answers.

CONTENT OUTLINE

CONCEPT	DETAIL	INSTRUCTOR'S NOTES

■ Using food models, ask participants to estimate the ounces of different-sized meat portions. Ask, "Are you surprised by any of the sizes of these portions?"

6.2 Weighing or measuring food is the way to know the amount you actually eat. Food labels give you the amount they consider to be a portion. This may be different from the amount you usually eat.

Introduce measuring as a tool to help participants become more aware of how much they eat now. Suggest that participants weigh or measure usual portions at home to get an idea of actual intake. The amount and the need for precision will vary from person to person and is reviewed in later sessions.

6.3 Use measuring cups and spoons to measure items that take the shape of the container, such as liquids and noodles.

Rice, noodles, soups, casseroles, vegetables, beverages, and condiments are usually measured by volume.

6.4 Use any easy-to-read food scale to weigh fruits, bread, baked goods, and meat.

If possible, demonstrate and allow time for participants to practice weighing and measuring.

6.5 Weigh and measure foods after cooking; the amount can change.

6.6 With practice, you will learn to estimate the amount of food in your dishes at home without measuring.

Most people do not weigh and measure all the time and do not need to do so.

6.7 You can also learn to estimate serving sizes.

■ A 1-cup serving of carbohydrates, including fruit, vegetables, pasta, or rice, is about the size of your fist.
■ One 3-oz serving of protein, such as meat, fish, or poultry, is equivalent to the size of a deck of playing cards or the palm of your hand.
■ A 1-oz serving of cheese is equal to the size of your thumb.
■ A teaspoon-size serving of

CONTENT OUTLINE

CONCEPT	DETAIL	INSTRUCTOR'S NOTES

mayonnaise or margerine is about the size of your thumb-tip.
- A 2-oz serving of a snack food is about the size of a handful.
- A 1-cup serving of yogurt or fresh greens is about the size of a tennis ball.

6.8 You may need to weigh and measure your foods when:
- you're just learning about portion sizes or are making a change in your meal plan
- you lose or gain weight
- your blood glucose goes out of target range
- you change your medication doses or exercise level
- you want to avoid "portion-size creep," when portion sizes gradually increase without you noticing.

Measuring helps you to be sure food intake is consistent so other changes can be better understood and you can make informed decisions.

7. Assessing how you eat now

7.1 You (and your health care team) need to know what you are eating now so you can see what changes could help. People are often not aware of what they eat during the day.

The fewer changes a person makes, the more likely he or she is to maintain those changes. Making fewer changes that can be sustained is more useful than short-lived radical or multiple changes.

7.2 A food diary shows exactly what you are eating. It shows you the kinds, times, and amounts of foods you eat.

Ask, "What is a food diary?" Distribute Handout #1, Food Diary Example.

7.3 A food diary is a record of what you eat during the day. It shows:
- what foods you eat and drink
- amounts of food
- the times you eat
- the way you usually eat
- foods you can and cannot live without.

Ask, "How do you think a food diary might help you?" A food diary can help both the patient and the health care team in several ways. Benefits may include understanding:
- total intake
- meal timing and location
- food preparation patterns
- food preferences
- emotional eating
Changes to improve blood

CONTENT OUTLINE

CONCEPT	DETAIL	INSTRUCTOR'S NOTES

glucose or reduce calories can be more easily determined.

7.4 Decide which days to keep the diary. Choose both weekdays and weekend days. Write down:
- ■ the food you eat and drink (even small bites)
- ■ the amount in teaspoons, tablespoons, cups, and ounces
- ■ the time
- ■ the place
- ■ your thoughts and feelings.

Acknowledge that the task has cost (work) and benefits (learning about yourself).

7.5 Write down the foods when you eat them so you don't forget. Keep the diary where you can see it, such as on the refrigerator.

7.6 Try writing down what you plan to eat and drink before you actually do—this may help with portion control.

Studies have shown this to be an effective weight loss and maintenance strategy.

7.7 Because many of us eat when we are "stressed, blessed, or depressed," writing down how you feel when you eat can help you better understand why you eat what you eat.

Ask, "Does this ever happen to you? Have you tried ways to deal with feelings other than food?" Write these on the board and discuss.

7.8 Include information about where you were and what you were doing and feeling. This helps to identify specific situations that are hard for you.

If possible, have participants practice recording their most recent meals or snacks.

7.9 Remember to write down the amount of each food you eat (the portion size). Include liquids. Remember that all the little bites of food you eat while you are cooking need to be recorded.

Remind them to record the parts of a sandwich as:
    1 sandwich:
    bread, 2 slices regular
    roast beef, 2 oz
    mayonnaise, 1 tsp lite
    lettuce, tomato

7.10 Note how the food was prepared.

7.11 Be sure to write down salad dressings, condiments, and any other added items (e.g., nondairy creamer to coffee).

Distribute Handout #2, Food Diary. Participants can use this to keep their own food diaries.

CONTENT OUTLINE

CONCEPT	DETAIL	INSTRUCTOR'S NOTES
	7.12 Keep the food diary for at least 3 days before the next nutrition session. The food diary will be most helpful if you try to eat in your usual way while keeping it.	Write the date of that session on the chalkboard. The days selected should be typical of their eating pattern and reflect weekdays and weekend days.
	7.13 Keep in mind that a food diary is information, not a judgment.	Stress the importance of data for learning and informed decision-making.
8. Getting started	8.1 Lasting eating changes usually come in steps, not all at once. Steps are actions you can measure. For example, you could: ■ carry lunch to work one day ■ drink 1/2 cup instead of 1 cup of juice for breakfast ■ test before and after a snack if you would like to see how that snack affects your blood glucose.	
	8.2 Choose one thing you will do this week to care for your diabetes.	Close the session by asking participants to identify one action step they will take this week.

SKILLS CHECKLIST

Each participant will be able to weigh and measure food and keep a food diary.

EVALUATION PLAN

Knowledge will be evaluated by achievement of learning objectives and by responses to questions during the session. The ability to apply knowledge will be evaluated by the development of personal meal-planning goals, by implementation of changes in the amount or timing of food intake, and through program outcome measures.

DOCUMENTATION PLAN

Record class attendance and achieved objectives as appropriate using the Diabetes Self-Management Record, the Participant Follow-Up Record, or another form.

SUGGESTED READINGS

American Diabetes Association: Eating Healthy with Diabetes. Alexandria, VA: American Diabetes Association, 1998

Chalmers KH, Peterson AE: *16 Myths of the Diabetic Diet.* Alexandria, VA: American Diabetes Association, 2007

D'Arrigo T. Build your bones. *Diabetes Forecast* 59(9):62–65, 2006

Franz MJ, Wylie-Rosett J: The 2006 American Diabetes Association nutrition recommendations and interventions for the prevention and treatment of diabetes. *Diabetes Spectrum* 20:49–52, 2007

Geil PB, Holzmeister LA: *101 Nutrition Tips for People with Diabetes.* Alexandria, VA: American Diabetes Association, 2006

Hammond J: Mindful eating. *Diabetes Self-Management* 4(2):36–40, 2007

Kleefstra N, Houweling ST, Jansman GA, Groenier KH, et al.: Chromium treatment has no effect in patients with poorly controlled, insulin-treated type 2 diabetes in an obese western population. *Diabetes Care* 29:521–525, 2006

Liu S, Song Y, Ford ES, Manson JE, Buring JE, Ridker PM: Dietary calcium, Vitamin D, and the prevalence of metabolic syndrome in middle aged and older U.S. women. *Diabetes Care* 28:2926–2932, 2005

Pastors JG, Arnold MS, Daly A, Franz M, Warshaw HS: *Diabetes Nutrition Q&A for Health Professionals.* Alexandria, VA: American Diabetes Association, 2003

Pittas AG, Dawson-Hughes B, Li T, Van Dam RM, et al.: Vitamin D and calcium intake in relation to type 2 diabetes in women. *Diabetes Care* 29:650–656, 2006

Shahar DR, Abel R, Elhayany A, Vardi H, Fraser D: Does dairy calcium intake enhance weight loss among overweight diabetic patients? *Diabetes Care* 30:485–489, 2007

Spano M: Choosing a multivitamin. *Diabetes Self-Management* 24(3):46–54, 2007

Wansink B: What really determines what we eat? *Diabetes Self-Management* 23(6):44–51, 2006

Watts S, Anselmo J: Nutrition for diabetes: all in a day's work. *Nursing* 36(6):46–48, 2006

Webb R: B vitamins are vital. *Diabetes Forecast* 59(5):27–29, 2006

➲ Reasons for Meal Planning

- ■ Maintain blood glucose as close to your target range as possible.

- ■ Maintain cholesterol (blood fats) as close to your target range as possible.

- ■ Maintain blood pressure as close to your target level as possible.

- ■ Prevent, delay, or treat diabetes-related complications.

- ■ Improve health through food choices.

- ■ Meet individual nutritional needs.

⏺ Food Diary Example

Time	Place	Thoughts and Feelings	Foods and How Prepared	Amount
8:15 am	Home (kitchen, at table, in front of tv)	Hungry, in a hurry	Egg, poached Orange juice Toast Margarine	1 1/2 cup 1 slice 1 tsp
10:00 am	Work		Coffee	1 cup

12:30 pm	Home	Hungry, ate alone	Sandwich:
			  Bread
			  Roast beef
			  Mayonnaise
			  Lettuce, tomato
			Sugar cookies
			Low-fat (1%) milk
				
				2 slices reg.
				2 oz
				1 Tbsp lite
				
				2
				1 1/2 cups

6:00 pm	Restaurant (fast food, take out, sit down)	Enjoyed friends, got too full	Fried chicken Coleslaw Mashed potatoes Gravy Apple pie Lemonade	1 leg and thigh 1/2 cup 1 cup 1/4 cup 1 piece 1 1/2 cups
10:00 pm	Movie	Tired, popcorn smelled good	Buttered popcorn Diet cola	2 cups 2 cups (16 oz)

➡ Food Diary

_____   _____   _____
NAME   DAY   DATE

Time	Place	Thoughts and Feelings	Foods and How Prepared	Amount

| #4 | Food and Blood Glucose |

▶ ▶ ▶ ▶ ▶

STATEMENT OF PURPOSE

This session is intended to provide an understanding of how different foods affect blood glucose levels and lay the groundwork for approaches to meal planning. Participants are asked to review their food diaries and look for relationships between their food intake and blood glucose levels. To help participants predict the likely impact of individual foods, the general effects of carbohydrate, protein, and fat on blood glucose are presented; food groups are introduced; and the nutrients present in foods from each group are identified. Participants are encouraged to use blood glucose monitoring to evaluate the actual effects of different foods on their blood glucose levels. The need for all nutrients and the benefits of including all food groups to promote overall health are stressed. This approach to diabetes nutrition education emphasizes outcomes and encourages experimentation. Access to blood glucose monitoring is helpful. Select the material from this outline that is appropriate for your audience.

The impact of food on weight and the cardiovascular system is expanded in Outline #17, *Food and Weight* (p. 367), and Outline #18, *Eating for a Healthy Heart* (p. 379). Encourage the participants to bring the person who prepares their food to this session. If participants have not kept a food diary, ask that they write down what they ate the previous 2–3 days so that they can refer to it during class.

PREREQUISITES

It is recommended that participants have attended Session #3, *The Basics of Eating* (p. 37), or have achieved those objectives. Ask participants to bring their completed food diaries to this session. If participants have not kept a food diary, ask that they write down what they ate the previous week so that they can refer to it during class.

OBJECTIVES

At the end of this session, participants will be able to:

1. discuss what they learned from keeping a food diary;

2. name the six basic groups of food;

3. name several foods in each group;

4. state that the body needs foods from all the groups to stay healthy;

5. name the three nutrients in food that contain calories and affect blood glucose;

6. describe how each nutrient affects blood glucose;

7. develop an initial understanding of their personal food habits;

8. state that blood glucose monitoring is a way to find out how specific foods affect blood glucose;

9. name the foods they eat that are highest in carbohydrate, protein, and fat.

CONTENT

Incorporating nutritional management into lifestyle.

MATERIALS NEEDED

VISUALS PROVIDED	ADDITIONAL
1. Reasons for Meal Planning	■ Food models
2. Nutrients in Food	■ Commercial food product containers or labels that illustrate types of food
	■ Chalkboard and chalk/Board and markers
Handouts (one per person)	■ *The First Step in Diabetes Meal Planning,* 2nd Edition, *or Healthy Food Choices,* 2nd Edition
1. Food Groups	■ *Choose Your Foods: Exchange Lists for Diabetes* (available from the American Diabetes Association, www.diabetes.org, or 800-232-6733)
2. Nutrients in Food Groups	■ *Guide to Good Eating* (one-page flyer with color pictures of foods in each of five groups; available from the National Dairy Council)

METHOD OF PRESENTATION

Start by introducing yourself and telling what you do. Ask participants to introduce themselves. Explain that the purposes of this session are to provide information about different groups of foods, the nutrients in each group, and the effects these nutrients have on blood glucose and overall health. The information can be used by participants to make food choices that help them reach personal targets.

Begin by asking how they did with their short-term goal and what they learned from it. Present material in a question/discussion format, using the first question as a starting point. Provide appropriate content outlined below in response. Ask if there are additional questions, and respond, repeating the process for the entire session. Use the questions in the Instructor's Notes section to generate discussion if no questions are forthcoming after a period of silence. Keeping track of the content discussed in each session, using the Diabetes Self-Management Record, the Participant Follow-up Record, or another form, helps you to evaluate if all needed content has been discussed.

CONTENT OUTLINE

CONCEPT	DETAIL	INSTRUCTOR'S NOTES
1. Review	1.1 The purpose of meal planning is to help you reach blood glucose, weight, and other long-term goals.	Review reasons for meal planning using Visual #1, Reasons for Meal Planning. Ask participants to identify the reason that is most important to them. Ask, "What questions or concerns do you have about meal planning for diabetes?"
2. Food diary	2.1 Keeping a food diary can help you become more aware of how you eat.	Ask participants to look over their food diaries and discuss what they find. Ask questions like, "Did you discover anything? How far apart were the times you ate? Were there some days you ate later than others? Did you eat large amounts at some meals or on some days and much smaller amounts other times? How did your feelings affect your food choices? Did keeping a record affect your food choices?"
	2.2 If you notice what you eat and monitor your blood glucose, you can discover how food choices affect your blood glucose.	Ask, "Did you notice any differences in your blood glucose when you ate differently?" Explore this neutrally; allow participants to find (or not find) links between their eating and blood glucose levels.
	2.3 Your food diary can help you figure out what is easy and hard for you about food choices and what foods you want to keep in your plan and which foods you can easily do without.	Assessment is essential before making plans for change. Ask, "Did you identify any changes you want to make based on your food diaries?"
	2.4 Learning about food and how it affects you can also help.	

CONTENT OUTLINE

CONCEPT	DETAIL	INSTRUCTOR'S NOTES
3. What are food groups?	3.1 For decades, foods with similar nutritional values have been sorted into groups.	Some people will remember the Basic 4 or even the Basic 7 food groups. The food guide pyramid and the exchange systems for meal planning build on the use of food groups.
	3.2 Grouping foods can make it easier to think about how different foods affect your blood glucose, weight, heart, and overall health.	
	3.3 At the present time, foods are divided into six groups: ■ starch ■ vegetable ■ fruit ■ meat ■ milk ■ fat.	Ask, "What are the six food groups used today?" List the six groups on the chalkboard. Acknowledge different ways to group foods.
	3.4 Foods in each group include: ■ **Starch.** Bread, rolls, pasta, rice, cereal, and dried beans and starchy vegetables such as potatoes, corn, peas, and winter squash. ■ **Fruit.** Apples, oranges, bananas, and all other fruits—fresh, frozen, canned, or juice (even unsweetened).	Ask, "What foods in your diary belong in the starch group?" Use food models or pictures to illustrate which foods belong to each group. Allow time for participants to practice assigning their foods to groups. For a more complete listing, refer to *Choose your Foods: Exchange Lists for Diabetes*. Use Handout #1, Food Groups, *The First Step in Diabetes Meal Planning*, 2nd Edition, or the *Guide to Good Eating* from the National Dairy Council.
	■ **Vegetable.** Carrots, green beans, broccoli, beets, greens, and other crunchy vegetables.	Fat added to vegetables needs to be counted as fat.
	■ **Milk.** All milk and some yogurts.	Plain or sweetened with non-nutritive sweeteners yogurt has about the same nutrients as a glass of milk. Extra sugar may be added to fruit-flavored and frozen yogurts.

CONTENT OUTLINE

CONCEPT	DETAIL	INSTRUCTOR'S NOTES

| | | Some diet hot chocolate mixes may fit in this group. |

■ **Meat.** Beef, fish, poultry, cheese, cottage cheese, eggs, tofu, and wild game.

Instructor's Notes: Note that the meat group includes fish, meat substitutes, and other high-protein foods.

■ **Fat.** Butter, margarine, cream, oils, salad dressings, sour cream, cream cheese, fatback, bacon, nuts, olives, and avocados. Alcohol is included in this group.

Instructor's Notes: Some foods do not obviously fit in one of these groups. The grouping rationale is addressed later.

3.5 Your body needs food from all six groups. Each group contains different nutrients.

Instructor's Notes: The amount of food needed from each group is discussed in Outline #5, *Planning Meals* (p. 69).

4. Nutrients in food

4.1 Your body needs many types of nutrients to live and be healthy. You have to take in nutrients because your body cannot make them.

Instructor's Notes: Ask, "What questions do you have about nutrition?"

4.2 Some foods make your blood glucose go up higher and faster than others. Knowing about the nutrients in food can help you predict what different foods will do to your blood glucose.

4.3 Nutrients in food are carbohydrate, protein, fat, vitamins, minerals, and water.

Instructor's Notes: Ask, "What are the major nutrients in food?" As the class names the nutrients, list them on the chalkboard, or use Visual #2, Nutrients in Food Groups.

4.4 Carbohydrate, protein, and fat contain calories. Only carbohydrates directly affect blood glucose levels.

Instructor's Notes: Ask, "What have you noticed about how different nutrients affect your blood glucose levels?"

4.5 Vitamins, minerals, and water do not contain calories or raise blood glucose but are necessary for optimal health.

Instructor's Notes: Some vitamins and minerals are required for the body to be able to use glucose for energy. Ask, "What vitamins and minerals do you take?"

CONTENT OUTLINE

CONCEPT	DETAIL	INSTRUCTOR'S NOTES
5. What is carbohydrate?	5.1 Carbohydrate is another term for sugar, starch, and fiber. Starch is a chain of sugar molecules. All starch is broken down into sugar. Starch is like a string of beads, where each single bead is sugar.	In terms of glycemia, the total amount of carbohydrate is more important than the source or type.
	5.2 Your body burns carbohydrate for energy and needs more of this nutrient than any other.	Clarify the difference between starch as a nutrient (one component of food) and starch as a food group.
	5.3 Starch, fruit, and milk are the food groups high in carbohydrate. Small amounts of carbohydrate are present in foods from the vegetable group.	See Handout #2, Nutrients in Food Groups. To illustrate that sugar is not inherently bad for people with diabetes, note that the carbohydrate in fruit and milk is in the form of a sugar.
	5.4 Foods that include ingredients from those three food groups contain carbohydrate. Some examples are casseroles, soups, stews, pizza, and snacks (chips, pretzels, and french fries). Sweets (ice cream, cake, cookies, and pie) and some alcoholic beverages (beer and sweet wine) also contain carbohydrate.	Ask, "Which foods in your diary contain carbohydrate?" Most of these foods contain fat and some also contain protein.
	5.5 The total carbohydrate equals sugar + starch + fiber. The human body cannot change fiber into blood glucose.	Animals can get energy from fiber.
6. What is protein?	6.1 Protein is also a nutrient in food. Protein builds and repairs muscles, skin, and every cell in the body.	Ask, "What foods in your food diary contain protein?"
	6.2 Protein breaks down into amino acids.	The body needs insulin to use protein.
	6.3 Nitrogen from the breakdown of amino acids must be filtered by the kidneys. Reducing protein is often recommended for people with diagnosed nephropathy.	The recommended daily allowance (RDA) for protein is 0.8 g/kg. For a 150-lb person, this is 55 g, which is provided by 4 oz meat, 1 cup milk, 6 slices of bread, and 1/2 cup vegetables.

CONTENT OUTLINE

CONCEPT	DETAIL	INSTRUCTOR'S NOTES
		Many people eat more protein than this each day.
	6.4 Milk and meat groups are high in protein. Smaller amounts are found in foods from the starch and vegetable groups. 1/2 cup milk and 3–4 oz meat per day, within a balanced diet, will provide the RDA for protein.	Refer to Handout #2, Nutrients in Food Groups. Ask participants to review their food diaries and find foods that contain protein. Note how cheese, eggs, and peanut butter can be substituted for meat. Point out that more milk products are needed to provide the RDA for calcium.
7. What is fat?	7.1 Fat is an essential nutrient that supplies energy, maintains healthy skin, and carries the fat-soluble vitamins A, D, E, and K.	A very small amount (1 tsp corn oil) is required to prevent fatty acid deficiency. More fat (18% of calories) is needed to transport fat-soluble vitamins and maintain cells in the body. Ask, "Which foods in your food diary contain fat?"
	7.2 Fat contributes flavor and texture. Without fat, beef and lamb would taste about the same.	
	7.3 Too much saturated fat increases the risk for heart and blood vessel disease.	A low-fat, high-carbohydrate diet elevates triglycerides in some people. A diet with 20–40% calories from fat may be optimal. Saturated fat contributes most to cardiovascular disease. Types of fat are discussed in Outline #18, *Eating for a Healthy Heart* (p. 379).
	7.4 Fat is high in calories. Foods with fat contain more calories per bite than foods without fat. All fats have the same number of calories, even though some are better than others for your heart and blood vessels.	Each gram of fat has 9 calories. This is more than twice the 4 calories per gram in carbohydrate and protein.
	7.5 The nutrient fat is, of course, high in the fat food group. Several (but not all) foods in the milk and meat group also provide fat.	Refer again to Handout #2, Nutrients in Food Groups. Examples: A cup of whole milk contains 8 g of fat (equal to

CONTENT OUTLINE

CONCEPT	DETAIL	INSTRUCTOR'S NOTES
		about 1 1/2 pats of butter). Skim milk contains less than 1 gm of fat. Point out that caloric differences are due to different amounts of fat content.
	7.6 Fat is present in most combination, convenience, snack, and sweet items. These are often thought of as "comfort" foods.	Ask, "Can you think of other foods that contain fat? Have you ever tried to cut down on high-fat foods? How did it go?"
8. Effects of carbohydrates on blood glucose levels	8.1 As much as 100% of the carbohydrate you eat may be changed into glucose in your body.	You may want to use the word *metabolism*—the process by which energy is made available for body functions.
	8.2 All absorbable carbohydrate foods turn to sugar in the blood. In equal amounts, sugar and starch affect blood glucose in a similar way.	Starch, a string of glucose molecules, may be absorbed more quickly than sucrose (table sugar), a combination of glucose and fructose. Fructose is absorbed more slowly than glucose. Fiber is not observed as blood glucose.
	8.3 Most carbohydrate is digested and absorbed within 2 hours after eating.	Checking blood glucose levels 2 hours after eating shows you the effect of carbohydrates and how well your body used the food. Ask, "Do you ever check your blood glucose after meals? What have you noticed?"
	8.4 Other sweet liquids, such as regular soft drinks, lemonade, punch, and cider, will also raise your blood glucose quickly, as will sherbets and sorbets.	These items may be used to treat a low blood glucose reaction.
	8.5 Foods with added sugar, such as cookies and candy, contain a lot of carbohydrate per bite. It is easy to eat more carbohydrate than you think you are eating.	

CONTENT OUTLINE

CONCEPT	DETAIL	INSTRUCTOR'S NOTES
	8.6 Compact foods like granola or dried fruit are also higher in carbohydrate per bite than similar foods that contain more air and/or water. Eating the same amount of cereal every morning does not always mean eating the same amount of carbohydrate.	Compare the volume of different cereals with 30 g of carbohydrate. Ask, "Which cereal would you choose?" There is no "right" answer. Ask participants to pour out three different cereals in same-size bowls. Ask them to calculate the grams of carbohydrate based on the nutrition label information.
	8.7 If you divide carbohydrate among all your meals and snacks, your body can use the glucose more easily and keep your blood glucose levels more even. This does not necessarily mean eating less total carbohydrate.	Ask participants to use food models to show a day's menu that does (and does not) distribute carbohydrate-containing foods throughout the day. If there are no food models, ask that they write menus on the board.
	8.8 Fat takes longer to be digested and absorbed. Because fat leaves the stomach more slowly, it slows down how fast carbohydrate (including sugar) reaches the bloodstream.	High-sugar, high-fat foods like regular ice cream may not cause an immediate or noticeable postprandial increase in blood glucose.
9. Finding balance	9.1 Your body needs all the nutrients to feel good, repair itself, and fight disease. We all need carbohydrate, protein, and fat every day.	Meals that include carbohydrate plus protein and/or fat delay the absorption of glucose into the bloodstream and may delay hunger.
	9.2 But too much carbohydrate makes blood glucose too high, too much fat contributes to weight gain and heart and blood vessel disease, and too much protein may increase the chance for kidney problems. Eating too much food of any kind can give your body more carbohydrate, protein, fat, and calories than it needs.	
	9.3 Eating meals that contain carbohydrate, protein, and fat helps keep your blood glucose levels more even.	Point out that substituting a low-fat or fat-free food may cause blood glucose levels to rise more quickly.

CONTENT OUTLINE

CONCEPT	DETAIL	INSTRUCTOR'S NOTES

9.4 A sample meal would include:
■ 2–3 starch choices (such as 2–3 slices of bread or 1–1 1/2 cups of potato, or 1 cup pasta or rice)
■ 1 small piece of fruit and/or 1 cup of plain vegetables
■ 1 cup of milk and/or 1–3 oz of meat, poultry, fish, or cheese.

Help the class develop several meals that fit these criteria. One possibility is to write a meal on the chalkboard and ask the class what is missing.

9.5 Foods with added sugar or fat can make your meal plan more enjoyable. Knowing the nutrients in food can help you make choices about how much and how often you want to eat these foods.

Ask, "How do you handle cravings for these foods?" Some people find eating a little bit helps, while others can't "eat just one."

9.6 In general, everyone also benefits from:
■ spacing meals and eating regularly
■ managing portion sizes
■ eating at least three meals per day
■ eating breakfast every day.

Refer to Outline #3, *The Basics of Eating* (p. 37).

10. Planning for change

10.1 The following are food choices that could help you lower your blood glucose after a meal:
■ Eat less carbohydrate at the meal and include some fat or protein in the meal.
■ Eat more fiber at the meal.

Ask, "What is your blood glucose target? At what times of the day is your blood glucose higher or lower than you want it to be? What food changes might help you lower or raise your blood glucose at that time?"

10.2 To eat less carbohydrate at a meal:
■ Choose fewer high-carbohydrate foods. You could have orange juice, toast, and peanut butter instead of orange juice, cereal, milk, and banana. Or, choose baked potato, green beans, and tossed salad instead of baked potato, corn, and a roll.
■ Eat smaller portions. Drink 1/2 cup juice instead of 1 cup, or have one roll instead of two.

Ask, "What are ways to eat less carbohydrate at a meal?" Refer to concept 8 in this outline. *Note:* Substituting carbohydrate foods with items from the meat or fat group is a way to reduce postprandial blood glucose levels and still satisfy hunger and meet caloric needs.

CONTENT OUTLINE

CONCEPT	DETAIL	INSTRUCTOR'S NOTES

■ Eat foods with less carbohydrate per bite. Choose 1 cup of Cheerios instead of 1 cup of granola, or 1 cup of broccoli instead of 1 cup of peas.
■ Drink a diet soft drink instead of a regular one.
■ Skip dessert or eat a small portion.
■ Eat a less sweet dessert. Choose plain ice cream instead of a hot fudge sundae.

10.3 Check blood glucose regularly to see if you are reaching your targets and to see how different foods affect your blood glucose.

Check at varying times throughout the day, including post-meals.

10.4 Treat a low blood glucose reaction with the right amount of carbohydrate needed to bring your blood glucose level up to the target level without going too high.

Refer to Outline #11, *Managing Blood Glucose* (p. 231), for information about treating hypoglycemia.

10.5 Choose one thing you will do this week to care for your diabetes.

Although overall health is not the primary focus in this session, some participants may be interested in adding foods from a food group (such as milk or vegetables) they currently omit.

SKILLS CHECKLIST

None.

EVALUATION PLAN

Knowledge will be evaluated by achievement of learning objectives and by responses to questions during the session. The ability to apply knowledge will be evaluated by development of personal meal-planning goals to improve blood glucose levels and through program outcome measures.

DOCUMENTATION PLAN

Record class attendance and achieved objectives as appropriate using the Diabetes Self-Management Record, the Patricipant Follow-up Record, or another form.

SUGGESTED READINGS

American Diabetes Association and American Dietetic Association: *Choose Your Foods: Exchange Lists for Diabetes.* Alexandria, VA: American Diabetes Association, 2007

American Diabetes Association and American Dietetic Association: *Choose Your Foods: Exchange Lists for Weight Management.* Alexandria, VA: American Diabetes Association, 2007

American Diabetes Association and American Dietetic Association: *Official Pocket Guide to Diabetic Exchanges.* Alexandria, VA: American Diabetes Association, 2003

Atkinson FS, Foster-Powell K, Brand-Miller JC: International tables of glycemic index and glycemic load values. *Diabetes Care* 31:2281–2283, 2008

Balay JL: Glycemic index update. *Diabetes Self-Management* 25(1):34–40, 2008

D'Arrigo T: Meal replacements: safe and effective? *Diabetes Forecast* 60(8):18, 2007

D'Arrigo T: Emotional eating. *Diabetes Forecast* 60(7):23, 2007

Franz MG: The glycemic index: useful or not? *Practical Diabetology* 26(2):11–16, 2007

Freeman J, Hayes C: Low-carbohydrate food facts and fallacies. *Diabetes Spectrum* 17:137–140, 2004

Sheard NF, Clark NG, Brand-Miller JC, Franz MJ, Pi-Sunyet FZ, Mayer-Davis E, Kulkarni K, Geil P: Dietary carbohydrate (amount and type) in the prevention and management of diabetes: ADA position statement. *Diabetes Care* 27:2266–2271, 2004

➲ Reasons for Meal Planning

■ Maintain blood glucose as close to your target range as possible.

■ Maintain cholesterol (blood fats) as close to your target range as possible.

■ Maintain blood pressure as close to your target level as possible.

■ Prevent, delay, or treat diabetes-related complications.

■ Improve health through food choices.

■ Meet individual nutritional needs.

➲ Nutrients in Food

Nutrient	Contains Calories
Carbohydrate	☒
Protein	☒
Fat	☒
Vitamins	☐
Minerals	☐
Water	☐

⊖ Food Groups

Starch	Bread, rolls, bagels, English muffins, tortillas, pita bread, naan, crackers, matzoh
	Rice, pasta, noodles, spaghetti, macaroni
	Cereal, dry or cooked
	Legumes: lentils, dried or canned beans (garbanzo, kidney, black, or butter beans), dried peas (split peas or black-eyed peas), miso
	Starchy vegetables: potatoes, corn, green peas, squash, taro root, yams
Fruit	Apples, oranges, bananas, and all other fruits except avocado— fresh, frozen, canned, or juiced
Milk	All milk products
	Yogurt (plain or artificially sweetened)
Vegetable	Carrots, green beans, wax beans, broccoli, beets, greens, okra, and all other crunchy vegetables
Meat	Beef, pork, lamb, chicken, turkey, fish
	Peanut butter, cheese, cottage cheese, eggs, tofu
Fat	Butter, margarine, cream, oil, salad dressing, mayonnaise
	Sour cream, cream cheese, coffee creamer
	Bacon, lard, fatback, nuts, seeds, avacado

➲ Nutrients in Food Groups

Food Group	Nutrient(s)	Effect on Blood Glucose	Rate of Effect on Blood Glucose
Starch	**Carbohydrate** Protein	Large	Fast
Fruit	**Carbohydrate**	Large	Fast
Milk	**Carbohydrate** Protein Fat	Large	Fast (slower if reduced fat [2%] or whole milk)
Vegetable	**Carbohydrate** Protein	Small	Fast
Meat	**Protein** Fat	—	—
Fat	**Fat**	—	—

#5   **Planning Meals**

▶ ▶ ▶ ▶ ▶

STATEMENT OF PURPOSE

This session builds on the information in Outline #3, *The Basics of Eating* (p. 37), and Outline #4, *Food and Blood Glucose* (p. 53), and provides information and practice in planning menus using *Healthy Food Choices, Eating Healthy with Diabetes, Healthy Food Choices,* 2nd Edition, *Basic Carb Counting,* and the plate method. Information about the basics of carbohydrate counting is also included in this outline. The purpose of this session is to present a variety of options for meal planning. Omit discussion of approaches that do not meet the needs of your audience. Sections on eating out, the use of alcohol, and selecting cookbooks are included. More advanced carbohydrate counting is covered in Outline #19, *Carbohydrate Counting* (p. 399).

The choice of the meal-planning approach depends on the personal goals, abilities, and lifestyle needs of each participant and the type and status of his or her diabetes. Encourage participants to consider which approach they could most easily use on a consistent basis.

PREREQUISITES

This session will be more useful for those who complete and bring a food diary to the session. It is recommended that each participant have attended sessions #3, *The Basics of Eating* (p. 37), and #4, *Food and Blood Glucose* (p. 53), or have achieved those objectives. If they have a meal plan, ask that participants bring it to class with them.

OBJECTIVES

At the end of this session, participants will be able to:

1. using the food diary, compare their food choices with the basic guidelines;

2. describe five different approaches to planning meals;

3. use one of these approaches to plan a menu for 1 day;

4. plan one restaurant meal that fits with their usual plans;

5. describe how alcohol may affect a person with diabetes;

6. identify three guidelines for the use of alcohol (if they use alcohol);

7. identify personal benefits and barriers for their chosen meal planning method;

8. identify strategies to incorporate meal planning into their lives;

9. explain how at least three cookbook recipes will fit into their meal plans.

CONTENT

Incorporating nutritional management into lifestyle.

MATERIALS NEEDED

VISUALS PROVIDED

1. Reasons for Meal Planning
2. Free Foods
3. Plate Method: Breakfast
4. Plate Method: Lunch/Dinner
5. Food Groups
6. Nutrients in Food Exchange Groups

Handouts (one per participant)
1. Counting Carbohydrate Servings
2. Tips for Counting Carbohydrate Servings
3. Eating Away From Home
4. Guidelines for Use of Alcoholic Drinks
5. Cookbooks for People with Diabetes

ADDITIONAL

■ Chalkboard, chalk/Board, markers
■ Food models or pictures of food
■ *The First Step in Diabetes Meal Planning* and *Eating Healthy with Diabetes* (booklets available from the American Diabetes Association, www.diabetes.org, or 800-232-6733)
■ The *Month of Meals* series (books available from the American Diabetes Association— use several)
■ *Basic Carbohydrate Counting* (booklet available from the American Diabetes Association)
■ *Choose Your Food: Exchange Lists for Diabetes* (booklet available from the ADA)
■ Restaurant menus (obtain from restaurants popular with the participants)
■ Examples of diabetes cookbooks, including appropriate ethnic cookbooks

METHOD OF PRESENTATION

Start by introducing yourself and telling what you do. Ask participants to introduce themselves. Begin by asking about their short-term goal and what they learned from it. Ask participants to review their food diaries by asking if they made any discoveries while they were keeping it.

Family members and significant others, especially those who shop or prepare meals for the person with diabetes, should be encouraged to attend. Present material in a question/discussion format. Include time for participants to practice meal planning by creating menus they could use at home and at a restaurant.

Begin by asking how they did with their short-term goal and what they learned from it. Present material in a question/discussion format, using the first question as a starting point. Provide appropriate content outlined below in response. Ask if there are additional questions, and respond, repeating the process for the entire session. Use the questions in the Instructor's Notes section to generate discussion if no questions are forthcoming after a period of silence. Keeping track of the content discussed in each session, using the Diabetes Self-Management Record, the Participant Follow-up Record, or another form, helps you to evaluate if all needed content has been discussed.

CONTENT OUTLINE

CONCEPT	DETAIL	INSTRUCTOR'S NOTES
1. Basic guidelines	1.1 These basic guidelines offer a starting point for meal planning: ■ Eat at least three meals and snacks spaced throughout the day. ■ Eat each meal and snack at about the same time each day. ■ Do not skip meals. ■ Eat about the same amount at each meal each day. ■ Pay attention to how much you eat.	Ask, "What questions or concerns do you have about planning meals?" Review the guidelines discussed in Outline #3, *The Basics of Eating* (p. 37). Allow time for participants to share their experiences and ask questions. Day-to-day variation leads to less even glucose patterns.
	1.2 The purpose of meal planning is to help you reach your personal blood glucose or weight goals. Some can reach their goals by spacing their food intake and limiting portion sizes. Others benefit from a more specific meal plan.	Review reasons for meal planning in Outline #3, *The Basics of Eating* (p. 37). Ask participants to identify their personal blood glucose and weight targets and reasons for meal planning. Ask, "Have you ever tried a very specific meal plan? Did it work for you? Why or why not?" Use Visual #1, Reasons for Meal Planning.
	1.3 Knowing what and when you eat now is the first step in deciding what changes might help you. Knowing why you eat certain foods and at certain times and situations, is equally important.	Assessment is essential to identify patterns, meal components, and areas of difficulty. Consider self-determined blood glucose, lipid, and weight goals; medical needs; weight history; food preferences; psychosocial and cultural needs; interest in change; how much flexibility you want and need in your diet; and available financial and other resources.
	1.4 Keeping a food diary can help you become more aware of how you eat now. It may also help you understand how certain foods affect your blood glucose when combined with your monitoring record.	Ask participants to look over their food diaries. Ask, "How did your choices compare with the basic guidelines? What did you learn about yourself and your eating habits? Did you find anything you would like to do differently? Anything you are willing to change?" It is

CONTENT OUTLINE

CONCEPT	DETAIL	INSTRUCTOR'S NOTES

| | | important to know both what you will and will not do. |

| | 1.5 There are many different ways to plan meals for diabetes. Approaches presented in this session are:
■ healthy food choices
■ preplanned menus
■ the plate method
■ basic carbohydrate counting
■ the exchange system. | An overview of carbohydrate counting may be introduced in this session. It is discussed in more detail in Outline #19, *Carbohydrate Counting* (p. 399). A dietitian may work with someone to count calories or fat grams methods often used for weight loss), but these methods are not detailed in these outlines. |

| | 1.6 Different plans work for different people. You may use different approaches over time or in different situations. Think about which approaches might work for you. | Any method that helps participants to focus on meal planning is helpful. For a personal plan, refer participants to a dietitian who is experienced in diabetes or who is a diabetes educator. |

| | 1.7 If you see a dietitian, let him/her know how they can be of the most help to you. While they are experts in diabetes and nutrition, you are the expert on yourself and your diet. | |

| **2. Healthy Food Choices** | 2.1 *Healthy Food Choices* is a guide for simplifying diabetes meal planning. It has two main parts: "Healthy Food Choices" and "Food Servings," a meal planning section. | |

| | 2.2 "Healthy Food Choices" gives eight guidelines:
■ Eat a variety of foods.
■ Avoid skipping meals.
■ Eat healthy carbohydrates.
■ Watch serving sizes.
■ Eat less fat.
■ Be at a healthy weight.
■ Be physically active.
■ Choose a healthy lifestyle. | Ask participants to look at each section. Refer to their food diary or ask them to write down everything they ate since yesterday at this time or just think about the food they eat each day. Ask participants to think about how much exercise they get each week. |

| | 2.3 One idea under EAT HEALTHY CARBOHYDRATES says: "Avoid regular soft drinks. One can has 9 teaspoons of sugar." It also has 150–200 calories. | Other ideas include eating fewer sweet foods and using sugar-free soft drinks/powdered drinks, sparkling water, club soda, |

CONTENT OUTLINE

CONCEPT	DETAIL	INSTRUCTOR'S NOTES

sugar-free iced tea, or a slice of lemon in plain water. Ask, "Are there changes you can make to eat healthier carbohydrates?" List these on the board and add to the list as needed.

2.4 Then look at the ideas under EAT LESS FAT. The first idea talks about how meat is cooked. Another strategy is to choose lower-fat and very lean meat and other foods. Cook lean meats in small amounts of "good" fats like olive, peanut, canola, sunflower, and safflower oils so they are less dry, or use cooking methods such as stewing or braising.

Ask, "Are there ways you could eat less fat?" List these on the board and add to the list as needed. For example, if you eat 8 oz of meat at dinner, could you eat 5 or 6 oz instead? Other ideas include having a meatless meal a few times a week; buying veggie burgers, lean hamburger, or ground round; using less butter, cream, and salad dressing; and drinking skim or low-fat milk instead of whole milk.

2.5 The "Food Servings" section helps you to plan meals using foods from six food groups and two specialty sections. The six food groups are:
- starch
- fruits
- milk
- nonstarchy vegetables
- meat and meat substitutes
- fats.

The specialty sections are "Other Foods" and "Free Foods."

Space for developing menu ideas that fit into the participants' meal plan is given on the back of the pamphlet. Encourage participants to design a meal plan to fit personal food preferences and calorie needs. Any plan should include a variety of foods from each group. Eating a food high in vitamin C every day and a food high in vitamin A three or four times a week is recommended. Calcium requirements also need to be considered, particularly for postmenopausal women. Vitamin D (1,000 mg/day) is increasingly recommended for people with diabetes. Suggest that participants ask for a blood test of Vitamin D levels to determine if additional Vitamin D is needed.

CONTENT OUTLINE

CONCEPT	DETAIL	INSTRUCTOR'S NOTES

2.6 *Eating Healthy with Diabetes* is a resource that participants can use to design a meal plan. You can design your own meal plan or work with a dietitian to help you plan the number of servings from each group. Each person's needs (calories, nutrients), likes, and dislikes are different.

Refer to *Eating Healthy with Diabetes*. Point out the sections of each meal and snack and how to count mixed meals. Ask, "Do you think having a meal plan would be helpful for you? Would you prefer to develop it on your own or work with a dietitian?"

2.7 In each food group, each food listed is one serving. For example:

1 serving of starch = 1/3 cup pasta (noodles), **or** 1 small potato, **or** 1 slice of bread, **or** 3 cups popcorn

Read the foods listed in each group. If there are foods you like that aren't listed, ask your dietitian how to count them.

If your plan has four servings from the starch group, you could either choose four different foods or eat four servings of one food (such as four slices of bread).

Note the spaces to write in menu ideas. Some of your favorite foods may be combination foods (one, two, or more different food groups in one serving), such as pizza or casseroles.

Exchange values of foods are available in *Choose Your Foods; Exchange Lists for Diabetes* and other books. Calorie, carbohydrate, protein, and fat values for additional foods are available in commercial product information, such as Pennington and Church's *Food Values of Portions Commonly Used* and on food labels.

2.8 Here are some tips about food groups:

■ **Fruits**. No sugar or syrup is added. Unsweetened fruit juice.
■ **Milk**. 1% and 2% milk counts as reduced fat. Skim and 1/2% milk count as low fat. Plain yogurt counts as milk.
■ **Vegetables**. Use without sauce or added fat. (Choose from fat group, if desired.)

Note that calories vary in different kinds of milk, but the amount of carbohydrate, protein, and calcium are the same. If syrup or juice from canned fruit is used in cooking, it is counted as fruit juice.

CONTENT OUTLINE

CONCEPT	DETAIL	INSTRUCTOR'S NOTES

■ **Protein**. Servings are given in ounces. Add up the total ounces per day. One egg or 1/4 cup tuna counts as 1 oz of protein.

Protein servings are likely to be smaller than participants usually eat. Illustrate with models.

■ **Fats**. Most people enjoy foods that are high in fat. "Spend" your fats carefully on foods that you truly enjoy.

Other examples of high-fat foods are bacon and powdered coffee creamer.

2.9 At the bottom of the "Food Servings" page, "Other Foods" shows how to count combination foods, which count more than one food group in a single serving.

Examples:
Casserole (1 cup) = 2 starch servings + 2 protein servings + 0–2 fat servings
Cream soup (1 cup) = 1 starch serving + 1 fat serving

2.10 "Free Foods" lists foods with less than 20 calories per serving that can be eaten with meals or between meals. Remember that even low-calorie foods can add up to weight gain if you eat a lot of them. If you need a lot of free foods to feel full, talk with your dietitian about how to adjust your plan.

Ask, "Do you eat a lot of 'free foods'? Do you find them helpful?"

Examples:
1 stick diet gum = 5–10 calories
1/2 cup diet Jell-O = 8 calories
1 Tbsp diet syrup = 10 calories
1 Tbsp diet salad dressing = 6–16 calories

Use Visual #2, Free Foods. Too many free foods can slow weight loss. A meal plan that is too hard to stay on without eating a lot of free foods won't last long and may not provide adequate nutrients.

2.11 Use the "Menu Ideas" space on the back to write the times of your meals/snacks and menu ideas.

When discussing meal times, keep in mind that consistency is more important for people who take insulin than for those who don't. It is desirable for all participants to spread foods out over the day. For participants who take insulin, the number of servings planned for each meal can be included to the left of the sample meals to help ensure consistency.

CONTENT OUTLINE

CONCEPT	DETAIL	INSTRUCTOR'S NOTES
	2.12 Now that you have some ideas about food choices, it is time to think about your goals. Choose what is important to you and do what is possible. Write down your goals.	Suggested steps: ■ Choose one way to change eating habits to work toward goals. ■ Write a sample menu using *Healthy Food Choices,* 2nd edition.
3. Preplanned	3.1 Using preplanned menus is another way to structure eating. The *Month of Meals* series presents menus with 28 breakfasts, 28 lunches, and 28 dinners. The pages of the books are divided so that each breakfast can go with any lunch and dinner.	Show a book from the *Month of Meals* series, and demonstrate the variety of menus that could be planned. These menus offer a resource for participants who say, "Just tell me what to eat," and others interested in using preplanned menus and recipes.
	3.2 The three meals plus a planned snack provide 1,500 calories. Instructions are included to increase or decrease the calorie level to match your needs.	Point out the snack lists in the back of the book. Show how to adjust the calorie level. Ask, "Does this appeal to you? Have you ever tried using preplanned menus? How did it work for you? Why or why not?"
	3.3 Simple recipes are printed with the menus. Most recipes make one to four servings.	In groups (depending on the number of copies of *Month of Meals* books available), ask participants to plan a menu for a day that they would be willing to prepare and eat.
4. The plate method	4.1 The plate method is a way to plan meals and manage carbohydrates with no measuring. You fill your plate to match the amount of vegetables, starch, and meat in a sample picture, then add a piece of fruit and/or glass of milk.	This is a simple method used first in Europe. It is especially useful for older adults, those with limited literacy, or numeracy skills, and those who do not want to use more structured or counting methods. Some patients who use other approaches may find this method helpful when eating away from home (e.g., at potlucks, restaurants, or dinner parties).

CONTENT OUTLINE

CONCEPT	DETAIL	INSTRUCTOR'S NOTES
	4.2 Divide your plate into fourths. At breakfast, 1/2 is for starches and 1/4 for meat. No vegetables are eaten and protein is optional, so the entire plate is not used.	Use Visual #3, Plate Method: Breakfast. Using food models, ask participants to create breakfast meals using Visual #3 as a guide. If participants eat cereal for breakfast, mark a disposable bowl they can take home, with a line showing a serving size of the cereal they like.
	4.3 At lunch and dinner, use 1/4 for starches, 1/4 for meat, and 1/2 for vegetables. Keep in mind that this method does not account for fat.	Use Visual #4, Plate Method: Lunch/Dinner. Create other lunch and dinner meals (including a potluck or restaurant meal) using Visual #4 as a guide. Use food models on a plastic plate with sections or a marked paper plate. For those unable to eat a lot of vegetables, use 1/2 of the plate for the fruit serving instead of vegetables.
	4.4 Filling a dinner (9-inch) plate without snacks will provide 1,200–1,500 calories per day, depending on serving sizes and fat portions.	Ask, "Does the plate method appeal to you? How do you think it would work for you? Are there strategies you could use to make it easier?"
5. Basic carbohydrate counting	5.1 Carbohydrate counting is another meal-planning approach. As you remember, carbohydrate affects blood glucose more than any other nutrient.	Review the effects of carbohydrate, protein, and fat on blood glucose from Outline #3, *The Basics of Eating* (p. 37), as needed Ask, "Have you ever tried counting carbohydrates? did it work for you? Why or why not?"
	5.2 The starch, fruit, milk, and sweets and desserts groups have similar amounts of carbohydrate. Even when the amount of carbohydrate is the same, the amount of fiber can affect how a food impacts your glucose level. Many foods have fiber added.	Use *Basic Carbohydrate Counting* or review carbohydrate-containing foods from Outline #4 as needed. Ask the group to practice identifying which foods do and do not contain carbohydrate. Note that vegetables contain 5 g carbohydrate, but that amount

CONTENT OUTLINE

CONCEPT	DETAIL	INSTRUCTOR'S NOTES

is so small it can be ignored unless three or more servings are eaten. Provide information about how to deal with fiber, either by subtracting half the total fiber or by subtracting the total fiber from the number of carbohydrates when there are more than 5 grams of fiber.

5.3 Each serving of starch, fruit, or milk is counted as one carbohydrate serving.

5.4 Each carbohydrate serving provides about 15 g carbohydrate. You can count either carbohydrate servings or grams. If you know the carbohydrate content, all foods can be worked into this plan.

Use food labels or reference books to determine the amounts of foods often eaten by participants that equal 15 g carbohydrate.

5.5 You first need to decide how many servings or grams of carbohydrates to have at each meal. You can then make choices about the specific carbohydrate foods you will eat to match the number of servings. This provides flexibility and variety in your meals.

The carbohydrate level and distribution is determined by each person, based on food preferences, blood glucose records, caloric needs, and triglyceride levels. Stress the importance of pre- and postmeal blood glucose monitoring. As a general guideline, use 3–4 carbohydrate servings per meal for women and 4–5 carbohydrate servings per meal for men.

Examples of meals providing four carbohydrate servings each:
- 1 sandwich
- 1 small apple
- 1 oz potato chips
   OR
- 1 cup spaghetti
- 1/2 cup pasta sauce
- 1 oz slice garlic bread
   OR
- 1 cup oatmeal
- 2 Tbsp raisins
- 1 slice toast

Using food models, show how to use different carbohydrate food items to create different meals with similar carbohydrate content. Use the *Basic Carbohydrate Counting* booklet and Handouts #1 and #2 to reinforce these concepts.

CONTENT OUTLINE

CONCEPT	DETAIL	INSTRUCTOR'S NOTES
6. The Exchange System	6.1 Review reasons for meal planning. Your most important personal goal may be to improve blood glucose levels, cholesterol levels, or weight.	Ask, "What questions or concerns do you have about the exchange system? How many of you use it."
	6.2 Meal planning using the exchange system provides a consistent balance of carbohydrate, protein, and fat to keep blood glucose stable. Regular timing of meals also helps to keep blood glucose in the target range.	Ask "How has the exchange system worked for you?" Blood glucose monitoring results can help determine your response to various foods.
	6.3 Using an exchange plan can help people with diabetes obtain the variety of foods needed for good health and the calories needed to reach or maintain a desired body weight. It can also help lower blood fats and regulate blood glucose.	Use Visual #1, Reasons for Meal Planning. Note that using the exchange system can help with all the reasons for meal planning.
	6.4 The meal plan is like a food budget with a certain number of food choices to "spend" at each meal.	
	6.5 Food choices are from six basic groups of food. The food or exchange groups are starch, fruit, vegetables, milk, meat, and fat. These are the same food groups used in the MyPyramid; however, some foods may be grouped differently in the MyPyramid.	Ask, "What are the six food groups?" Use Visual #5, Exchange Groups.
	6.6 The food groups are listed so that all of the carbohydrate-containing groups are together: starch, fruit, sweet, desserts, and other carbohydrates and nonstarchy vegetables.	
	6.7 The absorption of carbohydrate will be slowed by the presence of fat in a mixed meal and decreased by fiber.	

CONTENT OUTLINE

CONCEPT	DETAIL	INSTRUCTOR'S NOTES

6.8 Note the major nutrients in each group. The foods in each group contain similar amounts of carbohydrate, protein, fat, and calories. This means that each food in one group will affect blood glucose in a similar way when used in the amount listed.

Use Visual #6, Nutrients in Food Groups. You may want to note that nutrient values for different foods in a group are similar, not identical. Using food models or the *Choose Your Food: Exchange Lists for Diabetes* booklet, review foods from each group.

6.9 Exchange means that any food in one group can be exchanged for any other food in the same group because foods in the same group affect blood glucose similarly.

6.10 The exchange system allows for many choices.

Give examples of choices (for 1 fat exchange, you could use 1 tsp margarine, 1 Tbsp cream cheese, or 2 Tbsp sour cream). Use Visuals of each food group or, using food models, set up a dinner plate that includes 1 vegetable exchange. Show how different vegetables can be "exchanged" to provide 1 vegetable exchange. Repeat with other groups until the concept of exchanging is clear. Note that exchanges are for measured amounts.

6.11 Your personal meal plan includes the number of choices or exchanges from each food group and the meal or snack for which they are planned.

6.12 You and your dietitian will calculate your personal meal plan, based on your likes and dislikes, personal eating habits, activity level, and diabetes medications. You need to help develop a meal plan that you can use in real life. Tell your dietitian about foods that are important to include or omit. Remember, it's your meal plan.

Ideally, insulin programs are adjusted to fit the meal plan and activity level. It takes trial and error to work out the best plan. Also, note that some adaptation of this system is needed for those with special dietary needs.

CONTENT OUTLINE

CONCEPT	DETAIL	INSTRUCTOR'S NOTES
7. Eating away from home	7.1 Many people enjoy eating in restaurants, but the food is different than you might fix at home.	Ask, "Do you enjoy eating at restaurants? Why?" Discuss reasons for eating out (other than food).
	7.2 Review reasons for meal planning. Your most important personal goal may be to improve blood glucose levels, cholesterol levels, or weight.	Ask participants to identify their most important nutritional goal.
	7.3 Possible barriers to eating in a restaurant: ■ temptation to overeat ■ foods don't fit your meal plan ■ methods of food preparation make it hard to tell what's in the food ■ mealtime may be early or later	Ask, "Do you expect any problems taking care of your diabetes when eating away from home? What strategies have you used to deal with those barriers?" Write these on the board and discuss.
	7.4 Tips for eating out: ■ Know what is important to you about eating out. ■ Remember the reasons you use a meal plan. ■ Know your meal plan. ■ Choose kinds and amounts of food that best fit into your meal plan. ■ Choose plain food. Limit foods that have been sweetened, breaded, or fried or are in sauces or gravies. It is harder to predict the nutrient value of combination foods.	Distribute Handout #3, Eating Away from Home. Review content and answer questions. Ask, "Are there particular restaurants or types of restaurants that you find more difficult? Are there strategies you can use to handle those situations?" Plain foods have fewer calories per bite so you can eat more without overeating.
	■ Collect sample menus to review at home or look online. ■ Substitute an extra starch for a fruit or milk choice if milk or fruit are not available. ■ Look for free foods or plain vegetables to increase the amount of food without raising blood glucose. ■ Ask how foods are prepared—	Plan ahead—call the restaurant or bring up the menu online if you are unsure of the menu. Bread or rolls are often more available than unsweetened fruit or fat-free (skim) milk, and the carbohydrate content is similar. Raw or plain cooked vegetables should not greatly affect blood glucose or calorie levels. Ask, "How comfortable are you

CONTENT OUTLINE

CONCEPT	DETAIL	INSTRUCTOR'S NOTES

breaded, fried, sugar added?
■ Ask if foods are available even if they are not listed on the menu: fresh fruit, juice, fat-free (skim) milk, vegetables, margarine, and diet drinks.

with asking questions or asking for an item that's not on the menu?" Role-playing may help people becomes more assertive in asking for what they want in a restaurant.

7.5 The following are requests you might make:
■ Serve salad dressing, sour cream, and butter on the side so you can control your portion.
■ Prepare vegetables and meat without added fat.

■ Substitute plain vegetables, starch, or fruit for a sweetened menu item.

Ask, "What item might you request?" Write answers on the board and discuss.

Examples: broiled fish instead of fried fish; baked potato instead or french fries.
Examples: fresh fruit instead of cocktail; toast instead of a sweet roll.

7.6 Activity: Select a restaurant dinner using the plate method and/or carbohydrate counting. Choose the main dish first. Notice the foods that would most easily fit into a meal plan.

Distribute the restaurant menus. Use the plate method as a guide to choosing foods from the menu, not a literal, "filling-the-plate" unless selecting from a buffet.

7.7 It is possible to adjust insulin to cover increases in food if you know the amount of carbohydrate in the food.

8. Guidelines for altered mealtimes

8.1 If the meal is delayed:
■ 1 hour—eat a piece of fruit or bread from dinner at the regular time; subtract from dinner.
■ 2–3 hours—eat the evening snack at dinnertime and dinner at snacktime.
Each person responds differently to changes in meal timing, depending on insulin, activity, etc. Blood glucose monitoring can help you adjust your meal schedule

Delayed meals may cause hypoglycemia if you take medicine (particularly certain types of insulin) for diabetes.

CONTENT OUTLINE

CONCEPT	DETAIL	INSTRUCTOR'S NOTES

and keep your blood glucose level where you want it to be.

8.2 If the meal is early:
■ 1 hour—follow regular eating pattern (or use next option)
■ 2–3 hours—save one carb from meal and eat it as a snack at your regular mealtime.

Stress that guidelines for delayed and early meals will vary depending on the participant's therapy.

9. Use of alcoholic drinks

9.1 Alcohol is not a food. It does not provide carbohydrate, protein, fat, or vitamins. It does provide 7 calories per gram.

Ask, "How does drinking alcohol affect your blood glucose level?"

9.2 Alcohol is treated like a poison by the body. Your liver works first to get rid of the alcohol and is less able to help regulate your blood glucose. You may have a low blood glucose reaction after drinking alcohol. This effect can last 8–12 hours.

The liver cannot counterregulate during hypoglycemia because alcohol blocks gluconeogenesis. This is of particular concern for people who take insulin or certain diabetes medicines.

9.3 Alcohol is a depressant. You may not be able to tell the difference between early effects of alcohol and early symptoms of hypoglycemia.

Alcohol itself does not improve cholesterol. It is other compounds in the ingredients of an alcoholic beverage that can be beneficial.

9.4 Alcohol during pregnancy can harm the developing baby.

9.5 Alcohol is not recommended with some types of medication. Alcohol changes the action of many drugs.

9.6 Because it provides calories without other nutrients and stimulates appetite, alcohol can make weight control more difficult.

The additional calories in alcoholic beverages are counted as fats in the exchange system. One regular beer (12 oz) has 150 calories and counts as 1 starch and 2 fat exchanges. One regular nonalcoholic beer (12 oz) has 60 calories and counts as 1 starch exchange.

9.7 Guidelines for using alcohol include:
■ Alcohol can be safely used only when your blood glucose is in

Distribute Handout #4, Guidelines for Use of Alcoholic Drinks. Ask, "What do you do

CONTENT OUTLINE

CONCEPT	DETAIL	INSTRUCTOR'S NOTES
	the target range. Discuss its use with your provider to be sure it is safe for you.	to make sure you are safe when you drink alcohol?"
	■ Because alcohol can lower blood glucose, drink only with meals or snacks containing carbohydrate.	Name some carbohydrate snacks. Note that peanuts, cheese, or boiled eggs do not provide carbohydrate.
	■ Drink in moderation. ■ Avoid sweet wine, liqueurs, and sweetened mixed drinks because of their high sugar content.	Moderation is defined as one equivalent for women and two for men per day. Equivalent = ■ 1 1/2 oz distilled spirits ■ 4 oz dry wine ■ 12 oz beer
	■ Mixers such as water, soda water, and sugar-free carbonated drinks are free; unsweetened fruit or vegetable juices can be counted as fruit or vegetable exchanges. ■ Sip slowly. ■ Do not drink before, during, or after vigorous exercise.	Wine spritzer made with club soda is a better choice than a wine cooler, which is made with fruit juice or sweetened mixers. Both alcohol and exercise can lower blood glucose. In combination, reactions are more likely.
10. Recipes	10.1 Most recipes can be adapted to provide low-fat, low-sugar foods that still taste similar.	As an activity, ask for favorite recipes and work with the group to adapt them.
	10.2 Try reducing the amount of fat you add to your favorite recipe, or substitute a nonfat or lite product. The sugar in baked products can often be reduced by 1/4 to 1/2 of the original recipe without major changes in taste.	Ask, "Have you tried to lower the fat or sugar content of a familiar recipe? How did it work?"
	10.3 Several cookbooks provide low-fat, low-sugar recipes and provide information about nutrient content.	Distribute Handout #5, Cookbooks for People with Diabetes. Show sample cookbooks. *Note:* Not all recipes from a cookbook for people with diabetes fit all meal plans.
	10.4 Keep in mind that no single food or dish is good or bad. There is nothing you cannot eat and you can learn to include all foods in your plan.	Practice by selecting recipes and stating how that dish might fit into an overall plan.

CONTENT OUTLINE

CONCEPT	DETAIL	INSTRUCTOR'S NOTES
11. Planning	11.1 Food and meal planning are often the areas of greatest struggle for people with diabetes.	Ask, "What is hardest or the most difficult aspect of planning meals for you? Are there things you can do to make it easier?" Write on the board and discuss with the group.
	11.2 Choose a method that you believe you can and will use on a regular basis. You can take charge of your diabetes one meal and one day at a time.	
	11.3 Be careful not to judge yourself as good, bad, or "cheating" based on your food choices.	Distinguish between making choices and cheating. As an adult you have the right to make choices about the food you eat. You also have the right to choose when and how you will use your meal plan.
	11.4 Choose one thing you will do this week to care for your diabetes.	Close the session by asking participants to identify one action step they will take this week.

SKILLS CHECKLIST

Participants will be able to create a menu that helps to meet their goals and will be able to identify items on a restaurant menu that fit with their meal plans.

EVALUATION PLAN

Knowledge will be evaluated by achievement of learning objectives and by responses to questions during the session; skills will be evaluated by observation. The ability to apply knowledge will be evaluated by the development of personal meal-planning goals, by development and implementation of a plan to achieve those goals, and through program outcome measures.

DOCUMENTATION PLAN

Record class attendance and achieved objectives as appropriate using the Diabetes Self-Management Record, the Participant Follow-up Record, or another form.

SUGGESTED READINGS

Bellens JWJ, Stolk RP, van der Schoouw YW, Grobbee DE, et al.: Alcohol consumption and risk of type 2 diabetes among older women. *Diabetes Care* 28:2933–2938, 2005

Buethe M: CountCarbs: a 10 step guide to teaching carbohydrate counting. *The Diabetes Educator* 34:67–74, 2008

King AB: Alcohol consumption and diabetes. *Practical Diabetology* 27(1):27–30, 2008

Kulkarni K: Carbohydrate counting: a practical meal-planning option for people with diabetes. *Clinical Diabetes* 23:120–124, 2005

Papanas N, Mallezos: Education for dietary freedom in type 1 diabetes. *The Diabetes Educator* 34:54–58, 2008

Povey RC, Clark-Carter D: Diabetes and healthy eating: a systematic review of the literature. *The Diabetes Educator* 33:931–959, 2007

Richardson T, Weiss M, Thomas P, Kerr D: Day after the night before: influence of evening alcohol on risk of hypoglycemia in patients with type 1 diabetes. *Diabetes Care* 28:1801–1804, 2005

Roberts S: Carb counting: a flexible way to plan meals. *Diabetes Forecast* 60(5):25–27, 2007

Shal I, Wainstein J, Harman-Boehm I, Raz I, Fraser D, Rudich A, Stampfer MJ: Glycemic effects of moderate alcohol intake among patients with type 2 diabetes. *Diabetes Care* 30:3011–3016, 2007

Sheard NF, Clark NG, Brand-Miller JC, Franz MJ, Pi-Sunyet FZ, Mayer-Davis E, Kulkarni K, Geil P: Dietary carbohydrate (amount and type) in the prevention and management of diabetes: ADA statement. *Diabetes Care* 27:2266–2271, 2004

◐ Reasons for Meal Planning

■ Maintain blood glucose as close to your target range as possible.

■ Maintain cholesterol (blood fats) as close to your target levels as possible.

■ Maintain blood pressure as close to your target level as possible.

■ Prevent, delay, or treat diabetes-related complications.

■ Improve health through food choices.

■ Meet individual nutritional needs.

⬤ Free Foods

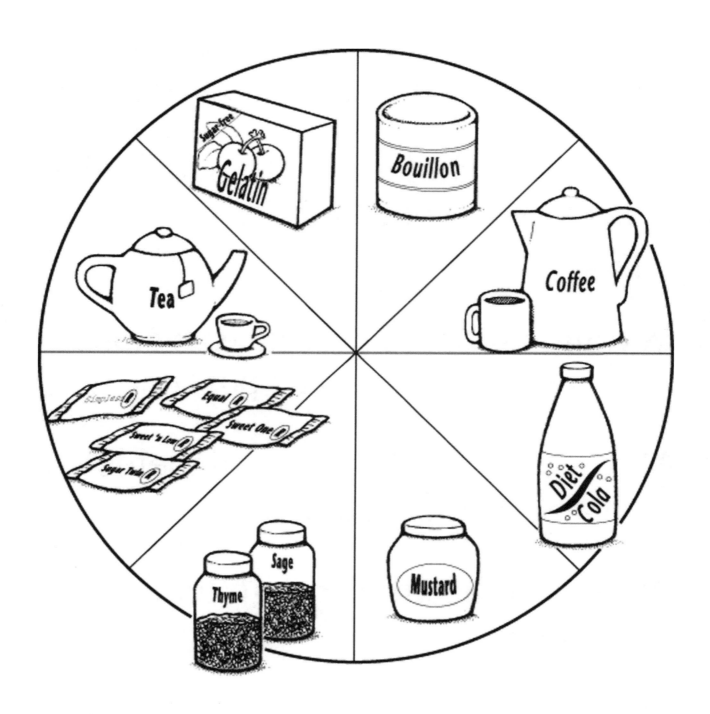

➲ Plate Method: Breakfast

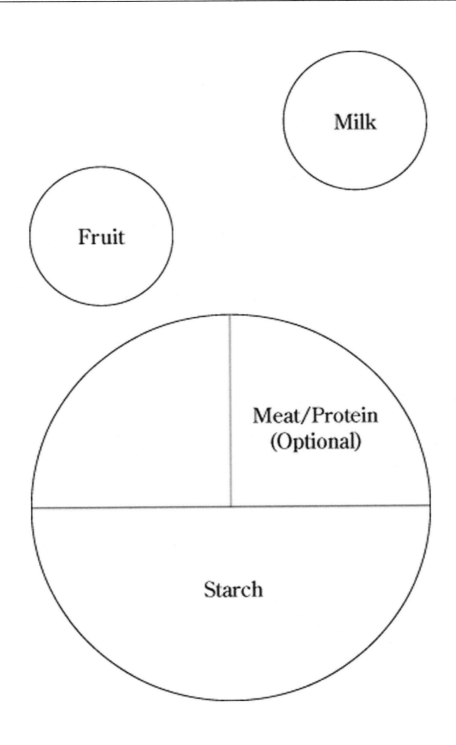

➡ Plate Method: Lunch/Dinner

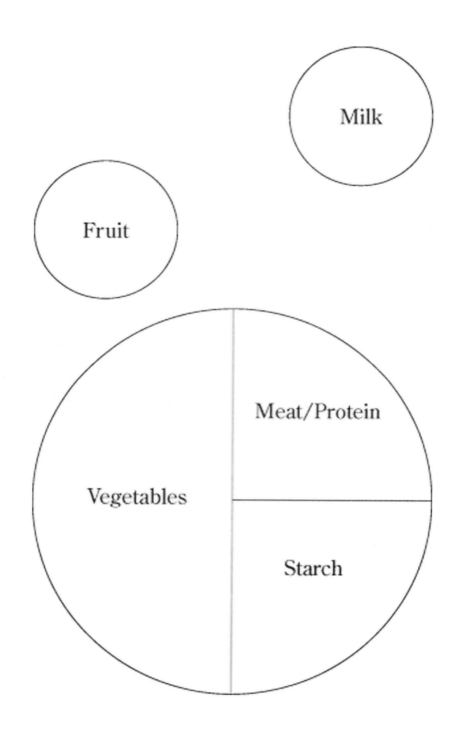

Food Groups

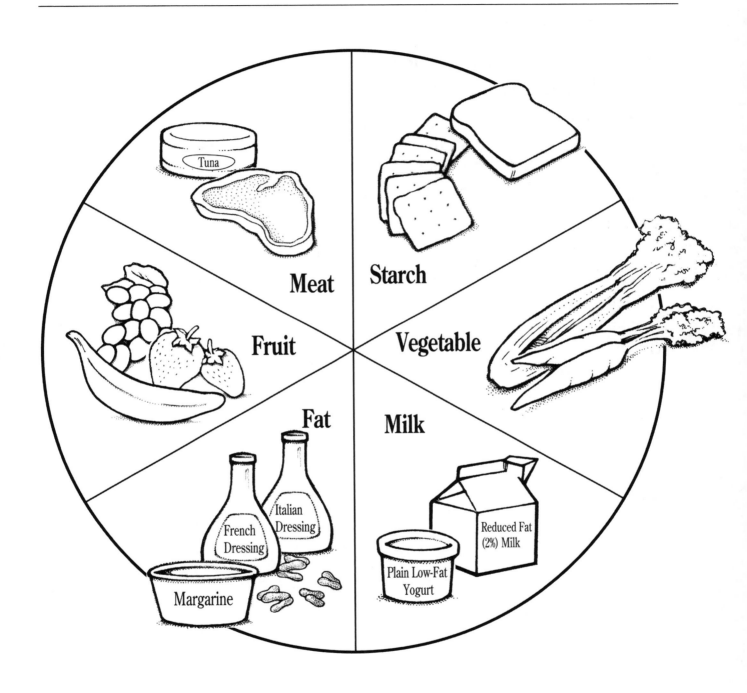

⬤ Nutrients in Food Groups

Group	Carbohydrate (g)	Protein (g)	Fat (g)	Calories
Carbohydrate				
Starch	15	3	1 or less	80
Fruit	15	—	—	60
Milk				
Fat-free (skim)	12	8	0–3	90
Low-fat (1%)	12	8	5	120
Whole	12	8	8	150
Nonstarchy Vegetables	5	2	—	25
Other Carbohydrates	Varies	Varies	Varies	Varies
Meat/Meat Substitute				
Very lean	—	7	0–1	35
Lean	—	7	3	55
Medium fat	—	7	5	75
High fat	—	7	8	100
Fat	—	—	5	45
Monounsaturated	—	—	5	45
Polyunsaturated	—	—	5	45
Saturated	—	—	5	45
Hydrogenated	—	—	5	45

➲ Counting Carbohydrate Servings

Meal Time _____:_____

_____ carbohydrate servings OR

_____ grams carbohydrate

_____ meat or meat substitutes

_____ fats

Snack Time _____:_____

_____

_____

Meal Time _____:_____

_____ carbohydrate servings OR

_____ grams carbohydrate

_____ meat or meat substitutes

_____ fats

Snack Time _____:_____

_____

_____

Meal Time _____:_____

_____ carbohydrate servings OR

_____ grams carbohydrate

_____ meat or meat substitutes

_____ fats

Snack Time _____:_____

_____

_____

© 2009 American Diabetes Association

◑ Tips for Counting Carbohydrate Servings

Grams of usable carbohydrate	Count as
0–5 g	Do not count
6–10 g	1/2 carbohydrate serving or 1/2 starch, fruit, or milk serving
11–20 g	1 carbohydrate serving or 1 starch, fruit, or milk serving
21–25 g	1 1/2 carbohydrate servings or 1 1/2 starch, fruit, or milk servings
26–35 g	2 carbohydrate servings or 2 starch, fruit, or milk servings

Know what you are eating. Measure or weigh your foods to help you learn what carbohydrate servings look like. The foods I will measure are:

_____

The food labels I will check are:

_____

Feel good about what you already do. If you decide to make food changes, choose only one or two changes to make. This is what I will do:

_____

_____

Counting carbohydrate in your food allows you more flexibility in food choices and helps keep your blood glucose levels within target range.

➡ Eating Away From Home

- ■ Know what is important to you about eating out.
- ■ Know your goals and your meal plan.
- ■ Choose the kinds and amounts of food that best fit your meal plan.
- ■ Plan ahead—call the restaurant or host/hostess if unsure of the menu.*
- ■ Consider using the plate method as a guideline.

EATING IN RESTAURANTS

Choose

■ *Appetizers*
Broth or bouillon, unsweetened fruit or vegetable juice, fresh fruit, or raw vegetables

■ *Salads*
Tossed vegetable or fresh fruit salads served with low-fat dressing or dressing that is on the side

■ *Main Course*
Any main dish item that does not contain large amounts of gravy, cream sauce, breading, or fat and contains ingredients that can be easily identified

■ *Vegetables*
Stewed, steamed, or boiled

■ *Starches*
Baked potatoes, plain noodles, rice, hard rolls, melba toast, bread sticks, matzoh, or other plain breads

■ *Desserts*
Fresh fruits or artificially sweetened Jell-O

■ *Drinks*
Water, unsweetened coffee or tea, fat-free (skim) milk, juices, diet soft drinks, or soda or sparkling waters

---

* This is especially important for vegetarians looking for nonmeat menu items.

EATING AWAY FROM HOME *continued*

Request

- Salad dressings, butter, sour cream, gravies, or sauces to be served on the side so you can control how much you use

- Vegetables and main dishes to be served plain, without butter, margarine, or sauces

- Tomato or other juice (usually available if the restaurant has a bar or serves breakfast)

- Low-calorie salad dressing and artificially sweetened Jell-O, if available

- Fresh fruit and fat-free (skim) milk (usually available even though not listed on the menu)

Choose less often

- Cream soups[1]

- Salads with dressing already added, such as potato salad or cole slaw[1]

- Foods that are breaded, deep-fat fried, creamed, or scalloped[1, 2]

- Casseroles or mixed dishes, unless you can easily identify the types and amounts of ingredients[1, 2]

- Desserts, pastries, sweetened fruits or juices, and regular gelatin desserts or salad[1, 2]

---

[1] These items contribute extra fat that interferes with control of weight and blood fats.

[2] These items contribute large or hard-to-measure amounts of carbohydrate that interfere with blood glucose control.

➲ Guidelines for Use of Alcoholic Drinks

■ Discuss use of alcohol with your health care team. Consider drinking only if your diabetes is well controlled and you are not pregnant. Alcohol can make some problems worse.

■ Alcohol initially lowers your blood glucose level. If you use insulin or certain diabetes medications, you are more likely to have a low blood glucose reaction when you drink alcohol.

■ Drink alcohol with meals or snacks containing carbohydrate, such as pretzels, bread sticks, or crackers.

■ Alcohol makes insulin reactions harder to recognize. It also interferes with some medicines.

■ Use alcohol in moderation (up to 1 equivalent for women and 2 for men per day).

> Equivalent = 1 1/2 oz distilled spirits
> 4 oz dry wine
> 12 oz beer

■ Mix alcohol with:

Free
- water
- club soda*
- seltzer*
- diet soft drinks

Fruit/Vegetable Exchange
- fruit juice (1 fruit)
- tomato juice (4 oz = 1 vegetable)
- V8 juice (4 oz = 1 vegetable)

■ Avoid sweet wine, liqueurs, and sweetened mixed drinks. Try a wine spritzer made with club soda rather than a wine cooler, which is usually made with a sweetened, fruit-flavored mix.

■ Drink with someone who recognizes and knows how to treat a low blood glucose reaction.

■ Note the differences in calories and carbohydrates among alcoholic drinks.

---

* Carbonation makes alcohol enter the bloodstream more quickly.

GUIDELINES FOR USE OF ALCOHOLIC DRINKS *continued*

ALCOHOLIC DRINKS

Beverage	Amount	Calories	Carbohydrates
Beer:			
regular	12 oz	150	13
light	12 oz	100	5
nonalcoholic	12 oz	75	16
Cocktails:			
Distilled spirits (80 proof): gin, rum, scotch, vodka, whiskey	1 1/2 oz	100	trace
Martini	5 oz	310	4
Wines			
Red	4 oz	80	2
White	4 oz	80	1
Hard lemonade	12 oz	250	37

⟳ Cookbooks for People with Diabetes

Cookbooks written for people with diabetes may add variety to your meal planning. Choose a cookbook that:

■ lists the serving size and number of servings per recipe

■ lists the carbohydrate content and food exchange value for each serving

■ contains recipes with acceptable ingredients (evaluate each recipe before you use it)

Many diabetes cookbooks are available. Check your local bookstore or library. The following cookbooks can be obtained from the American Diabetes Association by calling 800-232-6733 or by visiting http://store.diabetes.org.

Diabetes & Heart Healthy Meals for Two
by American Diabetes Association and American Heart Association

Diabetes Meal Planning Made Easy, 4th Edition
by Hope Warshaw

Diabetic Cooking for Latinos (Cocinando para Latinos con Diabetes)
by Olga V. Fuste

Diabetic Meals in 30 Minutes—or Less!, 2nd Edition
by Robyn Webb

More Diabetic Meals in 30 Minutes—or Less!
by Robyn Webb

One Pot Meals for People with Diabetes, 2nd Edition
by Ruth Glick and Nancy Baggett

Quick & Easy Diabetic Recipes for One, 2nd Edition
by Kathleen Stanley and Connie Crawley

The 4-Ingredient Diabetes Cookbook
Nancy Hughes

COOKBOOKS FOR PEOPLE WITH DIABETES *continued*

The Big Book of Diabetic Desserts
by Jackie Mills

The Diabetic Chef's Year-Round Cookbook
by Chris Smith

The Healthy Carb Diabetes Cookbook
by Jennifer Bucko and Lara Rondinelli

Holly Clegg's Trim & Terrific Diabetic Cooking
by Holly Clegg

The New Soul Food Cookbook for People with Diabetes, 2nd Edition
by Fabiola Demps Gaines and Roniece Weaver

Also by the American Diabetes Association:
The Diabetes Food & Nutrition Bible
Guide to Healthy Restaurant Eating, 4th Edition
Guide to Healthy Fast-Food Eating, 2nd Edition
Mix 'n Match Meals in Minutes for People with Diabetes, 2nd Edition
Mr. Food's Quick & Easy Diabetic Cooking, 2nd Edition
The Complete Quick & Hearty Diabetic Cookbook, 2nd Edition

▶ ▶ ▶ ▶ ▶

#6	Stocking the Cupboard

STATEMENT OF PURPOSE

This session is intended to help participants plan grocery lists that include the foods they need to use their meal plans discussed in session #5, *Planning Meals* (p. 69). Label reading and the use of food products modified to be low in sugar, fat, or salt (including the use of sugar and fat substitutes) are discussed.

PREREQUISITES

It is recommended that participants have attended sessions #3, *The Basics of Eating* (p. 37), and #5, *Planning Meals* (p. 69), or have achieved those objectives. Ask participants who have them to bring their meal plans to class. Ask participants to bring food labels for a few items they like to eat.

OBJECTIVES

At the end of this session, participants will be able to:

1. plan a shopping list that includes the foods needed to use their meal plans;

2. read a food label to find the ingredients, the serving size, and the carbohydrate, fat and salt content of each serving;

3. use a food label to decide where, if, and how the food fits into their meal plans;

4. name the sugar and fat substitutes available and how they might be used in their meal plans;

5. identify foods that they do and do not want to keep on hand;

6. state the guidelines for choosing free foods and how they might be used in their meal plans.

CONTENT

Incorporating nutritional management into lifestyle.

MATERIALS NEEDED

VISUALS PROVIDED	ADDITIONAL
1. Reasons for Meal Planning 2. Nutrition Facts Label 3. Choosing Free Foods **Handouts** (one per participant) 1. Shopping Guide 2. Money-Saving Shopping Tips 3. Nutrient Claims	■ Pencils for participants ■ Chalkboard and chalk/Board and markers ■ Commercial food product containers or labels from a variety of products, including dietetic foods and those that participants bring from foods they use frequently ■ *Reading Food Labels* (booklet available from the American Diabetes Association, www.diabetes.org, or 800-232-6733)

METHOD OF PRESENTATION

Start by introducing yourself and telling what you do. Ask participants to introduce themselves. Explain that the purpose of this session is to provide information on how to shop for foods that fit their meal plans. It will include label reading and an update on artificial fats and sweeteners. This information may be taught as part of the *Planning Meals* session. Because recommendations for and availability of special products change often, it is necessary to stay up-to-date to provide accurate information.

Begin by asking how they did with their short-term goal and what they learned from it. Present material in a question/discussion format, using the first question as a starting point. Provide appropriate content outlined below in response. Ask if there are additional questions, and respond, repeating the process for the entire session. Use the questions in the Instructor's Notes section to generate discussion if no questions are forthcoming after a period of silence. Keeping track of the content discussed in each session, using the Diabetes Self-Management Record, the Participant Follow-up Record, or another form, helps you to evaluate if all needed content has been discussed.

CONTENT OUTLINE

CONCEPT	DETAIL	INSTRUCTOR'S NOTES
1. Choosing food	1.1 Having the food items or ingredients available is the first step in using your meal plan. It helps make using a plan less of a chore and allows you to be more flexible and spontaneous. Choosing not to buy, or buying smaller amounts of foods you are trying to limit can also help.	Ask, "What concerns or questions do you have about using a meal plan? Is the food you need for your meal plan available in your home? Are there foods you no longer want to keep in your home? Who does the grocery shopping?"

CONTENT OUTLINE

CONCEPT	DETAIL	INSTRUCTOR'S NOTES
		Ask, "What is your meal plan? What is the most important reason you use your meal plan?" Use Visual #1, Reasons for Meal Planning.
	1.2 Foods that you prepare yourself fit easily into meal plans used by people with diabetes.	Cooking from scratch is the least expensive way to prepare food, but many people choose to spend their time in other ways.
	1.3 Most people also use products that have been partly prepared by someone else. Prepared foods are more likely to contain extra sugar, salt, and fat. The package label can help you decide if a product will fit with your plan and help you meet your targets.	Review the publication *Reading Food Labels,* with participants or labels that participants have brought.
	1.4 Including food items low in sugar, fat, sodium, and calories may also help you meet your nutrition goals.	Many convenience foods are lower in sugar, salt, and sodium than they used to be. Check the label for designations of low sodium, low sugar, low fat, etc.
2. Planning a shopping list	2.1 A shopping list can help you buy the foods you need.	Ask, "How many of you make a shopping list before you go to the grocery store? How does it help you?"
	2.2 Look at your meal plan and think about the foods you will need. For example, to use the MyPyramid, you need to buy at least 14 servings of fruit per person each week (fresh or canned).	Ask, "How many servings of fruit do you eat each day? How many pieces of fruit do you need to buy to last one week?" Note that 14 pieces of fruit for one person adds up to 56 for a family of four.
	2.3 The MyPyramid recommends 2 cups of milk per day, which adds up to a gallon per person, per week, or 1/2 gallon of milk and seven, 6 oz containers of sugar-free yogurt per person.	Ask, "How many servings of milk do you plan to drink each day? How much milk or dairy products do you need to buy to last a week?"

CONTENT OUTLINE

CONCEPT	DETAIL	INSTRUCTOR'S NOTES
	2.4 You also need to buy vegetables and meat. The MyPyramid recommends 3–5 servings of vegetables; 6 or more servings of bread, cereal, or starches; and 4–6 oz of meat each day.	Repeat with other food groups to demonstrate the planning needed to purchase the food that fits their plan. Amounts needed per person per week to meet minimum serving recommendations: ■ vegetables 4 lb frozen ■ meat 2–3 lb
	2.5 This shopping guide lists foods that can help you use your meal plan. Different foods help reach different nutrition goals.	Use Handout #1, Shopping Guide. Ask, "What items on this list do you usually buy?"
	2.6 These items are examples of foods that are low in fat, saturated fat, calories, or added sugar or high in fiber.	The meats contain ≤ 3 g of fat per ounce. Low-fat meat and dairy products are low in saturated fat.
	2.7 No single food is "good" or "bad." All foods can be included in your meal plan. You may need to eat smaller amounts of some foods if you want to reach your nutrition and blood glucose goals.	Ask, "What items would you add to the shopping guide to make it fit with your meal plan and the way others in your family eat?"
	2.8 Many people worry that it costs more for food when you have diabetes. It may mean spending more on some items (such as low-fat meats and fresh fruits) and less on others (such as snacks and convenience foods). Eating with diabetes does not need to cost more than it does for other people.	Ask participants to brainstorm ideas for saving money on food. Distribute Handout #2, Money-Saving Shopping Tips. Bring in a grocery flyer and ask participants to evaluate how foods on sale fit with their meal plans.
	2.9 No special products are needed to use a meal plan for diabetes, although artificial sweeteners and diet soft drinks may make your diet more enjoyable and easier to use.	
3. Label information	3.1 Food labels give information to help you decide if a food fits into your meal plan.	Use Visual #2, Nutrition Facts Label, or distribute product labels brought by participants

CONTENT OUTLINE

CONCEPT	DETAIL	INSTRUCTOR'S NOTES

and help them locate the information.

3.2 The U.S. Food and Drug Administration (FDA) requires almost all foods in the United States to have a standard nutrition label.

Restaurant menus are exempt. Nutrition information is required for any food that makes nutritional claims and is voluntary on produce, fresh meat, and poultry.

3.3 The main parts of a food label show:
- nutrition facts
- list of ingredients.

3.4 The nutrition facts panel tells you:
- serving size
- number of servings per container
- nutrient content.

Ask, "What do you need to know about a food product before you know if and how to include it among your food choices?" List responses on the chalkboard. Ask, "Where can you find this information?"

3.5 The percentage of daily values is also included. This tells how a food fits into a 2000-calorie diet.

Point out that these guidelines are based on the needs of an 18-year old male and may not be appropriate for them based on their gender, calorie needs, etc.

3.6 Compare the serving size on a food label with the amount you usually eat.

The serving sizes are given in household measurements. They may not be the same as your usual portion. Use a label on a snack food (e.g., chips, popcorn) to illustrate this point.

3.7 The following nutrients must be included on the label:
- total fat
- saturated fat
- cholesterol
- sodium
- total carbohydrate
- vitamins A and C
- fiber
- sugar
- protein
- iron
- calcium.

Point out the location of the amount in grams next to each nutrient. Other nutrients such as unsaturated fats or other vitamins and minerals may be added. Foods that contain only a few of these nutrients or are in a small package may use a shortened label.

3.8 It's important to look at grams of total fat as well as saturated fat. Saturated fat is most likely to clog blood vessels because the liver

The percentage of total fat in a food item can be calculated by dividing the calories of fat by the total calories. It is the percentage

CONTENT OUTLINE

CONCEPT	DETAIL	INSTRUCTOR'S NOTES

	makes cholesterol from saturated fat.	of fat in the *total diet* that is important, and the goal varies from person to person. This material is not usually emphasized for pediatric patients. (See Outline #18, *Eating for a Healthy Heart,* p. 379).
	3.9 Total carbohydrate includes dietary fiber, sugar, and starches. The total amount of carbohydrate (starch and sugar) is what affects blood glucose levels. The amounts listed are all based on serving size. The amount you get is based on the size of your portion.	Because fiber is not absorbed and does not affect blood glucose, total carbohydrate minus fiber is the most accurate measure for carbohydrate counting. This is clinically relevant only when someone eats foods very high in soluble fiber, such as legumes or oat bran. You can either subtract half of the amount of fiber from the total carbohydrate or, if there is more than 5 grams of fiber, it is subtracted from the total carbohydrate count.
	3.10 People who count carbohydrates as their method of meal planning use the total carbohydrate number on the nutrition facts label.	
	3.11 Some labels tell the number of calories in a gram of fat, carbohydrate, and protein.	Find this information on different labels. Ask a participant to read through each of the categories on their label while you write this information on the board. Then, ask the group to evaluate how it would fit into their meal plans. Choose labels of foods that they may and may not think of as "good."
4. Foods with special claims	4.1 More and more food products are reducing their sugar, fat, calorie, and sodium contents. More foods are adding fiber as well.	Ask, "Which 'special' foods do you use?" Point out that they still need to read the labels on those products to evaluate whether they are useful for

CONTENT OUTLINE

CONCEPT	DETAIL	INSTRUCTOR'S NOTES
		them. Caution them that they need to pay particular attention to fiber if they are adjusting insulin doses based on grams of carbohydrates.
	4.2 A product must be reduced by a certain amount of sugar or fat to claim that it has less sugar or is low in fat.	See Handout #3, Nutrient Claims.
	4.3 Cautions in selecting food items with special claims: ■ low-sugar items may be high in fat ■ low-fat items may be high in sugar ■ low-fat and low-sugar items may not be any lower in calories ■ low-calorie items may be a small portion of a high-fat/high-sugar product ■ products may be expensive ■ items sweetened with concentrated fruit juice may affect your blood glucose the same as table sugar.	Examples: ■ Nutrasweet-sweetened ice cream bars ■ Fat-free coffee cake Some of these may be higher in calories. ■ Very thinly sliced bread or small frozen dinners ■ Cookies and fruit spreads sweetened with fruit juice tend to be expensive and just as high in sugar.
5. Dietetic foods	5.1 "Dietetic" refers to a food prepared or processed for a special diet. Commercial dietetic foods are prepared for a variety of special diets—not just for use in a diabetes diet. For example, dietetic foods made for people with kidney problems may contain a lot of sugar.	Ask, "Do you use any dietetic foods? Which ones?" A particular ingredient may be: ■ Reduced—in sodium, sugar (light fruit), fat, or protein ■ Altered—corn oil substituted for milk fat in dietetic cheese ■ Eliminated—sugar in many diet soft drinks.
	5.2 Foods that contain less than 20 calories per serving and less than 5 g carbohydrate may be used as free foods. Two to three servings spread throughout the day will probably not raise blood glucose.	Use Visual #3, Choosing Free Foods. Ask, "Which of the products shown could be a free food?"

CONTENT OUTLINE

CONCEPT	DETAIL	INSTRUCTOR'S NOTES
	5.3 Recipes for dietetic foods or foods with special claims may contain a sugar or fat substitute. Sugar alcohols raise blood glucose levels, although more slowly than table sugar.	Note that sugar-free products may still contain sugar alcohols.
6. Sugar substitutes	6.1 Sugar substitutes can help satisfy the inborn taste for sweetness without increasing blood glucose.	Ask, "What sugar substitutes do you use?" Discuss only relevant ones. Ask, "Do you have any concerns about sugar and fat substitutes?" Refer to *Fitting Foods with Sugar Substitutes and Fat Replacers into Your Meal Plan.*
	6.2 *Saccharin* is 300–400 times sweeter than sugar, although some users report a bitter aftertaste. It contains no calories. For information and recipes: www.sweetnlow.com Sweet 'N Low Hotline 800-221-1763	The FDA 1995 guidelines for saccharin safety are 500 mg (25–35 packets) per day for children and 1000 mg (50–70 packets) per day for adults. Cancer risk with moderate use has not been shown. Heavy use during pregnancy is discouraged.
	6.3 *Aspartame* (Nutrasweet or Equal) is a protein and has no bitter after-taste. As a protein, aspartame provides 4 kcal/g, but since it is 180–200 times sweeter than sugar, the very small amounts used do not contribute significant calories. High temperatures destroy its sweetening power and taste; thus, aspartame cannot be used for extended cooking (>15 minutes). For information and recipes: www.equal.com The Equal Information Center 800-323-5316 www.nutrasweet.com 800-323-5323	Aspartame is made of the amino acids L-phenylalanine and L-aspartic acid. The FDA has established the acceptable daily intake (ADI) at 50 mg/kg (12–17 cans diet soda or 71 packets Equal for a 50-kg adult). Optional: Have participants calculate their own ADI. *Warning:* No safe limits have been established for children less than 2 years old. Aspartame causes mental retardation among all people with PKU.

CONTENT OUTLINE

CONCEPT	DETAIL	INSTRUCTOR'S NOTES

6.4 *Acesulfame K* (Sweet One by Sunette) is advertised to taste more like sugar. It can be used for cooking and baking. Like other artificial sweeteners, acesulfame K increases the sweetening power of other sweeteners, so it can be used with others to reduce the overall amount of sweetener needed in a product.

For information and recipes:
www.sweetone.com
Sweet One Hotline
800-544-8610

Acesulfame K was approved by the FDA in 1988 after 50 studies over 15 years showed no ill effects. It is 200 times sweeter than sucrose, is a derivative of vinegar, and is excreted without being metabolized. The ADI is 15 mg/kg (18 packets for a 60-kg person). Each packet contains 11 mg potassium.

6.5 *Sucralose* (Splenda) is made from sugar (sucrose). The body does not recognize it as a source of sugar or carbohydrate. Sucralose passes through your body quickly after you eat it. It has no calories. It is stable at all temperatures and has a long shelf-life.

For information and recipes:
www.sucralose.com
Sucralose McNeil Specialty Products
800-777-5363

This product was approved by the FDA in 1998. It is considered safe for all population groups.

6.6 Stevia is a plant-based product that is about 300 times sweeter than sugar. Stevia's taste has a slower onset and longer duration than sugar, although some people say that it has a bitter or licorice aftertaste. It is not currently added to foods you buy.

The FDA has not approved stevia as a food additive, but did approve it as a sugar substitute.

6.7 Packets of artificial sweeteners contain dextrose or lactose as a carrier and provide 4 calories of carbohydrate per package. It is recommended that use be limited to five packets per serving (20 extra calories).

Using a variety of alternative sweeteners rather than one type is recommended. New sugar substitutes are in development and may soon be available.

CONTENT OUTLINE

CONCEPT	DETAIL	INSTRUCTOR'S NOTES
7. Alternative sugars	7.1 *Sorbitol* and *mannitol* are alcohols of sugar. Because they are absorbed slowly, blood glucose rises more slowly. Because these sugars are only half as sweet as table sugar, twice as many calories are used to provide the same sweetening power. These sugars may cause diarrhea and gas.	Ask, "Have you heard of sorbitol or mannitol?" Show dietetic products that contain sorbitol and mannitol, such as hard candy.
	7.2 *Fructose* is a sugar made from cornstarch. It has as many calories as table sugar. In pure crystalline form (expensive), it raises blood glucose more slowly than table sugar, but as high-fructose corn syrup (less costly), it affects blood glucose the same as table sugar.	Fructose may taste slightly sweeter than sucrose in cold or acidic foods, such as lemonade. In insulin deficiency, crystalline fructose may be used for glucose synthesis, causing an increase in blood glucose.
8. Fat substitutes	8.1 Two of the fat substitutes that have been developed are Simplesse and Olean.	The goal of a fat substitute is to provide the feel and flavor of fat with fewer calories.
	8.2 Simplesse is finely whipped milk whey and egg white. It contains 1–2 calories per gram and can only be used in cold products. The product causes gastrointestinal symptoms among some individuals. If you are allergic to egg whites or milk, you may also be allergic to Simplesse. For more information: www.cpkelco.com/simplesse/ 800-535-2687	Simplesse is used in frozen desserts, cheese, and other dairy products, mayonnaise, and salad dressings. It is used in foods that will not be heated. Suggest to participants that they monitor their responses to any new product.
	8.3 *Olestra* (Olean) is made from soy-bean oil and table sugar. The molecule is too large to be absorbed, so it provides no calories. The product causes GI symptoms among some individuals. For more information: www.olean.com Proctor & Gamble Co. 800-543-7276	Olestra was approved by the FDA in 1996. It is used to replace part of the fat in shortenings and oils used for deep frying. Olestra is a way to cut calories from snack foods such as chips and crackers.

CONTENT OUTLINE

CONCEPT	DETAIL	INSTRUCTOR'S NOTES
9. Planning for change	9.1 Activity: Examine labels from a variety of low-sugar, low-fat, and dietetic foods. If possible, taste some of these products. Monitor your blood glucose to identify your own response to foods.	Ask participants to explain why they might use a certain product (or why not).
	9.2 Make a list of foods to include on your next grocery shopping list. Write down special products or new items you want to try.	Choose a short-term goal to try before the next session.

SKILLS CHECKLIST

Each participant will be able to use food label information to evaluate carbohydrate, fat, and calorie content of a product.

EVALUATION PLAN

Knowledge will be evaluated by achievement of learning and by responses to questions during the session; skills will be evaluated by observation. The ability to apply knowledge will be evaluated by the participants' abilities to buy food that meets their meal plan goals and through program outcome measures.

DOCUMENTATION PLAN

Record class attendance and achieved objectives as appropriate.

➡ Reasons for Meal Planning

■ Maintain blood glucose as close to your target range as possible.

■ Maintain cholesterol (blood fats) as close to your target levels as possible.

■ Maintain blood pressure as close to your target level as possible.

■ Prevent, delay, or treat diabetes-related complications.

■ Improve health through food choices.

■ Meet individual nutritional needs.

➲ Nutrition Facts Label

Nutrition Facts

Serving Size   1 cup (228g)
Servings Per Container   2

Amount Per Serving

Calories   260   Calories from Fat   120

% Daily Value*

Total Fat 13g	20%
Saturated Fat 5g	25%
Trans Fat 2g	
Cholesterol 30mg	10%
Sodium 660mg	28%
Total Carbohydrate 31g	10%
Dietary Fiber 0g	0%
Sugars 5g	
Protein 5g	

Vitamin A 4%	•	Vitamin C 2%	
Calcium 15%	•	Iron 4%	

*Per cent Daily V alues ar e based on a 2,000 calorie diet. Y our Daily V alues may be higher or lower depending on your calorie needs.

	Calories:	2,000	2,500
Total Fat	Less than	65g	80g
Sat Fat	Less than	20g	25g
Cholesterol	Less than	300mg	300mg
Sodium	Less than	2,400mg	2,400mg
Total Carbohydrate		300g	375g
Dietary Fiber		25g	30g

Calories per gram:
Fat 9   •   Carbohydrate 4   •   Protein 4

⊃ Choosing Free Foods

READ THE LABEL!

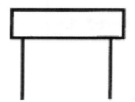

Free Foods:

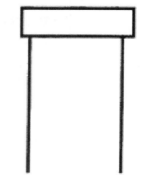

Contain less than 20 calories per serving
Total no more than 60 calories per day

DIETETIC SALAD DRESSING

Calories: 6/Tablespoon

INGREDIENTS: Water, vinegar, corn sweetener, salt, citrate, dill, lemon juice, pectin, carrageenan, dried red pepper, guar gum

DIETETIC SALAD DRESSING

Calories: 40/Tablespoon

INGREDIENTS: Water, soybean oil, cultured low-fat buttermilk, corn syrup, monosodium glutamate, xanthan gum, onion, spices

➲ Shopping Guide

Produce Aisle

Fresh fruit

★ apples

★ bananas

★ berries

★ cantaloupe

★ grapefruit

★ oranges

★ peaches

★ pears

★ strawberries

★ watermelon

_____

_____

Fresh vegetables

★ broccoli

★ cabbage

★ carrots

★ celery

★ corn

★ cucumber

★ green pepper

★ greens

★ kohlrabi

★ lettuce

★ mushrooms

★ okra

★ onions

★ potatoes

★ squash

★ tomatoes

_____

_____

Frozen Food Aisle

★ vegetables, plain

★ entrees, low-fat or lean

★ dinners, low-fat or lean

★ waffles

★ ice cream

★ juices

_____

_____

Bakery Aisle

★ bread

★ rolls

★ hamburger/hot dog buns

★ bagels

★ english muffins/muffins

★ pita pockets

★ tortillas

★ naan

★ angel food cake

★ sponge cake

_____

_____

Starch Aisle

★ whole-grain flour

★ plain dry cereals

★ plain cooked cereals

★ noodles/macaroni

★ rice (brown for more fiber)

★ dried beans

★ dried peas

★ graham crackers

★ saltine crackers

★ low-fat crackers (whole grain for more fiber)

★ pretzels

★ popcorn

_____

_____

Dairy Aisle

★ fat-free (skim) milk

★ yogurt (plain or artificially sweetened nonfat fruit)

★ cheese (reduced-fat)

★ cottage cheese (low-fat)

★ margarine

★ eggs

★ egg substitute

_____

_____

Meat Aisle

★ chicken, no skin

★ turkey, no skin

★ fish

★ round or sirloin steak

★ ground round or sirloin

★ beef round roast

★ flank steak

★ chipped beef

★ leg of lamb

★ lean lamb chops

★ pork loin roast

★ pork tenderloin

★ center loin pork chop

★ ham

★ Canadian bacon

★ tofu

★ 97% fat-free lunch meat, hot dogs, or sausage

_____

_____

SHOPPING GUIDE *continued*

Canned Goods Aisle

* fruit
* fruit juice
* low-sodium vegetables
* low-sodium vegetable juice
* mushrooms
* water chestnuts
* tomato sauce and paste
* tomatoes
* beans (kidney, pinto, northern, garbanzo, black, black-eyed peas)
* broth-based soups
* no-fat or low-fat cream soups
* dried soups
* evaporated skim milk
* tuna canned in water
* salmon
* peanut butter
* bouillon

_____

_____

Miscellaneous

* spices and herbs
* catsup
* mustard

* mayonnaise (lite or no-fat)
* salad dressing (lite or no-fat)
* vinegar
* lemon juice
* olive oil
* canola oil

_____

_____

Special Products

* artificial sweeteners
* artificially sweetened jelly/jam
* artificially sweetened pudding
* artificially sweetened Jell-O
* artificially sweetened syrup
* Butter Buds
* nonstick cooking spray
* Beano
* salt-free seasonings
* diet soft drinks

_____

_____

➲ Money-Saving Shopping Tips

1. Shop only with a list.

2. Shop only once or twice a week. You'll spend more if you go more often.

3. Buy only items you really need, unless something you use often is on sale. If something you use often is on sale and can be stored, consider buying enough for a few weeks.

4. Check grocery ads for sale items and the Sunday newspaper inserts for coupons.

5. Compare discounted items with similar products at the regular price to see if you really are saving.

6. Eat before you go shopping.

7. Check unit pricing (the price per ounce or pound, usually listed on the shelf below the item). This helps you compare sizes and brands, to decide which is the least expensive.

8. Look for store brands or generic brands—they are often cheaper than national brands.

9. Prepared foods cost more than the plain ingredients from which they are made.

10. Plain cereal costs less per ounce than sugar-coated cereal.

11. Fat-free (skim) milk is less expensive than reduced-fat (2%) or whole milk.

12. Buy only the amount you will use. An item that costs less per serving will not save money if it spoils.

13. Whole, unwashed produce usually costs less than washed and cut up items.

14. Buying salad makings at the store salad bar might be less expensive than buying all the various items separately—especially for one or two people.

MONEY-SAVING SHOPPING TIPS *continued*

15. Soups, stews, and casseroles stretch a little meat to serve more people.

16. Buy plain ice cream instead of premium ice cream or sherbet.

17. Limit use of pickles, relishes, and olives. They are high in cost but low in nutrients.

18. Limit use of chips, cookies, and other snack foods. They are high in calories and cost, but low in nutrients.

◑ Nutrient Claims

Nutrients per Serving	Free	Low	Reduced/Less	Light (Lite)
Calories	Less than 5 calories	40 calories or less	At least 25% fewer calories	At least 1/3 fewer calories
Fat	Less than 0.5 g fat	3 g or less fat	At least 25% less fat	At least 50% less fat
Saturated Fat	Less than 0.5 g saturated fat	1 gm or less saturated fat and no more than 15% of calories from saturated fat	At least 25% less saturated fat	Not used
Cholesterol	Less than 2 mg cholesterol and 2 g or less saturated fat	20 mg or less cholesterol and 2 g or less saturated fat	At least 25% less cholesterol and 2 g or less saturated fat	Not used
Sodium	Less than 5 mg sodium	140 mg or less sodium	At least 25% less sodium	At least 50% less sodium
Sugar	Less than 1.2 g sugars	Not a legal claim	At least 25% less sugar	Not used

Adapted from *Label Facts for Healthful Eating.* National Food Processors Association, Washington, DC, 1993.

#7   Physical Activity and Exercise

▶ ▶ ▶ ▶ ▶

STATEMENT OF PURPOSE

This session is intended to provide information about the effects of physical activity on blood glucose and the necessary dietary adjustments for changes in activity. It also provides the opportunity to create a plan for an exercise program, if the participant desires.

PREREQUISITES

It is recommended that participants have basic knowledge about diabetes and self-care, from either personal experience or attending previous sessions.

OBJECTIVES

At the end of this session, participants will be able to:

1. list three benefits of regular activity or exercise;

2. describe the difference between aerobic and anaerobic exercise;

3. state effects of activity/exercise on blood glucose level;

4. state the benefits of a consistent exercise program;

5. determine target heart rate;

6. state possible signs and symptoms of hypoglycemia during and after exercise;

7. describe how to make adjustments in food intake or insulin doses to balance increases in physical activity;

8. develop a personal exercise plan and strategies to overcome barriers.

CONTENT

Incorporating physical activity into lifestyle.

MATERIALS NEEDED

VISUALS PROVIDED	ADDITIONAL
1. Target Heart Rates	■ Pencils for participants
	■ Chalkboard and chalk/Board and markers
Handouts (one per participant)	■ Information about local exercise programs, including those that are low-cost or free
1. Recommended Activity Level	■ Videotape of simple exercises
2. Treatment of Low Blood Glucose	■ "Small Steps, Big Rewards" resource kit [available
3. Calories Spent in Various Exercises	from the National Diabetes Education Program
4. Sample Activity Snacks	(NDEP), www.yourdiabetesinfo.org or the Ameri-
5. Planning Your Exercise Program	can Diabetes Association at 1-800-232-6733 or
	www.diabetes.org]
	■ Pedometers
	■ Videotape of simple or chair exercises

METHOD OF PRESENTATION

Start by introducing yourself and telling what you do. Ask participants to introduce themselves and tell about their own activity programs, if any. Explain that the purposes of this session are to provide information about physical activity and, if desired, to develop a personal plan for regular exercise or increased activity level.

Begin by asking how they did with their short-term goal and what they learned from it. Present material in a question/discussion format, using the first question as a starting point. Provide appropriate content outlined below in response. Ask if there are additional questions, and respond, repeating the process for the entire session. Use the questions in the Instructor's Notes section to generate discussion if no questions are forthcoming after a period of silence. Keeping track of the content discussed in each section, using the Diabetes Self-Management Record, the Participant Follow-up Record, or another form, helps you to evaluate if all needed content has been discussed.

If possible, start the class with a walk, simple stretching, or an easy exercise videotape, using appropriate precautions for patients with diabetes complications or other health problems. Discuss only the areas that are appropriate for the participants based on their treatment, exercise needs, desires, and abilities. At the end of the class, invite participants to complete the Planning Your Exercise Program handout.

CONTENT OUTLINE

CONCEPT	DETAIL	INSTRUCTOR'S NOTES
1. Benefits of regular exercise	1.1 Exercise can lower blood pressure and cholesterol levels. Exercise strengthens your heart and circulatory system. It can decrease body fat and increase muscle tone.	Ask, "What are your experiences with regular exercise? What questions do you have? What are some benefits of exercise? What are some barriers/negatives for exercise?" If not mentioned,

CONTENT OUTLINE

CONCEPT	DETAIL	INSTRUCTOR'S NOTES
		point out that people usually look better and feel better, have more stamina, and are better able to deal with stress. Finding time to exercise, finding a place to exercise, and coming up with enjoyable activities are often barriers.
	1.2 Exercise can help you feel more relaxed. It relieves tension and stress and can be enjoyable. Exercise can also help prevent treat depression.	Some people eat to cope with stress, but with regular exercise, they may find that they are less likely to eat when stressed and distressed.
	1.3 While calories are burned with any exercise, regular exercise increases metabolism so more calories are burned all the time, even at rest.	Exercise supports weight loss and helps to sustain weight loss.
2. Effects on blood glucose	2.1 Generally, activity will lower your blood glucose because body cells take in glucose more efficiently.	Ask, "What effects on your blood glucose have you noticed with exercise?" Some patients may have noticed an increase in blood glucose initially or with short bursts of exercise because of the response of the liver.
	2.2 In type 2 diabetes, exercise may increase cells' sensitivity to the effects of insulin. It will also help reduce the amount of glucose released by the liver.	The duration of improvement is generally 12–72 hours. For improved control, exercise needs to be done at least every other day and preferably 5 days per week.
	2.3 Regular exercise may reduce insulin requirements.	
	2.4 Initially, exercise may make blood glucose control more difficult, because exercise needs to be balanced with your meal plan and medicines. Try not to get discouraged; planning, monitoring, and working with your health care team can help achieve this balance.	Hypoglycemia is less likely in people with type 2 diabetes and not at all likely in those treated with meal planning and exercise.

CONTENT OUTLINE

CONCEPT	DETAIL	INSTRUCTOR'S NOTES
3. Choosing an exercise program	3.1 There are two types of exercise: aerobic and anaerobic. Aerobic exercise uses oxygen to help release energy from fat cells. Anaerobic exercise does not use oxygen to burn fuel. Ideally, your exercise program will include both types of exercise.	Ask, "What kinds of exercise programs have you tried? What do you think will work for you?" Anaerobic exercise may not be safe or feasible for some participants. Resistance exercise improves insulin sensitivity at about the same rate as aerobic activity. Refer to Handout #1, Recommended Activity Levels.
	3.2 The recommendation for people with diabetes is 30 minutes of moderate aerobic exercise 5 times per week or 20 minutes of vigorous activity 3 times per week. For people with diabetes, anerobic exercise is recommended 3 times a week.	Ask, "What aerobic activities appeal to you? What anaerobic activities?" The best exercise is the one you will do and will be able to continue to do. The moderate and vigorous can be combined; for example, walk 2 days for 30 minutes and run 2 other days for 20 minutes.
	3.3 Choose an exercise you are willing and able to do regularly.	Ask, "What have you tried to make exercise more enjoyable? How did it work?" List ideas generated by the group on the board.
	3.4 One approach to exercise is the lifetime activity model. In this model, you accumulate a total of 30 minutes of moderately intense physical activity each day. Lower intensity activity (e.g., light housework) can be done more often and/or for a longer period of time.	This is helpful, even if you have an aerobic program. The goal is to use 3–4 kcal/kg/day. This level of activity provides cardiovascular benefits but 30 minutes of continuous exercise has more effect on weight.
	3.5 The idea is to fit 10 minutes of aerobic physical activity into your usual routine, three different times every day.	Ask, "What are ways you have tried to increase your daily activity?" Examples: Park so you have to walk farther, take the stairs, walk the golf course. Distribute "Small Steps, Big Rewards" materials.

CONTENT OUTLINE

CONCEPT	DETAIL	INSTRUCTOR'S NOTES

3.6 Another approach is the 10,000 Steps Program; 10,000 steps is equal to 5 miles. Using a pedometer helps make walking a daily contest with yourself. Keep in mind that 10,000 steps is a goal. Start with your current level of activity and add to it. Pedometers have been shown to help people take more steps per day.

Distribute pedometers if available. Remind participants to start slowly and to gradually increase the number of steps per day. Other guidelines recommend: For women age 18–40, 12,000 steps; age 40–50, 11,000 steps; age 50–60, 10,000 steps; and age 60+, 8,000 steps. For men, age 18–50, 12,000 steps; age 50+, 11,000 steps.

3.7 Another approach is a planned aerobic exercise program. Aerobic exercise is steady exercise for at least 12 minutes that increases the heart rate to at least 50–70% of maximum. This increases oxygen use.

Ask, "What are some aerobic exercises you have tried?" (e.g., walking, bicycling, cross-country skiing, swimming, or dancing.) Walking is a low-cost, safe way that many people find helps them to be more active.

3.8 Aerobic exercise burns glucose and fat and provides the greatest benefit for blood glucose and weight management. It also helps you to cope with stress and decreases hunger.

3.9 Activities such as bowling and baseball are not aerobic, because long periods of inactivity occur between short spurts of activity.

Ask, "What are other examples of anaerobic exercise?" Golf is generally not aerobic unless players walk briskly and do not use a cart.

3.10 Anaerobic or resistance exercise helps build muscle tissue. It can cause stiff and sore muscles and hunger after exercise.

Some anaerobic exercises can increase blood glucose and intraoccular pressure. Participants with diabetes complications need a medical evaluation before beginning this type of program.

4. Level and duration

4.1 Level of exercise is described as light, moderate, or strenuous. What is light exercise for one person may be moderate exercise for someone else, depending on the person's level of fitness. Your own response to exercise will change as you grow stronger.

Encourage participants to start with light exercise and work up to more strenuous levels to prevent injuries and to maintain motivation and self-efficiency.

CONTENT OUTLINE

CONCEPT	DETAIL	INSTRUCTOR'S NOTES
	4.2 Light exercise does not make you breathe heavily, but your pulse rate may increase slightly.	Light exercise done for less than 10 minutes will not affect blood glucose; if done for longer than 10 minutes, it can lower blood glucose.
	4.3 Moderate exercise involves noticeably heavier breathing, with a pulse rate increase to more than 100 beats per minute.	Teach patients how to take their pulse rates. Count for 6 seconds and add a zero to the number to find the rate per minute. Moderate exercise done for less than about 10 minutes may raise blood glucose (the liver releases stored glucose); done for longer, it lowers blood glucose.
	4.4 Strenuous exercise involves rapid breathing with a pulse rate between 125 and 160 beats per minute, depending on age.	Strenuous exercise done for less than 10 minutes may raise blood glucose. If done for longer than 10 minutes, it will lower blood glucose for a sustained period of time (if blood glucose is well controlled).
	4.5 Another way to evaluate exercise is to determine your perceived level of exertion. Perceived exertion is a method of rating how hard you are working during an activity. As you exercise, decide what you believe your rate of exertion is, using a scale of very, very light to very, very hard. Aim to work out in the somewhat-hard to hard range.	The rate of perceived exertion (RPE) scale is also known as the Borg scale. Exercise ratings range from 6 (very, very light) to 19 (very, very hard). Aim for aerobic exercise in the 12–16 range.
	4.6 You can also use the "talk test." If you cannot comfortably carry on a conversation, then you are exercising harder than you need to.	
	4.7 If taking insulin, any level of exercise done routinely will probably require a change in your treatment program. Ask your health care team to work with you on a plan.	Ask, "Do you adjust your insulin dose or food intake on your exercise days?"

CONTENT OUTLINE

CONCEPT	DETAIL	INSTRUCTOR'S NOTES
	4.8 A complete exercise program includes aerobic activity, stretching, and weight-bearing activity. Exercise continuously for 20–40 minutes.	Stretching helps to maintain flexibility and range of motion, which are important as we age.
	4.9 The recommended duration is 20–60 minutes. Lower-intensity exercise needs to be done for a longer period of time than higher-intensity exercise to get the most benefit.	
5. **Planning your exercise program**	5.1 See your health professional. Have any tests done that are recommended.	A history and physical exam are needed to look for signs of complications. In the presence of PDR or severe NPDR, vigorous aerobic or resistance exercise may be contraindicated. In the presence of severe peripheral neuropathy, non-weight bearing activities may be safer. Participants with autonomic neuropathy should undergo cardiac investigation before beginning any physical activity that is more intense. There are no restrictions of participants with diabetic kidney disease. Exercise testing may be recommended for patients at moderate or high risk of cardiovascular disease (CVD) depending on the intensity of the exercise program.
	5.2 Determine your target heart rate. Your target heart rate range is 60–85% of your maximum heart rate. To calculate your maximum heart rate, subtract your age from 220. Multiply by 0.60–0.85 to find your target heart rate range.	Figure an example on the chalkboard (220 – age × 0.70, depending on the fitness level). Have participants calculate their own target heart rate. Point out that their health care team may recommend a different target heart rate. Use Visual #1, Target Heart Rates. Ask, "What is your target heart rate?"

CONTENT OUTLINE

CONCEPT	DETAIL	INSTRUCTOR'S NOTES
	5.3 To achieve the greatest benefit for your heart, exercise at your target heart rate for at least 20 minutes three to five times a week.	Five or six exercise sessions per week may be needed for weight loss.
	5.4 People with other medical problems, such as heart disease or hypertension, or diabetes complications, such as retinopathy, need personally developed exercise programs.	For example, jogging may make retinal detachment or renal perfusion worse. Lifting weights is contraindicated in retinopathy. People with heart problems may not be able to use the target heart rate method.
	5.5 You may need different meal plans or insulin doses for different levels of activity on different days. Seasonal changes in activity levels may also require a change in insulin dose or a snack.	For example, use one plan for exercise days, and one for rest days; or use one plan for work days and one for weekends.
	5.6 Choose footwear to protect your feet. Use of silica gels or air midsoles as well as polyester or blended socks to keep feet dry may help minimize trauma.	Remind participants to check for blisters or other injuries before and after exercise.
6. Starting to exercise	6.1 Check your blood glucose. If your blood glucose is low (less than 70 mg/dl) before you begin to exercise, treat the hypoglycemia and do not exercise at that time. If your blood glucose is less than 100 mg/dl, eat additional carbohydrate.	Wait until blood glucose is up to at least 100 mg/dl before starting to exercise.
	6.2 If you have type 1 diabetes and your blood glucose is high (above 250 mg/dl), check your urine for ketones. Do not exercise if your blood glucose is over 250 mg/dl and you have ketones in your urine.	Ketones in the urine indicate insulin deficiency. Hyperglycemia due to insulin deficiency may increase with exercise. Your blood glucose levels may rise even further. These recommendations are specific to type 1 diabetes.
	6.3 Gradually warm up your muscles. Do low-intensity aerobic exercise such as walking or marching in place for 5–10 minutes, then stretch for 5–10 minutes before you begin more	Warm-up periods may also help to prevent postexercise hunger. Ask, "What have you tried as a warm-up activity?" List these on the board.

CONTENT OUTLINE

CONCEPT	DETAIL	INSTRUCTOR'S NOTES
	intensive exercise. This helps prevent muscle cramps and injury.	
7. During aerobic exercise	7.1 Wear diabetes and personal ID, wear appropriate shoes to avoid skin breakdown, and take coins or a phone in case of emergency.	Ask, "What safety precautions do you take?"
	7.2 Take your pulse every 10–15 minutes to be sure you are working at your target heart rate.	
	7.3 Do not overexert. You should be able to talk easily as you work out.	"No pain, no gain" is not true. If you are out of breath, you are not exercising aerobically.
	7.4 Avoid dehydration. Drink fluids every 30 minutes during your workouts.	
	7.5 Know the signs and symptoms of overexertion: increased shortness of breath, nausea or vomiting, irregular heartbeat, excessive fatigue, feeling faint or lightheaded, and pain or pressure in the chest or arm.	Stop exercising and contact your provider if you feel any of these symptoms.
8. After aerobic exercise	8.1 Gradually decrease your intensity, do low intensity aerobic activity for 5–10 min, and then finish your exercise period with about 5–10 minutes of stretching exercises. This is called a cooldown. It will help to prevent aches and muscle cramping later.	Ask, "What have you tried as a cool-down activity?" List these on the board.
	8.2 Check to determine the effect of exercise on your blood glucose level. Everyone has his or her own response to different types of exercise.	Remind participants to monitor more frequently postexercise.
9. Hypoglycemia and exercise	9.1 Exercise uses up glucose in your blood and helps insulin work better. Because of this, exercise usually lowers your blood glucose.	Distribute Handout #2, Treatment of Low Blood Glucose. Ask, "Have you ever had a low blood glucose during or after exercise? What was it like? What did you do about it?"

CONTENT OUTLINE

CONCEPT	DETAIL	INSTRUCTOR'S NOTES
	9.2 Know the signs and symptoms of hypoglycemia **during exercise:** undue anxiety or shakiness, as well as changes in gait, coordination, ability to think, or vision.	If possible, check your blood glucose level if you think you may be having an insulin reaction. If not possible to monitor, treat as a reaction.
	9.3 Carry a source of carbohydrate to treat low blood glucose.	Pin a sugar packet or package of glucose tablets to your clothes if you don't have a pocket.
	9.4 Effects of activity on your blood glucose can last for many (over 12–48) hours. It is possible to have a reaction up to 48 hours after exercising. Taking less of the insulin that is most active during/after exercise or eating a snack after exercise may help prevent postexercise late-onset hypoglycemia (PEL).	PEL is defined as a reaction >4 hours after exercise. It usually occurs in people with type 1 diabetes who exercise at a moderate-to-high intensity for more than 30 minutes. Remind participants to monitor more frequently postexercise.
	9.5 If you take insulin or a secretagogue, you may need extra food for extra activity. Extra activity means the body is working harder and/or longer than usual. You may need extra food when you are involved in any activity that is not a usual part of your day (i.e., raking leaves, washing windows, structured exercises). Just being more active in the summer may require a change in medication or meal plan.	Any activity (e.g., walking to the store) may be usual activity (requiring no snack) for one person and an unusual activity (requiring a snack) for another. Ask the group for other examples or their experiences, such as yard work or cleaning. Stress using monitoring results for making adjustments. Exercising after a meal may not be enough to prevent hypoglycemia. Some participants may prefer to take a lower medication dose rather than eat extra food. Work with participants to develop a personal plan based on their treatment program, blood glucose levels, and response.
	9.6 People who manage their diabetes with diet alone do not need extra food before exercising.	
10. Making adjustments for activity	10.1 If you exercise regularly and take insulin, you may need to decrease your insulin dose on	Ask, "What questions do you have about making adjustments for exercise? What concerns do

CONTENT OUTLINE

CONCEPT	DETAIL	INSTRUCTOR'S NOTES
	exercise days or eat an exercise snack. Exercising around the same time each day will make planning insulin changes and snacks easier and more consistent.	you have?" Insulin adjustments are most relevant for participants who intensively manage their diabetes and/or strenuously exercise.
	10.2 The decision about whether to eat additional food or adjust your medication is based on your goal for exercise.	Ask, "What is your goal for exercise? How consistent is your exercise program?"
Insulin adjustments	10.3 Reducing insulin doses is particularly helpful for those who exercise routinely, as part of weight management and/or to improve blood glucose levels.	
	The decision about which insulin to decrease is based on the timing and type of exercise and the insulin treatment plan.	
	10.4 The risk for hypoglycemia is less when the level of insulin in your body is lower. ■ Avoid planning your exercise program for the time when your insulin is peaking. ■ Avoid exercise for 1–2 hours after injecting rapid- or short-acting insulin. ■ Exercise before the morning insulin dose. ■ Exercise 1–3 hours after eating.	This may require insulin adjustments to accommodate the participant's schedule.
	10.5 The risk for nocturnal hypoglycemia is greater when you exercise in the evening.	
	10.6 Hypoglycemia is also a risk during pump therapy. Strategies for prevention include reducing the basal rate, eating an exercise snack, or removing the pump during exercise.	Another option is to reduce the bolus dose for planned postmeal activity.
Carbohydrate adjustments	10.7 The harder your body works during exercise, the more glucose it uses. The amount and timing of exercise snacks depends on the intensity of	**Optional:** Distribute Handout #3, Calories Spent in Various Exercises. This chart is a relative measure of energy

CONTENT OUTLINE

CONCEPT	DETAIL	INSTRUCTOR'S NOTES

the exercise, the duration of the exercise, your pre-exercise blood glucose, and your individual response.

expended. It may be used to estimate the extra calories needed to replace those spent in exercise.

10.8 Carbohydrate foods, such as fruit, juice, skim milk, and bread, turn to glucose the quickest. The harder your body works during exercise, the more carbohydrate it needs.

Distribute Handout #4, Sample Activity Snacks. Review material from Outline #4, *Food and Blood Glucose* (p. 53), as needed. Carbohydrate adjustments are most relevant for participants who intensively manage their diabetes and/or strenuously exercise. Ask, "What questions or concerns do you have about adjusting your carbohydrate intake for exercise?"

10.9 The timing of snacks varies from person to person and with different lengths and intensities of exercise.

10.10 If your blood glucose is less than 100 mg/dl, eat additional carbohydrate before you begin.

This is a guideline to use as a starting point. Each participant will need to monitor and adjust accordingly. Current guidelines recommend additional carbohydrate only when the pre-existing blood glucose level is <100 mg/dl and the patient is taking insulin or a secretagogue.

10.11 Eat additional carbohydrate before and during exercise as needed to prevent low blood glucose.

10.12 Several small carbohydrate snacks taken about every 30 minutes during exercise may be needed if exercise is very vigorous or strenuous.

10.13 It isn't always possible to stop every 30 minutes to eat during exercise. To avoid low blood glucose, eat additional carbohydrate 1–4 hours before starting, and extra carbohydrates after finishing very vigorous or strenuous exercise.

CONTENT OUTLINE

CONCEPT	DETAIL	INSTRUCTOR'S NOTES
	10.14 You may need to eat extra carbohydrates several hours after you have exercised. The longer and more intense the exercise, the longer that glucose will be lowered after exercise has stopped.	Monitoring your blood glucose after exercise will help to evaluate how well the extra food is meeting your needs.
11. Balancing food and insulin with activity	11.1 Everyone has his or her own response to exercise. Monitoring blood glucose levels helps you understand your response to any adjustments that you make. You will probably need to adjust for each activity.	Encourage participants to work closely with their health care team when making adjustments.
	11.2 The best way to know if the adjustments are adequate is to check your blood glucose before and after exercise. If the activity lasts longer than 30 minutes, check your blood glucose during the activity to monitor response.	
12. General information	12.1 Drink plenty of water before, during, and after exercise, especially if you sweat a lot. You can lose up to 2 liters of fluid per hour of exercise.	Ask, "What do you do to make sure you do not get dehydrated when you exercise?" For example, drink fluids 2 hours before exercise.
	12.2 For long periods of strenuous exercise, such as running, drinks with 60–80 calories (15–20 g carbohydrate) per 8 oz provide the best solution for fluid and carbohydrate absorption. Most sports drinks (such as Gatorade) meet this criterion, but juices and soft drinks may not.	Drinks with more than 25 g carbohydrate per 8 oz are hypertonic and may cause dehydration and diarrhea. Juice and soft drinks generally need to be diluted 50:50 with water to achieve the proper fluid/carbohydrate ratio.
	12.3 Alcohol and exercise don't mix well. Less glucose is available (effect of alcohol) and more is used (effect of exercise). Alcohol consumed before, during, or after exercise can cause a low blood glucose reaction.	Because alcohol decreases the liver's ability to release glucose, and exercise enhances the muscles' ability to take up glucose, hypoglycemia can occur.

CONTENT OUTLINE

CONCEPT	DETAIL	INSTRUCTOR'S NOTES
13. Tips for staying with your exercise program	13.1 Sticking with exercise is harder than getting started. Choose an exercise you enjoy and can do.	Ask participants to describe exercise programs they've tried and what helped and what hindered their efforts. List strategies on the board. If appropriate, work through Handout #5, Planning Your Exercise Program, as a group.
	13.2 Start slowly. Work up to more strenuous activity as you become more fit.	Walk one block the first day, and then gradually walk longer each day (e.g., add 1–2 min per session).
	13.3 If possible, exercise with your spouse or a friend. It helps you both to stay motivated and makes the time go by faster.	
	13.4 Set aside the same time each day for your exercise. Make it a habit. Choose a time that does not coincide with the peak action of your insulin.	It is easy not to exercise if you try to do it "when I get a chance." Some find it helpful to put it on their calendar or planner.
	13.5 Take a class or join an exercise club. Many malls have walking clubs.	Give information on programs in your area. Include those most relevant for the participants (e.g., senior centers, free programs).
	13.6 Choose activities that don't depend on good weather, or plan activities for good and bad weather.	For example, you can walk inside and out or put on music and dance.
	13.7 Record your progress.	Give suggestions on how to monitor and record distance, time, and heart rate.
	13.8 Reward yourself for progress made.	Ask, "How can you reward yourself?" Examples are time for yourself, time with a friend, or going to a movie.
	13.9 Contact your health care team if you have questions, concerns, or problems. They can help you plan your activity, diet, or medication	Choose a short-term goal to try before the next session.

CONTENT OUTLINE

CONCEPT	DETAIL	INSTRUCTOR'S NOTES
	changes and solve any problems that might occur as you continue your exercise program.	
	13.10 Choose one thing you will do this week to care for your diabetes.	Close the session by asking participants to identify one action step they will take this week.

SKILLS CHECKLIST

Participants will be able to locate pulse points, count heart rates, and determine target heart rates. Select participants will be able to calculate an insulin adjustment or exercise snack.

EVALUATION PLAN

Knowledge will be evaluated by achievement of learning objectives and by responses to questions during the session. The ability to apply knowledge will be evaluated by the development of personal exercise goals, by the development and implementation of a plan to achieve those goals, and through program outcome measures.

DOCUMENTATION PLAN

Record class attendance and achieved objectives as appropriate using the Diabetes Self-Management Record, the Participant Follow-up, or another form.

SUGGESTED READINGS

Albright A: Moving ahead with physical activity. *Diabetes Spectrum* 18:86–118, 2005

Allen NA: Social cognitive theory in diabetes exercise research: an integrative literature review. *The Diabetes Educator* 30:805–819, 2004

Araiza P, Hewes H, Gashetewa C, Vella CA, Berger MR: Efficacy of a pedometer-based physical activity program on parameters of diabetes control in type 2 diabetes mellitus. *Metabolism* 33:1382–1387, 2006

Colberg SR: Encouraging patients to be physically active: what busy practitioners need to know. *Clinical Diabetes* 26:123–127, 2008

Colberg SR: Increasing insulin sensitivity. *Diabetes Self-Management* 24(2):47–50, 2007

Conn VS, Hafdahl AR, Brown SA, Brown LM: Meta-analysis of patient education interventions to increase physical activity among chronically ill adults. *Patient Education and Counseling* 70:157–172, 2008

Di Loreto, Fanelli C, Lucidi P, Murdoto G, et al.: Make your diabetes patients walk: long-term

SUGGESTED READINGS *continued*

impact of different amounts of physical activity in diabetes. *Diabetes Care* 28:1295–1302, 2005

Eriksen L, Dahl-Petersen I, Haugaard SB, Dela F: Comparison of the effect of multiple short-duration with single long-duration exercise sessions on glucose homeostasis in type 2 diabetes mellitus. *Diabeteologia* 20:2245–2253, 2007

Eves ND, Plotnikoff RC: Resistance training and type 2 diabetes. *Diabetes Care* 29:1933–1941, 2006

Fentress D: Life fit: a family-friendly guide to getting more physical activity. *Diabetes Forecast* 58(3):4–6, 2005

Geil P, Hieronymus L: Physical activity: the magic of movement. *Diabetes Self-management* 22(1):7–12, 2005

Harris GD, White RD: Exercise stress testing in patient with type 2 diabetes: When are asymptomatic patients screened? *Clinical Diabetes* 25:126–130, 2007

Haskell WL, Lee I-M, Pate RR, Powell KE, Blair SN, et al.: Physical activity and public health: updated recommendation for adults from the American College of Sports Medicine and the American Heart Association. *Circulation* 116:1081–1093, 2007

Hayes C, Herbert M, Marrero D, Martin CL, Muchnick S: AADE Position Statement: diabetes and exercise. *The Diabetes Educator* 34:37–40, 2008

Hill JO: Walking and type 2 diabetes. *Diabetes Care* 28:1524–1525, 2005

Jeon CY, Ookken RP, Hu FB, van Dam RM: Physical activity of moderate intensity and risk of type 2 diabetes: a systematic review. *Diabetes Care* 30:732–744, 2007

Kavookjian J, Elswick BM, Whetsel T: Interventions for being active among individu-

als with diabetes: a systematic review of the literature. *The Diabetes Educator* 33:962–988, 2007

Morrato EH, Hill JO, Wyatt HR, Ghushachyan V, Sullivan PW: Physical activity in U.S. adults with diabetes and at risk for developing diabetes, 2003. *Diabetes Care* 30:203–209, 2007

Nethercott T: Exercise: good questions and answers. *Diabetes Forecast* 62(7):44–50, 2009

Praet SF, Manders RJ, Lieverse AG, et al.: Influence of acute exercise on hyperglycemia in insulin-treated type 2 diabetes. *Med Sci Sports Exerc* 38:2037–2044, 2006

Rank JS, Li TY, Manson JE, Hu FB: Adiposity compared with physical inactivity and risk of type 2 diabetes in women. *Diabetes Care* 30:53–58, 2007

Roberts SS: Aerobic exercise: what it is and why it's good. *Diabetes Forecast* 60(3):15–17, 2007

Scheiner G: The great blood glucose balancing act. *Diabetes Self-Management* 23(5):48–52, 2006

Shahar J: Helping your patients become active. *Diabetes Spectrum* 21:59–62, 2008

Sigal RJ, Kenny GP, Boule NG, Wells GA, et al.: Effects of aerobic training, resistance training, or both on glycemic control in type 2 diabetes. *Annals of Internal Medicine* 147:357–369, 2007

Sigal RJ, Kenny GP, Wasserman DH, Castaneda-Sceppa C, White RD: Physical activity/exercise and type 2 diabetes: a consensus statement from the American Diabetes Association. *Diabetes Care* 29:1433–1438, 2006

Snowling NJ, Hopkins WG: Effects of different modes of exercise training on glucose control and risk factors for complications in type 2 diabetic patients: a meta-analysis. *Diabetes Care* 29:2518–2527, 2006

Target Heart Rates (1 Minute)

Age (Years)	Maximum Heart Rate	Percentage of Maximum Heart Rate		
		60%	70%	85%
20	200	120	140	170
25	195	117	137	166
30	190	114	133	162
35	185	111	130	157
40	180	108	126	153
45	175	105	125	149
50	170	102	119	145
55	165	99	116	140
60	160	96	112	136
65	155	93	109	132
70	150	90	105	128
75	145	87	102	123
80	140	84	98	119

➡ Recommended Activity Level

Recommended Activity Level for Adults, Ages 18–65

Activity Levels	Activity Examples	Activity Amount
Light (no major increase in pulse or breathing rates)	**Walking, sitting, standing, and normal daily activities)**	**Normal daily routine**
	AND	
Moderate (increase in pulse/heart rate and breathing but can comfortably engage in a conversation)	**Walking briskly, bicycling (flat surface), swimming (leisurely), basketball**	**30 minutes/day 5 days a week**
Vigorous (rapid pulse and breathing)	**Walking very briskly, jogging or running, shoveling, digging ditches, bicycling (hard, hilly), basketball, soccer, volleyball games, swimming (moderate/hard)**	**20 minutes/day 3 days/week**
	AND	
Strength and Endurance (substantial fatigue after 8–12 repititions	**Exercise with weights, crunches**	**8–10 exercises with 8–10 reps, each using major muscle groups— 2 nonconsecutive day/week**

Note: American College of Sports Medicine/American Heart Association physical activity recommended documents suggest all adults strive for a minimum amount of daily activity to include the above examples.

Sources: Haskell WL, Lee IM, Pate RR, et al.: Physical activity in public health: Updated recommendation for adults from the American College of Sports Medicine and the American Heart Association. *Circulation* 116:1081–1093, 2007

Nelson ME, Rejeski WJ, Blair SN, et al.: Physcial activity and public health in older adults: recommendation from the American College of Sports Medicine and the American Heart Association. *Circulation* 116:1094–1105, 2007

➲ Treatment of Low Blood Glucose

If your blood glucose test is:	The amount of food or drink to take is:
Between 50 and 69 mg/dl	15 g carbohydrate (1 carbohydrate serving **or** 1 cup fat-free [skim] milk)
Less than 50 mg/dl	30 g carbohydrate (2 carbohydrate servings)

You should feel better in 10–15 minutes after you treat yourself. If your blood glucose is still less than 70 mg/dl or you don't feel better 10–15 minutes after the treatment, take 1 more carbohydrate serving. Check your blood glucose an hour after the reaction to make sure that your blood glucose has gone above 70 mg/dl and stayed there.

▶ ▶ ▶ ▶ ▶

EXAMPLES OF TREATMENTS FOR LOW BLOOD GLUCOSE

(All equal about 15 g carbohydrate or 1 fruit serving)

If your blood glucose is between 50 and 69 mg/dl, take the amount listed. If your blood glucose is less than 50 mg/dl, take twice the amount listed.

Foods	Amount
Orange or apple juice	1/2 cup
Grape or cranberry juice	1/3 cup
Non-diet soft drink	1/2 cup
Honey or corn syrup	1 Tbsp
Sugar packets	3
Life Savers	3–8 pieces
Glucose tablets	3–4 tablets

An additional carbohydrate snack may be needed at night or after exercise to keep your blood glucose above 70 mg/dl.

⊜ Calories Spent in Various Exercises

	Calories/hour	Calories/minute
LIGHT ACTIVITY		
Light housework	150	2.5
Strolling, 1.0 mile/hour	150	2.5
Golf, using power cart	175	3.0
Level walking, 2.0 miles/hour	200	3.5
MODERATE ACTIVITY		
Cycling, 5.5 miles/hour	210	3.5
Gardening	220	3.5
Canoeing, 2.5 miles/hour	230	4.0
Cleaning windows, mopping, vacuuming	240	4.0
Lawn mowing, power mower	250	4.0
Lawn mowing, hand mower	270	4.5
Walking, 3.0 miles/hour	275	4.5
Bowling	300	5.0
Golf, pulling cart	300	5.0
Scrubbing floors	300	5.0
Rowboating, 2.5 miles/hour	300	5.0
Swimming, 0.25 miles/hour	300	5.0
Cycling, 8 miles/hour	325	5.5
Golf, carrying clubs	350	6.0
Badminton	350	6.0
Horseback riding, trotting	350	6.0
Square dancing	350	6.0
Volleyball	350	6.0

CALORIES SPENT IN VARIOUS ACTIVITIES *continued*

	Calories/hour	Calories/minute
Roller skating	350	6.0
Doubles tennis	360	6.0
Calisthenics and ballet exercises	360	6.0
Table tennis	360	6.0
Walking, 4.0 miles/hour	360	6.0

STRENUOUS ACTIVITY

	Calories/hour	Calories/minute
Vigorous dancing	320–500	5.5–8.5
Cycling, 10 miles/hour	400	6.5
Ice skating, 10 miles/hour	400	6.5
Ditch digging, hand shovel	400	6.5
Wood chopping or sawing	400–600	6.5–10.0
Walking, 5 miles/hour	420	7.0
Cycling, 11 miles/hour	420	7.0
Singles tennis	420	7.0
Waterskiing	480	8.0
Jogging, 5 miles/hour	480	8.0
Cycling, 12 miles/hour	480	8.0
Hill climbing, 100 feet/hour	490	8.0
Downhill skiing	550	9.0
Running, 5.5 miles/hour	600	10.0
Squash and handball	600	10.0
Cycling, 13 miles/hour	660	11.0
Running, 6–9 miles/hour	660–850	11.0–14.0
Cross-country skiing	600–1200	10.0–20.0
Running, 10 miles/hour	900	15.0

◐ Sample Activity Snacks

Intensity of activity	Examples	If blood glucose is	Then eat	Suggestions
Light	Walking a half mile or leisurely biking for less than 30 minutes	less than 100 mg/dl	10–15 g carbohydrate per hour.	1 fruit **or** bread serving (1/2 cup orange juice **or** 1/4 bagel)
		100 mg/dl or above*	No food needed	
Moderate	Tennis, jogging, swimming, leisurely biking, gardening, golfing, vacuuming for 30 minutes to 1 hour	less than 100 mg/dl	15–30 g carbohydrate before exercise, then 10–15 g per 30–60 minutes of exercise	1 milk and 1 fruit serving **or** 1 milk and 1 bread (1 cup plain yogurt and 1/2 banana **or** cereal and 1 cup milk)
		100 mg/dl or above	10–15 g carbohydrate per 30–60 minutes of exercise	1 fruit **or** 1 bread serving (1/2 banana **or** 8 saltine crackers)

* Test for ketones if blood glucose is over 250 mg/dl before or after exercise.

© 2009 American Diabetes Association

SAMPLE ACTIVITY SNACKS *continued*

Intensity of activity	Examples	If blood glucose is	Then eat	Suggestions
Strenuous	Football, hockey, racquetball, basketball, strenuous biking or swimming, shoveling heavy snow, raking leaves	Less than 100 mg/dl	30–45 g carbohydrate. Check blood glucose often.	2 bread servings with either 1 milk or 1 fruit (2 slices toast, with 1 cup fat-free [skim] milk or 1 small orange)
		100 mg/dl or above*	30 g carbohydrate (depends on intensity and duration)	1 milk and bread serving (1 slice bread and 1 cup skim milk) **or** 1 fruit and 1 bread

Be sure to monitor and record your blood glucose before and after exercise (and every 30 minutes during exercise). Each person responds to exercise and food differently—activity snacks need to be planned for each person with the help of a dietitian.

* Test for ketones if blood glucose is over 250 mg/dl before or after exercise.

➡ Planning Your Exercise Program

Write down the answers to the following questions:

1. What exercise programs or activities are safe and practical for you to do regularly?

2. Of these, which activities would you enjoy doing?

3. Are there any activities you plan to do?

4. Where will you do these activities?

5. What time of day will you do your program?

6. How often will you exercise?

7. How long will you exercise each time?

8. What will you do to reduce your risk for hypoglycemia?

PLANNING YOUR EXERCISE PROGRAM *continued*

    9. What stretching, aerobic, and weight-bearing activities will you do?

  10. What is your target heart rate?

  11. What is your goal for your heart rate?

  12. What is your goal for how often you will exercise once your exercise program is established?

  13. How will you keep track of your exercise?

  14. How will you reward yourself for your exercise program?

#8 Oral Medications and Incretin Mimetics

▷ ▷ ▷ ▷ ▷

STATEMENT OF PURPOSE

This session is intended to provide information about the purpose, action, use, and side effects of medications used to treat type 2 diabetes. Discuss only those therapies relevant to the participants.

PREREQUISITES

It is recommended that only people currently taking oral diabetes medications attend this session. Participants who take oral agents and insulin need information about both types of therapy.

OBJECTIVES

At the end of this session, participants will be able to:

1. define the purpose and action of oral diabetes medications (diabetes pills);

2. state that oral diabetes medications are not insulin;

3. state the name of their oral diabetes medication, the dose to take, and the time it should be taken;

4. identify one idea they will use in remembering to take the medication;

5. describe one side effect of oral diabetes medications;

6. define the purpose and action of incretin mimetics;

7. identify the progressive nature of the treatment of type 2 diabetes.

CONTENT

Using medications safely and for maximum effectiveness.

MATERIALS NEEDED

VISUALS PROVIDED	ADDITIONAL
1. Natural History of Type 2 Diabetes 2. Diabetes Pills	■ Samples of different diabetes medications ■ Sample pill bottle ■ Price information from local pharmacies ■ Compartmentalized container for medications ■ Injection pen devices

METHOD OF PRESENTATION

Start by introducing yourself and telling what you do. Ask participants to introduce themselves. Explain that the purpose of this session is to provide information about oral antidiabetes medications (pills) and incretin mimetics and how they work.

Begin by asking how they did with their short-term goal and what they learned from it. Present material in a question/discussion format, using the first question as a starting point. Provide appropriate content outlined below in response. Ask if there are additional questions, and respond, repeating the process for the entire session. Use the questions in the Instructor's Notes section to generate discussion if no questions are forthcoming after a period of silence. Keeping track of the content discussed in each session, using the Diabetes Self-Management Record, the Participant Follow-up Record, or another form, helps you to evaluate if all needed content has been discussed.

CONTENT OUTLINE

CONCEPT	DETAIL	INSTRUCTOR'S NOTES
1. Definition of oral medications	1.1 Diabetes pills are taken to lower blood glucose levels.	Ask, "What questions/concerns do you have about your diabetes medicines?"
	1.2 Diabetes pills are not insulin. Insulin cannot be taken orally—it would be destroyed by digestive enzymes.	Insulin is a protein and would be digested like other proteins. Ask, "What diabetes medications are you taking? What have been your experiences?" List medicines on the board. Discuss **only** the listed medications, unless there are questions about others.
	1.3 These pills are effective only when the pancreas still produces some insulin. Therefore, they are prescribed for people with type 2 diabetes.	
	1.4 As people get older and heavier, cells can become resistant to insulin so that the glucose remains in the bloodstream. At first, the pancreas	

CONTENT OUTLINE

CONCEPT	DETAIL	INSTRUCTOR'S NOTES
	makes more insulin; but after a time, it just isn't able to keep up. The glucose stays in the blood, and your level goes above the normal range. This is called *insulin resistance*.	
	1.5 The liver stores some glucose (sugar) to release when your blood glucose goes below normal, such as between meals and overnight. When the liver cells are resistant to insulin, the liver puts out too much glucose. This is one reason why you may have high blood glucose levels before breakfast.	Reassure participants that diabetes does not damage the liver. Ask, "Has this ever happened to you?"
	1.6 It is likely that your therapy will change over time. Typically, people with type 2 diabetes start with meal planning and exercise, often along with an oral medication, and then add additional oral medications, and then other injectables or insulin.	Stress the use of different and multiple therapies over time to keep blood glucose levels near normal. Newer guidelines call for the use of oral medications from the time of diagnosis.
	1.7 How quickly you progress through the therapies depends on how your body responds. Three to six months is usually a fair trial of a therapy.	Ask, "How has your treatment changed since you were first diagnosed?" Point out that changes in therapy do not mean that your diabetes is worse or that you have failed. Note that hearing that diabetes is a progressive disease is very upsetting to patients, so discuss progression of therapy in the context of the natural history of diabetes and inform the patient that, over time, the body needs more help to keep blood glucose levels on target. Use Visual #1, Natural History of Type 2 Diabetes, to illustrate this point.
2. Types of oral medications and injectables	2.1 Currently, there are six types of pills on the market. A prescription is needed for all six. These medications help your body make more insulin, help your body use insulin better, or keep your blood glucose from going too high after meals. There are also	Participants taking combination medications need information relevant for both agents. Combination medications need to be taken with meals and titrated gradually to reduce gastrointestinal upset, prevent hypoglycemia,

CONTENT OUTLINE

CONCEPT	DETAIL	INSTRUCTOR'S NOTES
	pills that combine two types of oral medications into one pill.	and determine maximum effective dose.
	2.2 Each of the six types has a different chemical structure and works differently. The types are: ■ sulfonylureas ■ biguanides ■ alpha-glucosidase inhibitors ■ thiazolidinediones ■ meglitinides ■ DPP-4 inhibitors.	Medications that help with weight loss are also on the market, although these are not specific for diabetes. Identify types of pills from the list on the board. Use the discussion as a way to review pathophysiology. Incorporate participant experiences into the discussion. Discuss synergistic effects of medications and the importance of taking all medications. Assist participants to correlate glucose monitoring schedules and results with medication schedule and action.
	2.3 There are also injectable medicines called incretin mimetics that can be used to treat type 2 diabetes.	
3. Types of oral medications— sulfonylureas	3.1 Sulfonylureas stimulate the pancreas to produce insulin and cause the body to respond better to the insulin it does produce. They help lower premeal blood glucose levels.	Use Visual #2, Diabetes Pills, or samples of different pills. Say each name so patients hear how it is pronounced. (Use either the brand name or generic name, or both.)
	3.2 There are three different sulfonylureas.	Elicit and discuss patient experiences.
	3.3 The different sulfonylurea pills work similarly but are not exactly the same and **cannot** be used interchangeably.	The action and effectiveness of older and newer sulfonylureas are similar.
	3.4 Sulfonylureas can be used alone or in combination with other medicines.	Sulfonylureas, like all drugs, must be used with caution by some patients or should not be used at all by others. Review the package insert to become familiar with the risks and benefits of each drug.
	3.5 Primary disadvantages are side effects, such as hypoglycemia and weight gain.	
4. Types of oral medications— meglitinide	4.1 Repaglinide (Prandin) and nateglinide (Starlix) cause the beta cells to release insulin. These are different	Repaglinide and nateglinide belong to a class of medications known as insulin secretagogues.

CONTENT OUTLINE

CONCEPT	DETAIL	INSTRUCTOR'S NOTES
	than sulfonylureas in that they work more quickly and their effects are glucose-dependent. They are designed to treat post-meal hyperglycemia.	Their effects decrease when the blood glucose is low. These are metabolized in the liver but their risk for accumulation is small because of their short half-life (1–1 1/2 hours).
	4.2 Repaglinide and nateglinide can be used with diet and exercise or with other agents, diet, and exercise.	Ellicit and discuss patient experiences.
	4.3 Because they only work for a short time, take just before or up to 30 minutes before each meal or large snack.	Stress the importance of not taking these medications if a meal is skipped.
	4.4 Disadvantages include side effects, possible drug interactions, and hypoglycemia.	These should not be combined with alpha-glucosidase inhibitors.
5. Types of oral medications— biguanides	5.1 Metformin (Glucophage) enhances the action of insulin on the liver and in the muscles. It works mainly by inhibiting the release of glucose from the liver. It also slows the absorption of glucose in the gut and enhances the absorption of glucose in other parts of the body. Its main effect is on fasting blood glucose.	Elicit and discuss patient experiences. Metformin is often the first oral agent used. It was approved for use in the United States in 1995 but had been used in other countries for many years. It was also tested as a drug to delay the onset of type 2 diabetes in the DPP.
	5.2 Metformin can be used with diet and exercise or with other agents, diet, and exercise.	If sulfonylureas alone are ineffective in accomplishing blood glucose targets, metformin should be added— not used in place of the sulfonylurea.
	5.3 Metformin may also decrease cholesterol and triglycerides and does not promote weight gain, as sulfonylureas and insulin do.	Review the package insert to become familiar with the risks and benefits of the drug.
	5.4 Disadvantages include side effects, possible drug interactions, and risk for lactic acidosis. It is not appropriate for people with liver or kidney damage or heart failure. Side effects are primarily gastrointestinal—loss of appetite, diarrhea, and an unpleasant	Review symptoms of lactic acidosis, surgical contrast dye, and alcohol precautions. Furosemide and cimetadine may interact with metformin. Because cimetadine is available over the counter, instruct participants

CONTENT OUTLINE

CONCEPT	DETAIL	INSTRUCTOR'S NOTES
	metallic taste. Taking the daily dose at supper may decrease stomach upset and taking it with food may decrease the metallic taste.	to use a different preparation (e.g., Pepsid AC).
6. Types of oral medications— thiazolidinediones	6.1 Rosiglitazone (Avandia) and pioglitazone (Actors) act primarily to reduce insulin resistance by improving target cell response (sensitivity) to insulin. They also decrease glucose output from the liver and increase glucose disposal in the skeletal muscles.	Elicit and discuss patient experiences. Rosiglitazone and pioglitazone were approved in 1999. A related drug, troglitazone (Rezulin), was removed from the market in 2000 and warnings about rosiglitazone and heart attacks were added in 2007.
	6.2 Rosiglitazone and pioglitazone may be taken with or without food.	
	6.3 These medicines do not cause hypoglycemia when used alone.	Edema may occur among some people.
	6.4 These medicines can take 2–12 weeks to become effective. They should be used with caution if you have liver and heart disease.	These agents may lower lipid levels. Like all drugs, these must be used with caution by some patients or should not be used at all by others.
	6.5 Watch for possible side effects, including jaundice, nausea and vomiting, stomach pain, and dark urine. Blood tests of liver function should be done before starting these drugs and periodically thereafter.	Refer to product literature for specific testing recommendations. Stress the importance of these tests for the participants' safety.
7. Types of oral medications— alpha-glucosidase inhibitors	7.1 Acarbose (Precose) and miglitol (Glyset) block the enzymes that break down starches so that they are more slowly absorbed. This blunts the increase in blood glucose that occurs after eating.	Elicit and discuss patient experiences. Acarbose was approved for use in the U.S. in 1996 and miglitol in 1999.
	7.2 They can be used with diet and exercise, with other oral agents, or with insulin, diet, and exercise.	These agents only affect post-prandial (not fasting) blood glucose levels. They should not be used with rapid-acting insulins They should also not be used with insulin secretagogues.

CONTENT OUTLINE

CONCEPT	DETAIL	INSTRUCTOR'S NOTES
	7.3 To be effective, take them with the first bite of food at all meals.	These agents, like all drugs, must be used with caution by some people or should not be used at all by others. Obtain the package insert to become familiar with the risks and benefits of the drug.
	7.4 Primary disadvantages are side effects, such as bloating, gas, and diarrhea. The side effects generally disappear after 6 months.	
8. Types of oral medication— DPP-4 inhibitors	8.1 The newest medicines for type 2 diabetes are related to the incretin hormones. The incretin hormones help insulin to work better.	Elicit and discuss patient experiences.
	8.2 Incretin hormones are made by the gut. They help to: ■ increase glucose-dependent insulin secretion ■ suppress glucagon secretion ■ slow rate of gastric emptying ■ decrease food intake/weight ■ decrease blood glucose levels ■ may help preserve beta cell function.	Although researchers have known about the incretin hormones for some time, therapeutic applications are relatively new and the area of much research.
	8.3 These hormones are quickly broken down by a substance (enzyme) called DPP-4. In addition, secretion of the incretin hormones is decreased among people with diabetes.	Discuss only as much of this information as is of interest and relevance to the participants.
	8.4 Therefore, to provide these hormones as medications, you have to either give larger than normal amounts of the incretin hormones or block the effects of DPP-4.	The incretin hormones are GLP-1 and GIP. People with diabetes are not responsive to GIP. They can be made to respond to GLP-1 by giving supraphysiologic doses or by inhibiting the action of DPP-4.
	8.5 DPP-4 inhibitors are a class of medicines that block the action of DPP-4.	
	8.6 Sitagliptin (Januvia) was the first DPP-4 inhibitor, and saxagliptin (onglyza) was the second. A combination of Januvia and metformin (Janumet) is also on the market.	Others are in the pipeline (e.g., vildagliptin [Galvus]).

CONTENT OUTLINE

CONCEPT	DETAIL	INSTRUCTOR'S NOTES
	8.7 DPP-4 inhibitors enhance the secretion of insulin and suppress glucagon secretion.	These medicines do not generally suppress appetite and are considered weight neutral.
	8.8 These pills are taken once or twice daily with or without food. They have very few side effects. They do not cause hypoglycemia if taken alone. Because they are newer medicines, they may be expensive.	Side effects may include allergic reactions, cold symptoms, sore throat, upset stomach, and headache.
	8.9 DPP-4 inhibitors can be used with diet and exercise or with other medicines, diet, and exercise.	
9. Types of injectables— incretin mimetics	9.1 There are also medicines that mimic the effects of these hormones. Exenatide (Byetta) was the first incretin approved in the U.S.	Elicit and discuss patient experiences. Others are in the pipeline (e.g., liraglutide) as are weekly dosages.
	9.2 Because these hormones are a protein, they must be taken by injection using a pen.	Compare this to insulin, which is also a proteineous substance. Demonstrate pen devices and point out needle size.
	9.3 You take exenatide in your abdomen, thigh, or upper arm, 60 minutes or less before your two main meals and at least 6 hours apart. If you forget to take your injection, skip that dose and take your next dose at your usual time.	
	9.4 Incretin mimetics can be used with diet and exercise or with other agents, diet, and exercise.	
	9.5 Side effects include satiety, nausea, vomiting, loss of appetite, dizziness, acid stomach, and feeling jittery. Incretin mimetics taken alone do not cause hypoglycemia. Weight loss is another side effect.	In order to maintain weight loss, these medicines may need to be taken indefinitely. Nausea usually diminishes after taking the medicine for a short time. Eating smaller portions can help prevent nausea.
10. Side effects	10.1 Oral diabetes may have side effects.	Ask, "What side effects have you experienced with medicines?"
	10.2 Side effects to look for include: ■ unpleasant metallic taste	Assure participants that sulfonylureas are no longer

CONTENT OUTLINE

CONCEPT	DETAIL	INSTRUCTOR'S NOTES
	■ diarrhea ■ nausea or vomiting ■ loss of appetite ■ abdominal discomfort ■ skin rash or itching ■ dizziness ■ flushing and nausea with alcohol intake (chlorpropamide).	thought to cause hypertension or heart disease. Glucatrol XL is contained in a nonabsorbable shell; participants should not be concerned if they occasionally notice the shell in their stool. Second-generation agents do not cause alcohol intolerance.
	10.3 Report side effects to your provider.	Encourage participants to report problems rather than discontinuing.
	10.4 It is a good idea to get all prescriptions filled at the same pharmacy, so the pharmacist can be alert for any drug interactions.	
11. Hypoglycemia	11.1 Hypoglycemia (low blood glucose reaction) can occur when taking sulfonylureas and glitinides.	Ask, "What are the signs and symptoms of hypoglycemia?" Refer to Outline #11, *Managing Blood Glucose* (p. 231).
	11.2 Metformin, acarbose, miglitol, DPP-IV inhibitors, and glitazones do not cause hypoglycemia if taken alone.	If taken with a sulfonylurea, a glitinide, or insulin, hypoglycemia may occur.
	11.3 Duration of action determines when hypoglycemia is likely to occur and how long it lasts.	Other medications (e.g., nonsteroidal anti-inflammatory drugs) potentiate hypoglycemia.
	11.4 Hypoglycemia from oral agents may need to be treated repeatedly. If taking acarbose or miglitol, hypoglycemia should not be treated with sucrose-containing products. Use milk or glucose tablets instead.	Ask, "How do you treat low blood glucose?" Hypoglycemia occurs less often but is more difficult to treat than for patients on insulin because of the long duration of action of the sulfonylureas. In addition, hypoglycemia may persist beyond the standard duration of action of these drugs. Hypoglycemia may recur anytime while the patient is taking sulfonylureas.
	11.5 If your hypoglycemia does not respond to treatment, contact your health care team right away.	Glucagon is generally not an appropriate treatment for hypoglycemia by patients with type 2 diabetes.

CONTENT OUTLINE

CONCEPT	DETAIL	INSTRUCTOR'S NOTES
12. Using diabetes medicines	12.1 Because the medicines work differently, the choice of which pill is best for you is based on your blood glucose goals, your costs and coverage, and your levels before and after you start taking the pill. Some people take one type of pill, some take two types of pills, and others take pills plus insulin because the medicines work well together.	Ask, "Have you found ways to cut the costs of your medicines?" Provide information about lower cost options and sources.
	12.2 Blood glucose monitoring helps you to know if the medicines are working.	Ask, "Do you check your blood glucose levels? What does it tell you?" Review their schedule and results in relation to their medications' actions and timing.
	12.3 Never take anyone else's diabetes medicine (or any other kind) or give anyone yours.	
	12.4 You need to know: ■ the name of your pills ■ how many pills to take ■ when to take your pills ■ the shape and color of your pills ■ why you take it ■ side effects ■ which blood glucose readings are affected.	Ask, "Do you keep a list of your medications and dosages in your wallet or purse?" Remind patients to read the label when they get a new bottle from their pharmacy, to be sure the name, dose, and times it should be taken are correct. Show these points on sample bottles.
	12.5 Prices for prescription medicines vary, so you may want to shop around.	Have price information available from several pharmacies, or ask participants to bring this information to the next session.
13. Duration of action	13.1 Duration of action refers to the length of time the pill is effective.	Use Visual #2, Diabetes Pills.
	13.2 Duration affects the dose and how often the pills need to be taken. Almost all last 6–24 hours.	Exceptions are chlorpropamide (48 hours), acarbose, miglitol, repaglinide, and nateglinide.
14. When to take diabetes medicines	14.1 You may need to take your pill(s) only once per day or as many as three times per day.	Frequency depends on duration of action and how the body responds to medication.

CONTENT OUTLINE

CONCEPT	DETAIL	INSTRUCTOR'S NOTES
	14.2 These medicines work best when you take them routinely, not only when your blood glucose is high.	
	14.3 It's helpful to take them at about the same time each day.	This helps the pancreas to establish a more consistent pattern and helps you to remember the medication.
	14.4 Most diabetes medicines are taken at mealtime, usually at breakfast. Glucotrol (glipizide) will work best if taken 30 minutes before your meal. Glitinides work best if taken 10–30 minutes before your meal. Alpha-glucosidase inhibitors should be taken only at meal time, with the first bite of food. If insulin is used with sulfonylureas or biguanides, the insulin is often taken at bedtime.	Emphasize that the timing of a medication dose can influence the medication's effectiveness and/or its side effects.
15. Remembering to take the medication	15.1 If you forget to take your **daily** dose but remember later in the day, go ahead and take the pill.	Ask, "How often do you forget to take your medicine? How do you handle it? What strategies do you use to help you remember your medicines?"
	15.2 If you take one pill each day and forget one day, do **not** take two pills the next day.	If you have any questions, call your health care team.
	15.3 If you take pills two times a day and forget your morning pill, do **not** take both doses in the evening.	Ask, "What helps you remember to take your medicines when you are not at home at mealtime? Traveling?"
	15.4 Missed doses of acarbose, miglitol, nateglinide, or repaglinide should not be made up at the next meal.	
	15.5 The following are tips for remembering to take your medicine: ■ Take it at the same time each day. ■ Take it at the same time you take other pills or do a routine activity (e.g., brushing teeth). ■ Store pills in plain sight, close to where you will take them.	Ask, "How do you remember to take other medicines?" Coupling a new behavior with an already established behavior increases the likelihood the new behavior will be done. Example: If it's hard to remember a pill at lunchtime at

CONTENT OUTLINE

CONCEPT	DETAIL	INSTRUCTOR'S NOTES
	■ Focus attention on times that are hard for you.	work, put a note in your lunch or set an alarm on your watch or phone.
	■ Make it easy to remember by giving yourself cues. ■ Devices are manufactured that can be set to buzz as a reminder of your pill times, or use your phone.	Load a compartmentalized container, either purchased or homemade, with pills for the day or week. Have one available to show.
16. Care and storage	16.1 Store oral medications at room temperature. Unopened boxes of incretin mimetics need to be stored in the refrigerator.	
	16.2 Do not use medicines after the expiration date.	Show a bottle and point out the expiration date.
	16.3 If pills are discolored, discard them.	
	16.4 Always keep your medicines with you when traveling (not in your suitcase). Take enough for the trip, plus extras.	A prescription and/or provider's letter is helpful for overseas travel.
17. Meal planning and exercise	17.1 Food raises blood glucose. The more you eat, the more insulin your body needs to lower blood glucose. Even with the medicines, your body can only make so much insulin.	It is a common misunderstanding that a meal plan is no longer needed once medicines are added. Medications may not be needed after weight loss.
	17.2 Your blood glucose will stay lower and more even if you divide your food into several small meals and snacks throughout the day. Too much food at once can raise blood glucose too high.	Ask, "Have you made any changes in your food choices or schedule since you started taking diabetes medicines?"
	17.3 Exercise helps burn calories, improves sense of well-being, increases insulin sensitivity, and lowers blood glucose levels.	Exercise snacks are usually only recommended for patients taking secretagogues and insulin.
18. Other facts	18.1 Oral agents should not be taken by women who are pregnant, lactating, or planning to become pregnant. They may be harmful to the baby.	Remind women to seek preconception counseling and work with their provider to create a new treatment plan prior to pregnancy.

CONTENT OUTLINE

CONCEPT	DETAIL	INSTRUCTOR'S NOTES
	18.2 If you are ill and unable to eat, you still need to take your diabetes pills.	Blood glucose may actually increase because of the infectious process.
19. Research	19.1 New medications are being tested and may be on the market in the near future.	Insulin-like agents are areas of great research interest.
	19.2 Ask your provider if any new treatments are available that would help you.	
	19.3 Choose one thing you will do this week to care for your diabetes.	Close the session by asking participants to identify one action step they will take this week.

SKILLS CHECKLIST

None.

EVALUATION PLAN

Knowledge will be evaluated by achievement of learning objectives and by responses to questions during the session. The ability to apply knowledge will be evaluated by appropriate use of oral medications and through program outcome measures.

DOCUMENTATION PLAN

Record class attendance and achieved objectives as appropriate using the Diabetes Self-Management Record, the Participant Follow-up Record, or another form.

SUGGESTED READINGS

Ahren B: DPP-4 inhibitors. *Insulin* 4:15–31, 2009

American Diabetes Association: Resource guide. Medications for type 2. *Diabetes Forecast* 62(1):37–40, 2009

Amori RE, Lau K. Pittas A: Efficacy and safety of incretin therapy in type 2 diabetes: systematic review and meta-analysis. *JAMA* 298:194–206, 2007

Blonde L, Klein EJ, Han J, Zhang B, Mac SM, Poon TH, Taylor KL, Trautmann ME, Kim DD,

Kendall DM: Interim analysis of the effects of exenatide treatment on A1C, weight and cardiovascular risk factors over 82 weeks in 314 overweight patients with type 2 diabetes. *Diabetes, Obesity, and Metabolism* 8(4):436–447, 2006

Blonde L, Leahy J, Haines ST, Siminerio L: A multidisciplinary approach in addressing novel mechanisms in the management of type 2 diabetes. *The Diabetes Educator* 33(Suppl 5): 100S–116S, 2007

SUGGESTED READINGS *continued*

Bloomgarden ZT: Gut hormones and related concepts. *Diabetes Care* 29:2319–2324, 2006

Cavaghan MK: Exenatide use in real life. *Practical Diabetology* 26(4):22–27, 2007

Edwards KL, Alvarez C, Irons BK, Fields J: Third-line agent selection for patients with type 2 diabetes mellitus uncontrolled with sulfonylureas and metformin. *Pharmacotherapy* 28:506–521, 2008

Fowler MJ: Oral agents for glycemic management. *Clinical Diabetes* 25:131–134, 2007

Gangji AS, Curkierman T, Gerstein HC, Goldsmith CH, Clase CM: A systematic review and meta-analysis of hypoglycemia and cardiovascular events: a comparison of glycuride with other secretagogues and with insulins. *Diabetes Care* 30:389–394, 2007

Goldstein BJ, Feinglos MN, Lungeford JK, et al.: Effect of initial combination therapy with sitagliptin, a depeptidyl peptidase-4 inhibitor, and metformin on glycemic control in patients with type 2 diabetes. *Diabetes Care 30:1979–1987, 2007*

Grant R, Adams AS, Trinacty CM, Zhang F, et al.: Relationship between patient medication adherence and subsequent clinical inertia in type 2 diabetes glycemic management. *Diabetes Care* 30:807–812, 2007

Grant RW, Devita NG, Singer De, Meigs JB: Polypharmacy and medication adherence in patients with type 2 diabetes. *Diabetes Care* 26:1408–1412, 2003

Hayes RP, Bowman L, Monahan PO, Marrero DG, McHorney CA: Understanding diabetes medications from the perspective of patients with type 2 diabetes. *The Diabetes Educator* 32:404—414, 2006

Hood R, Valentine V, Mac S, Polonsky WH: Uses of exenatide in patients with type 2 diabetes. *Diabetes Spectrum* 19:181–186, 2006

Koski RR: Practical review of oral antihyperglycemic agents for type 2 diabetes mellitus. *The Diabetes Educator* 32:869–876, 2006

Kruger D: Symlin and byetta. *Practical Diabetology* 25(1):49–52, 2006

Lin EHB, Ciechanowski P: Working with patients to enhance medication adherence. *Clinical Diabetes* 26:17–19, 2008

McKennon SA, Campbell RK: The physiology of incretin hormones and the basis for DPP-4 inhibitors. *The Diabetes Educator* 33:55–66, 2007

Neumiller JJ, Odegard PS, White JR, Jr., Setter SM, Campbell RK: Focus on DPP-4 inhibitors for the treatment of type 2 diabetes and emerging therapies. *The Diabetes Educator* 34:183–197, 2008

Nichols GA, Gomez-Caminero A: Weight changes following the initiation of new anti-hyperglycaemic therapies. *Diabetes Obes Meta* 9:96–102, 2007

Odegard PS, Capaoccia K: Medication taking and diabetes. *The Diabetes Educator* 33:1014–1029, 2007

Odegard PS, Setter SM, Iltz JL: Update in the pharmacologic treatment of diabetes mellitus. *The Diabetes Educator* 32:693–712, 2006

Riddle MC, Drucker DJ: Emerging therapies mimicking the effects of amylin and glucagon-like peptide 1. *Diabetes Care* 29:435–449, 2006

Roberts SS: Symlin and byetta. *Diabetes Forecast* 60(7):23–25, 2007

Ruder K: Take charge of your meds. *Diabetes Forecast* 59(5):52–54, 2006

Tsend C-W, Tierney EF, Gerzoff RB, Dudley RA, et al.: Race/ethnicity and economic differences in cost-related medication underuse among insured adults with diabetes. *Diabetes Care* 21:261–266, 2008

White JR: Changing paradigms in the pharmacological management of type 2 diabetes. *Diabetes Spectrum* 22:73–92, 2009

White JR: Dipeptidyl peptidase-IV inhibitors: pharmacological profile and clinical use. *Clinical Diabetes* 26:53–57, 2008

Natural History of Type 2 Diabetes

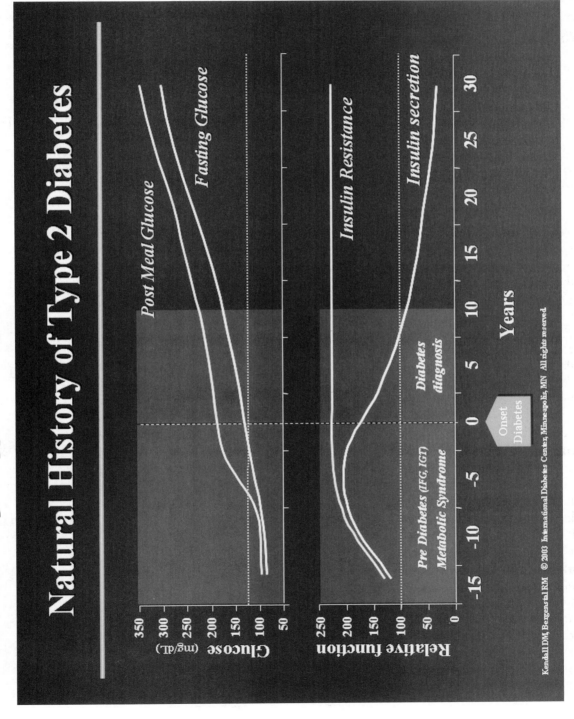

Natural History of Type 2 Diabetes

➲ Diabetes Pills

Class	Name	Description	Dosage (mg)	Number of Times per Day
Sulfonylureas	Micronase (glyburide)	Round, scored tablet: White Dark pink Blue	1.25 2.5 5.0	1–2
	Diabeta (glyburide)	Oval, scored tablet: White Pink Green	1.25 2.5 5.0	1–2
	Glynase PresTab (glyburide)	Oval, scored tablet: White Blue Yellow	1.5 3.0 6.0	1–2
	*Glucotrol (glipizide)	White, scored, diamond-shaped tablet	5.0 10.0	1–2
	Glucotrol XL (glipizide XL)	White, round tablet	5.0 10.0	1
	Amaryl (glimepiride)	Oval, scored tablet: White Pink Green	1.0 2.0 4.0	1
Biguanides	Glucophage (metformin)	White, round tablet White, round tablet White, oval tablet	500 800 1000	2–3
	GlucophageXL (metformin)	White capsule		1
Insulin sensitizers	Avandia (rosiglitazone)	Five-sided tablet: Pink Orange Red/brown	200 400 800	1–2

*Take 30 minutes before meals.

DIABETES PILLS *continued*

Class	Name	Description	Dosage (mg)	Number of Times per Day
	Actos (pioglitazone)	Tablets: White, round, convex White, round, flat White, round, flat	15 30 45	1
Glitinides Meglitinide	***Prandin (repaglinide)	Unscored, round tablet: White Yellow Pink	0.5 1.0 2.0	3–4
Phenylalanine derivative	***Starlix (nateglinide)	Pink, round tablet Yellow, oval tablet	60 120	3
Alpha-glucosidase inhibitors	**Precose (acarbose)	White, round, scored tablet	50	3
	**Glyset (miglitol)	White, round tablet	25 50 100	3
DPP-4 inhibitor	Januvia (sitagliptin)	Round tablet: Pink Light beige Beige	25 mg 50 mg 100 mg	1
	Onglyza (saxagliptin)	Round tablet: Yellow Pink	2.5 mg 5.0 mg	1
Incretin mimetic Exenatide	Byetta	Pre-filled injection pen device	5 or 10 mcg	2

**Take with the first bite of meal.   ***Take 1–30 minutes before meal.

DIABETES PILLS *continued*

Class	Name	Description	Dosage (mg)	Number of Times per Day

Sulfonylurea**** and biguanide combination	Glucovance (glyburide/ metformin)	Capsule shape:
		  Pale yellow
		  Pale orange
		  Yellow
			
			1.25/250
			2.5/500
			5/500
				1–2

	****Metaglip (glipizide/ metformin)	Oval tablet:
		  Pink
		  White
		  Pink
			
			2.5–250
			2.5–500
			5.0–500
				2

Insulin sensitizer and biguanide combination	***Avandamet (rosiglitizone/ metformin)	Oval tablet:
		  Pale yellow
		  Pale pink
		  Orange
		  Yellow
		  Pink
			
			1.0/500
			2.0/500
			4.0/500
			2.0/1000
			4.0/1000
				2

DPP-4 inhibitor and biguanide combination	Janumet (sitagliptin/ metformin)	Capsule shape:
		  Light pink
		  Red
			
			50/500
			50/1,000
				2

**Take with the first bite of meal.   ***Take 1–30 minutes before meal.   ****Take with meals.

#9	All About Insulin

▶ ▶ ▶ ▶ ▶

STATEMENT OF PURPOSE

This session is intended to provide information about insulin and other therapies, how they work, and how they are administered; intensive insulin therapy is also discussed.

PREREQUISITES

It is recommended that only participants starting insulin, other therapies, or currently using one of these therapies attend this session. Participants who take oral diabetes medications and insulin need information about both types of therapy.

OBJECTIVES

At the end of this session, participants will be able to:
1. define insulin, including where it comes from and what it does;
2. state that different kinds of insulin preparations differ as to source, strength, and duration of action;
3. state how to store insulin properly;
4. state how to tell if a particular bottle of insulin is useable;
5. list the equipment needed to administer insulin;
6. state the importance of accurate measurement of insulin dosage;
7. state the importance of accurate timing of insulin dosage;
8. identify personal concerns about insulin therapy;
9. define other therapies used with insulin;
10. list the steps for accurately administering these therapies;
11. state how to treat hypoglycemia;
12. state the purpose of intensive insulin therapy;
13. identify three circumstances that are indications for intensive insulin therapy;
14. describe treatment options available to achieve goals of intensive insulin therapy;
15. identify personal advantages of intensive insulin therapy;
16. identify personal disadvantages of intensive insulin therapy;
17. describe resources needed to implement an intensive insulin program.

CONTENT

Using medications safely and for maximum therapeutic effectiveness.

MATERIALS NEEDED

VISUALS PROVIDED	ADDITIONAL
1. Normal Blood Glucose and Insulin Levels	■ Chalkboard and chalk/Board and markers
2. Insulin Action Times	■ Samples of all types of insulin syringes and pens
3. Insulin Programs	■ Sample bottles of all types of insulin
4. Timing of Regular Insulin and Meals	■ Sample boxes of insulins
5. Injection Sites	■ Injection pen devices
	■ Price information from local pharmacies
Handouts (one per participant)	■ Samples of insulin pens and injection devices
1. Comparison of Insulins	■ Information about local syringe disposal policies
2. Insulin Programs	■ MedicAlert or other diabetes identification
3. Intensive Insulin Program	information
4. Giving an Insulin Injection	■ Insulin pump and tubing
5. Treatment of Low Blood Glucose	■ Injection aid devices
6. How to Use Glucagon	■ Glucagon kit
	■ Samples of glucose products

METHOD OF PRESENTATION

Start by introducing yourself and telling what you do. Ask participants to introduce themselves. Explain that the purpose of this session is to provide information about insulin and how it works and to describe different types of insulin programs. Actual injection technique is usually taught individually; however, a demonstration of the procedure may be useful as a review, at the appropriate point in the session.

Some participants attending this session will be initiating insulin for the first time. The first section of the outline provides information specifically for these participants and should be provided only if needed. It is essential to begin by addressing fears and concerns about insulin by asking participants to describe these fears. It is also important to reassure participants with type 2 diabetes that initiating insulin does not mean that they have failed. Participants who have experiences with insulin may be helpful to them as well. A discussion of the decision-making process they used may be a useful way to begin. It may also help alleviate fear by starting the class by having participants insert an insulin needle.

This outline provides information from initiating insulin through implementing intensive programs. Provide only the content that is appropriate for the audience. Begin by asking how they did with their short-term goal and what they learned from it. Present material in a question/discussion format, using the first question as a starting point. Provide appropriate content outlined below in response. Ask if there are additional questions, and respond, repeating the process for the entire session.

Use the questions in the Instructor's Notes section to generate discussion if no questions are forthcoming after a period of silence. Keeping track of the content discussed in each session, using the Diabetes Self-Management Record, the Participant Follow-up Record, or another form, helps you to evaluate if needed content has been discussed.

CONTENT OUTLINE

CONCEPT	DETAIL	INSTRUCTOR'S NOTES
1. Initiating insulin therapy	1.1 Beginning insulin therapy is often difficult. Most people have questions, fears, and concerns.	Ask, "What are your thoughts about insulin therapy? What questions or concerns do you have?" If some group members take insulin already, ask that they share their initial thoughts and current experiences. It is particularly important that participants hear from those whose experiences are not all positive to get a balanced perspective on what to expect. Keep in mind that facts may not be as effective for overcoming fears as hearing from those who have had experience with insulin.
	1.2 As with every other type of treatment, there are advantages and disadvantages. What disadvantages are there for you? What advantages are there for you? What have you heard about insulin?	Encourage participants to voice opinions without offering positive or negative comments. Write these on the board. What are advantages for some will be disadvantages for others. Common disadvantages are: fear of needles and pain with injections; weight gain; loss of flexibility in lifestyle and independence; fear of hypoglycemia; view insulin as a personal failure or sign of worsening diabetes; fear that insulin causes complications; and fear that they will lose support of family and friends. Common advantages are: insulin works; you feel better and more energetic; more flexibility in lifestyle; "not as bad as I thought"; can be more involved with care; prevent complications; better quality of life. Once the list is complete, ask participants who take insulin to address some of the concerns or provide information as appropriate. Providing

CONTENT OUTLINE

CONCEPT	DETAIL	INSTRUCTOR'S NOTES
		emotional support through active listening is likely to be more useful than information at this point.
	1.3 Weighing the advantages and disadvantages is something that only you can do.	Ask, "What do you think is the biggest barrier for you? What supports do you have?" Remind participants with type 2 diabetes that while their health care team, family, and friends can help, the final decision is up to them.
	1.4 The purpose of this session is to give you the information and support you need to begin insulin therapy.	Ask, "What information or other help would be the most useful for you as you begin insulin therapy?"
2. What is insulin?	2.1 Insulin is a hormone, a protein substance.	Ask, "What questions or concerns do you have about insulin? What insulin(s) do you take?" Write these on the board so you that you can discuss each of them more fully later.
	2.2 Insulin is made in the beta cells of the pancreas.	Insulin is produced in the beta cells of the pancreatic islets (islets are 1% of the pancreas).
	2.3 Insulin attaches to the outside of most body cells and allows glucose to enter those cells. This lowers blood glucose (glucose leaves the blood).	Ask, "How does insulin work? How does insulin affect blood glucose?"
	2.4 In diabetes, there is not enough insulin action. Insulin injections may be needed to lower blood glucose.	Review differences in types of diabetes related to insulin production.
	2.5 At this time, insulin cannot be taken as a pill because it would be destroyed by digestive enzymes before it could act to lower blood glucose levels.	Insulin is a protein and would be digested like other proteins.
	2.6 Insulin is a natural and very effective treatment for diabetes. People with type 1 diabetes take insulin from the	Early use of insulin therapy is now recommended for type 2 diabetes and does not represent

CONTENT OUTLINE

CONCEPT	DETAIL	INSTRUCTOR'S NOTES
	onset of their diabetes. For people with type 2 diabetes, it is one of the steps in the progression of therapy.	a failure on the part of patients. Point out that they did not fail, but that the medications they were taking failed them.
3. Types of insulin	3.1 Insulin is made by three companies in the United States and is available worldwide under various brand names.	Show examples of each. Patients may notice some blood glucose variability with different brands.
	3.2 All insulins are classified by general types: rapid-acting, short-acting, intermediate-acting, and long-acting.	Distribute Handout #1, Comparison of Insulins. Show examples of different insulins. Use the list of insulin taken by participants and identify the classification for each.
	3.3 Rapid-acting: insulin lispro (Humalog) and insulin aspart (Novolog) and glulisine (Apidra).	These insulin analogs are created when two amino acids on the human insulin chain are switched or altered.
	3.4 Short-acting: regular.	
	3.5 Intermediate-acting: NPH.	
	3.6 Long-acting: glargine (Lantus) and detemir (Levemir).	Other insulins are currently in development and will be available in the near future.
	3.7 Combinations of NPH and regular are available in a 70:30 ratio, NPL and lispro in a 75:25 ratio, aspart protamine and aspart in a 70:30 ratio, and NPL and lispro in a 50:50 ratio.	Protomine lispro (NPL) is an analog intermediate-acting insulin. Clarify that the smaller number is the rapid- or short-acting insulin.
	3.8 When purchasing insulin, be sure to buy the brand, type, and strength that has been prescribed for you.	
4. Insulin programs	4.1 In someone without diabetes, normal preprandial blood glucose is 70–110 mg/dl. (Preprandial means before eating.)	Use Visual #1, Normal Blood Glucose and Insulin Levels. Refer to Handout #2, Insulin Programs to discuss participants' insulin programs.

CONTENT OUTLINE

CONCEPT	DETAIL	INSTRUCTOR'S NOTES
	4.2 In someone without diabetes, a small amount of insulin is continuously released by the pancreas to maintain the blood glucose in this range. This is the basal level of insulin.	The word "fasting" is often used as a synonym for preprandial. Fasting means no eating for 8 or more hours, so it usually refers to the first morning blood test.
	4.3 In someone without diabetes, normal blood glucose two hours postprandial is less than 140 mg/dl. (Postprandial means after eating, usually 2 hours after the start of a meal.	Timing for postprandial glucose levels is based on when the meal begins.
	4.4 An additional burst of insulin is released by the pancreas in response to the rising blood glucose levels after eating, causing the blood glucose to go back to normal. This is called a bolus of insulin.	Ask, "Do you check your blood glucose after meals? What have you found?"
	4.5 Insulin programs attempt to imitate the pancreas by providing insulin in a basal and bolus pattern through insulin shots.	Both bolus and basal insulin action is needed, through a combination of insulins, oral agents, and/or pancreatic function (for people with type 2 diabetes).
5. Choosing an insulin program	5.1 Various types of insulin can be used alone or in combination to produce specific action effects. Some programs use only one type of insulin.	Point out that there is no best insulin program, just the one that will work best to help you reach your targets and fits with your life.
	5.2 Each type of insulin has its own characteristic onset, peak, and length of action and can be combined to mimic the body's normal pattern.	Refer to Handout #1, Comparisons of Insulins, and use the list on the board to discuss participants' insulins, including onset, peak, and action time. Define *onset*.
	5.3 Onset, peak, and length of action of a particular insulin vary depending on injection technique, physical activity, and the way the body uses insulin.	

CONTENT OUTLINE

CONCEPT	DETAIL	INSTRUCTOR'S NOTES
	5.4 This information helps you balance your insulin with your food and physical activity. It also helps you know when an insulin reaction is likely to occur.	Ask, "Based on the insulins you take, when are you most likely to have a reaction?"
	5.5 The basal insulin dose can be provided by: ■ intermediate-acting insulin (NPH/NPL) ■ long-acting insulin (glargine/ detemir), often used because of its long duration and relatively low peak.	Use Visual #2, Insulin Action Times, to show basal insulins. This mimics the constant output of insulin in people without diabetes. Rapid- or short-acting insulins are used for the basal insulin in a pump. Multiple basal rates can be given.
	5.6 The onset of action of the intermediate- and long-acting insulins is gradual and their effects last longer.	Point out which insulins have the greatest effect on blood glucose levels. Use examples from the participants' insulin programs.
	5.7 Rapid- or short-acting insulins are always used for bolus doses. Taking the bolus dose before eating allows the insulin to get into the bloodstream and begin to work before glucose levels rise.	Use Visual #2 to illustrate. The bolus dose can be given via an insulin pump or by injection. Insulin pens and other devices make it more convenient to give bolus doses.
	5.8 The rapid-acting and short-acting insulins begin to act very quickly and last a short time. They are usually given to prevent the rise in blood glucose after meals.	Define bolus dose. Use Visual #2 to illustrate. Discuss onset, peak, and length of action for each type of insulin participants are taking, and the need for basal and bolus medicines.
	5.9 The intensity of your insulin program refers to the number of injections and the number and type of adjustments you make.	Using a carbohydrate:insulin ratio and adjusting insulin based on blood glucose levels using a correction factor are often part of intensive insulin programs. Ask, "Have you had experience with carb:insulin ratios? How did it work for you?"
	5.10 The intensity of your program is based on your personal glucose	Stress the importance of their role in decision making about

CONTENT OUTLINE

CONCEPT	DETAIL	INSTRUCTOR'S NOTES
	targets and other goals, how often you are willing and able to inject and monitor, the amount of flexibility you want and need, cost, and how hard you are willing and able to work to manage your diabetes.	the type of insulin program they choose. Ask, "What are advantages of a more intensive insulin program for you?" Examples of advantages include greater flexibility in scheduling and food, more choices, more even blood glucose levels, more energy, improved well-being, and decreased risk for complications. Examples of disadvantages include: weight gain, increased risk for hypoglycemia, cost, time, and effort. Ask, "How will you handle taking injections in various situations (work, restaurant, traveling, with family, etc.). How will you handle the questions or responses from others? What strategies will you use to address personal barriers?"
	5.11 Intensive programs are often used by people with type 1 diabetes, women with diabetes who are pregnant or planning to become pregnant, or people who want to feel more in charge of their diabetes.	If appropriate, emphasize the importance of preconception care.
	5.12 Intensive programs usually include three or more shots per day along with frequent monitoring. Insulin pumps may also be used. Meal planning is often based on carbohydrate counting and insulin and carbohydrate ratios.	Clarify the difference between intensive insulin programs and optimizing control throughout therapies. See Outline #19, *Carbohydrate Counting,* (p. 399). Distribute Handout #3, Intensive Insulin Program, as appropriate.
6. Other therapies	6.1 Amylin is a hormone produced by the beta cells of the pancreas that is secreted along with insulin.	Amylin production is diminished among people with diabetes.
	6.2 Amylin helps to regulate postprandial blood glucose levels by slowing gastric emptying, suppressing post-meal glucagon secretion, and increasing satiety and reducing food intake.	Ask, "What have been your experiences with pramlintide?"

CONTENT OUTLINE

CONCEPT	DETAIL	INSTRUCTOR'S NOTES
	6.3 Synthetic amylin, pramlintide (Symlin) is an injectable medication that can be taken by people who inject insulin and who have either type 1 or type 2 diabetes.	Because pramlintide is a protein, it must be taken by injection.
	6.4 Pramlintide is injected before each meal that has at least 30 grams of carbohydrate or 250 calories.	If you forget to take your pramlintide, skip that dose and take your usual dose at your next meal. Do not take after your meal.
	6.5 Pramlintide comes in either a pre-filled pen or vial. Inject pramlintide in either your thigh or abdomen. Storage guidelines are the same as insulin.	Show samples if available. Unopened vials or cartridges are stored in the refrigerator. Open vials can be stored at room temperature for 30 days.
	6.6 Side effects include: nausea, hypoglycemia, and weight loss. The dose is titrated slowly to minimize side effects. Your insulin dose will also be reduced to prevent hypoglycemia.	When starting pramlintide, it is recommended that the mealtime insulin dose be cut in half.
7. Mixing insulins	7.1 Most commonly used mixtures are rapid-acting or short-acting plus NPH; these can be given in one syringe.	See insulin package insert for specific product guidelines regarding mixing insulins.
	7.2 Draw up the rapid- or short-acting insulin first.	If intermediate- or long-acting insulin is drawn up first, traces of the retarding agent on the needle may contaminate the short-acting insulin and slow down its action time.
	7.3 Lispro, aspart, and glulisine insulins are stable when mixed with NPH. These should be taken immediately after mixing. Regular insulin is stable when mixed with NPH.	Ask, "What have your experiences been with taking two types of insulin?"
	7.4 The diluent used in glargine and detemir has a lower pH and cannot be mixed in the same syringe with other insulins.	Some users note burning with injection. The absorption of these insulins is not affected by the injection site.

CONTENT OUTLINE

CONCEPT	DETAIL	INSTRUCTOR'S NOTES
	7.5 If it is necessary to have someone predraw mixed doses for later administration, combinations of NPH and regular insulins are generally recommended.	Studies suggest that predrawn NPH and regular insulins can be safely stored in syringes for 30 days. Premixed insulins or insulin pens may be helpful in these situations.
	7.6 Store these in the refrigerator; allow the insulin to come to room temperature before injecting.	
	7.7 Store predrawn syringes for at least 24 hours before use to allow them to stabilize.	Always have an extra day's worth of syringes ready, so that you don't have to use a freshly drawn syringe, which will have a different action time.
	7.8 Store syringes flat or upwards. Roll gently between palms before use to remix the solution.	Storing with the needles downward can cause them to clog.
	7.9 Various proportions of NPH and regular insulins can be mixed by a pharmacist. These are stable for 3 months when refrigerated and for 1 month at room temperature.	These are in addition to commercially prepared premixed insulins.
8. Source of insulin	8.1 You can buy synthetic human and analog insulins.	Show examples of different types of insulin. Use the vials during the discussion in sections 8–10. Point out where this information is located and what they need to check each time they buy insulin.
	8.2 Insulin is made in a laboratory. This type is called "human insulin," but it is not actually insulin from humans.	Human insulins are made using recombinant DNA technology, where bacteria are used to make parts of the human insulin molecule, which are then joined together. NPH and regular are human insulins.
	8.3 Insulin analogs are also made in a laboratory, but the sequence of the molecules is changed to tailor the timing of their onset, peak, and duration.	All rapid and long-acting insulins are insulin analogs.

CONTENT OUTLINE

CONCEPT	DETAIL	INSTRUCTOR'S NOTES
9. Strength of insulin	9.1 U-100 is the strength of insulin most commonly available. U-500 insulin is also available.	Show an example of the U-100 insulin bottle. U-500 insulin reaches peak blood levels more slowly because of its greater concentration. Insulin can be diluted to U-100 by a pharmacist. The syringe needs to match the strength of the insulin.
	9.2 U-100 means 100 units of insulin per cc (cubic centimeter).	Some countries still have other insulin strengths available. Caution participants who travel abroad to always check the strength of insulin purchased outside the U.S., and to be sure to use a syringe that matches the strength.
10. Purity of insulin	10.1 All commercial preparations of insulin have small amounts of additives.	Show examples of various insulins.
	10.2 These additives help prevent the growth of bacteria and keep the pH balanced. Intermediate and long-acting insulins may have additives to prolong their action.	Because insulin is a naturally occurring hormone, most insulin allergies are actually allergies to these additives.
11. Storing insulin	11.1 The insulin bottle in use can be kept at room temperature. Keep extra bottles in the refrigerator.	Ask, "How do you store your insulin at home? Away from home? Have you ever had insulin 'go bad' because it got too hot or cold?"
	11.2 Insulin vials generally remain stable at room temperature for 28–30 days after opening. Storage guidelines vary for cartridges and prefilled pens and range from 10 to 28 days.	Refrigerated, unopened vials can be used until the expiration date.
	11.3 Insulin can lose its potency at greater than 86°F (e.g., in a steamy bathroom) and at freezing temperatures. Do not use insulin that has been exposed to temperature extremes.	Do not store insulin in direct sunlight (e.g., a window sill). If insulin freezes, do not use it. Once frozen, it has zero potency.

CONTENT OUTLINE

CONCEPT	DETAIL	INSTRUCTOR'S NOTES
	11.4 Taking insulin at room temperature is more comfortable than taking chilled insulin and may cause fewer skin irritations.	
	11.5 You do not need to refrigerate insulin when traveling unless expecting temperatures over 86°F or below freezing; then pack insulin in an insulated container.	Caution participants about leaving insulin in a hot or very cold car. They can pack insulin in a thermos or plastic foam container to keep cool. Do not store on ice.
	11.6 When traveling in airplanes, trains, or buses, pack insulin and syringes in a carry-on bag. Do **not** put in checked luggage.	Luggage can be lost on public transportation, and luggage compartments on buses and planes are often very cold.
12. Usability of insulin	12.1 Check the expiration date on the box.	Show the date on the box.
	12.2 Usability is not guaranteed by the manufacturer after that date.	
	12.3 Plan so that the amount you buy will be used up by the expiration date.	Sometimes, insulin on sale is short-dated.
	12.4 Calculate dosages from one bottle. The number of days a bottle of a particular kind of U-100 insulin will last is calculated by determining the total number of units of that type used in a day and dividing that number into 1000 (the number of units in a bottle of U-100).	Remember that some insulin may be lost while drawing it up. Use a participant's dosage to illustrate how to do this on the board.
	12.5 Examine insulin for change in color or for "stringiness"; do not use the insulin if it doesn't mix or if color is abnormal.	Define "stringy," or show an example. NPH insulin should be cloudy and all others clear. Ask, "Have you ever noticed stringiness or discoloration in your insulin? What did you do?"
	12.6 If you use a mail-order pharmacy service, make sure that the insulin is delivered in an appropriate	If concerned, contact the company for a replacement.

CONTENT OUTLINE

CONCEPT	DETAIL	INSTRUCTOR'S NOTES
	container to prevent over-heating and freezing.	
13. Syringes and needles	13.1 Different sizes of syringes available are: ■ 1/3 cc (30 units) ■ 1/2 cc (50 units) ■ 1 cc (100 units) ■ 2 cc (200 units).	Mention that several companies make syringes. Show examples of different syringes. Use U-100 syringes with U-100 insulin.
	13.2 Consider insulin dose, ease of reading scale, accuracy, and convenience when deciding which kind to use.	Ask, "What syringes do you use? What are your experiences with them?"
	13.3 Very fine and short needles may be less painful to use. The higher the gauge, the finer the needle.	Very short needles may not be appropriate for very obese patients.
	13.4 Dispose of needles and syringes safely. A plastic detergent bottle or metal container with a screw top can be used for collecting and then capped before disposal. Dispose with the regular trash—do not recycle. Label the container as containing used syringes. Do not recap, bend, or break off the needle of a used syringe. This increases the risk for sticking yourself.	Provide information from the local health department about syringe disposal regulations. Disposal guidelines can vary. If none, use the procedures outlined in 13.4. Commercial disposal boxes are available that can be returned when full.
	13.5 Some people prefer to reuse syringes. Put the cap back on, being careful not to touch the needle. Move the plunger up and down after each use; this helps to prevent needle clogs. Store at room temperature. Needles get dull with re-use.	Wiping the needle with alcohol between uses is not needed. Alcohol removes the silicone and makes the injection more painful. Reusing syringes may lead to infections for some people.
	13.6 Various injection devices can be purchased, including injection ports, spring loaded devices in which a syringe is loaded, cartridge pen-type injectors, and jet-injector devices.	These may be helpful for some patients, particularly those with an aversion to needles or on intensive programs. Show examples of these products.

CONTENT OUTLINE

CONCEPT	DETAIL	INSTRUCTOR'S NOTES
	13.7 Insulin pens are preferred by many people with diabetes. A variety of insulins are available in pen devices, and insurance coverage is improving.	Stress the need for an "air shot" prior to injecting and holding the device in place for 5 seconds after injecting.
	13.8 Devices are also available to make the syringe easier to read and for those with visual impairments.	Show samples of their devices.
14. Cost of equipment	14.1 Cost of insulin and syringes varies from store to store. Shop around for the lowest prices.	Distribute a list of price information from different pharmacies in your area, or ask participants to find out and bring this information to the next session. Ask, "Where have you found the price to be lowest?"
	14.2 Most insurance plans will cover costs with a prescription.	
15. Preparing insulin for injection	15.1 Clear insulin is already in solution and does not need to be mixed.	
	15.2 Cloudy insulins must be mixed by rolling or shaking gently.	Show precipitate in bottle of unmixed insulin.
	15.3 Here's how to draw up one type of insulin or dial your dose on your pen.	Distribute Handout #4, Giving an Insulin Injection. Demonstrate, if appropriate.
	15.4 Here's how to draw up two types of insulin.	
16. Injecting insulin	16.1 Here's how to inject insulin.	Ask, "What questions or concerns do you have about injecting?" Demonstrate proper injection technique. The angle used depends on body build and subcutaneous tissue. The deeper the injection, the faster the absorption, in general.
	16.2 Bleeding at the site may occur, caused by the needle going through a capillary.	Distinguish between bleeding at the site and blood in the syringe.
17. Injection sites and rotation	17.1 The abdomen is the recommended site for injection except for thin	Because absorption varies for some insulins, rotating to

CONTENT OUTLINE

CONCEPT	DETAIL	INSTRUCTOR'S NOTES
	people, young children, or patients who cannot pinch a half inch of fat.	various parts of the body may lead to erratic blood glucose levels. Ask, "Where do you inject your insulin? Where do you prefer to inject? Have you ever noticed change in your blood glucose based on the injection site?"
	17.2 Other parts of the body (arms, thighs, or buttocks) can be used. These areas are used because they have fewer nerves and a pad of fat underneath.	Use Visual #5, Injection Sites, to show abdominal and other sites. The abdomen may not be appropriate for thin adults, young children, or patients who cannot pinch up 1/2 inch of fat.
	17.3 Do not use other places—there is not enough fat, and also nerve endings and blood vessels are closer to the surface.	
	17.4 Insulin is absorbed most rapidly when injected into the abdomen, followed by the arms, thighs, and buttocks for some insulins.	Review manufacturer guidelines for site recommendations.
	17.5 Use sites 1 1/2 inches apart. Rotate sites within one area of your body only.	If the abdomen is not used, choose another area and rotate injections around that area.
	17.6 Rotating sites will help to prevent fat hypertrophy (a thickening at the site associated with poor insulin absorption), probably caused by overusing a site or injecting superficially.	Fewer nerve endings in hypertrophied areas mean decreased pain, but these areas should not be used for injection because insulin absorption is affected and may be unpredictable.
	17.7 Rotating sites will help to prevent fat atrophy (a depressed area with loss of subcutaneous fat).	This can be treated by injecting a pure insulin subcutaneously into the periphery of the area.
	17.8 Ask your nurse or physician to check your injection sites if you think you have fat atrophy or hypertrophy.	
	17.9 Localized skin reactions may develop.	True insulin allergies are very rare. This is usually due to

CONTENT OUTLINE

CONCEPT	DETAIL	INSTRUCTOR'S NOTES
		additives in the insulin, not to the insulin.
18. Tips for taking insulin	18.1 Giving yourself an injection can be frightening. It does get easier with time.	Ask, "What makes giving injections easier for you?" Suggest taking a deep breath before injection. If others in class give insulin already, they may offer reassurance. Approach children with a matter-of-fact and confident attitude. Parents may want to practice on themselves or other adults before injecting a child.
	18.2 Timing the insulin dose with time of eating leads to more even blood glucose levels. Glucose levels begin to rise about 10 minutes after you begin to eat.	
	18.3 Rapid-acting insulins may begin to work within 5 minutes.	
	18.4 If rapid-acting insulin is used for the bolus, give your shot 15 minutes or less before eating. If given too early, low blood glucose may result. You can also take these insulins after eating.	Rapid-acting insulins are given to children at or just after the meal.
	18.5 Regular insulin takes at least 15 minutes to get into the bloodstream. The standard recommendation is to take any injection containing regular insulin 30 minutes before eating. This helps prevent the rise in blood glucose that occurs after meals.	Ask, "When do you give your insulin in relation to meals?" Have you noticed changes in your blood glucose level based on timing?"
	18.6 If taken too early, low blood glucose may result. If taken at mealtime, food will cause the blood glucose to rise before the insulin can begin working. This may result in a postprandial blood glucose level that is above your target.	Use Visual #4, Timing of Regular Insulin and Meals, to stress the importance of timing. For more precise management, if your blood glucose is: 50–69 take a bolus dose with your meal 70–119 wait 15 minutes before eating

CONTENT OUTLINE

CONCEPT	DETAIL	INSTRUCTOR'S NOTES
		120–180 wait 30 minutes before eating >180 wait 45 minutes before eating
	18.7 Take your long-acting insulin at about the same time(s) each day. This helps you to remember and will help keep your blood glucose levels more even.	Ask, "Have you noticed changes in your blood glucose levels levels based on timing?"
	18.8 Keep all supplies together near where you will give your injection.	
	18.9 When you first start taking insulin, you will need to plan a few extra minutes into your schedule. Take your shot at the time you do other routine activities (e.g., checking blood glucose or brushing your teeth).	
	18.10 Use visual cues like notes or signs, or other cues such as an alarm clock.	
	18.11 Putting off your shot doesn't make it easier. Sometimes you just need to set a time and stick to it.	
	18.12 Blood glucose monitoring provides the information you need to see how well the insulin program is working and to make adjustments for meals and activity, as needed.	Ask, "What are reasons you check your blood glucose?" Stress the importance of this information for daily decision-making.
	18.13 Some people gain weight when starting insulin. Individuals on an intensive insulin program may gain up to 8–15 lb in the first year. Work with your dietitian to create a meal plan that will help you prevent this.	Fewer calories are lost as glucose in the urine and more calories are stored as fat because of the insulin action.
	18.14 Insulin therapy takes more time and effort on the part of both the person with diabetes and the health care team.	The need for family involvement and support may also increase. Ask, "What kind of support do you need to successfully use insulin?"

CONTENT OUTLINE

CONCEPT	DETAIL	INSTRUCTOR'S NOTES
	18.15 At first, you will need a great deal of contact with your health care team as your program is developed and fine-tuned. You need to find a team of people who are knowledgeable, easily accessible, and with whom you can develop a collaborative relationship.	It is likely that participants will be in frequent telephone contact with their health care team members. Stress the need to contact health care providers if blood glucose levels are not at target levels with the prescribed insulin dose.
	18.16 Insulin therapy gives you the opportunity and responsibility to make many daily decisions about your treatment plan. By learning how different insulins work and how exercise and specific foods affect your blood glucose, and by using information from blood monitoring and working closely with your health care team, you can develop an intensive insulin plan that works for you.	Point out that continuing education will help them keep abreast of new findings, treatments, and technology. Ask, "What decisions do you make about your insulin dose? Other self-management behaviors?"
19. Miscellaneous	19.1 Accurate measurement of insulin is critical. Bubbles in an insulin-filled syringe contain no insulin. They take up space and decrease your insulin dose.	Show how small a unit is by squirting 5 units on the table.
	19.2 For safety, wear identification that states you have diabetes.	Provide information about diabetes identification resources.
	19.3 In most states, a prescription is required to purchase insulin.	Clarify laws in your state. Even if available, most insurance companies require a prescription for reimbursement.
	19.4 You need a prescription when traveling overseas and a letter from your provider.	
	19.5 Take your insulin even if you are ill and cannot eat.	Illness or infection can raise blood glucose levels.
	19.6 Avoid: ■ rubbing the site ■ long, hot baths right after a shot.	These both alter absorption rates.

CONTENT OUTLINE

CONCEPT	DETAIL	INSTRUCTOR'S NOTES
20. Hypoglycemia	20.1 Hypoglycemia can occur when using insulin.	Ask, "What are signs and symptoms of hypoglycemia?" Refer to Outline #11, *Managing Blood Glucose* (p. 231).
	20.2 It is most likely to occur at peak insulin action times.	Help participants determine when they would be most likely to have a reaction.
	20.3 Hypoglycemia must be treated with food or drink containing sugar.	Ask, "How do you treat an insulin reaction?" Distribute and review Handout #5, Treatment of Low Blood Glucose, and Handout #6, How to Use Glucagon. Remind participants who are lactose-intolerant to avoid using milk as a treatment.
21. Research	21.1 Insulin administration and new products are areas of much research. Ask your health care team if there are trials of these products in your areas in which you can participate.	Inhaled, nasal, and oral insulins and insulin patches are all being studied.
	21.2 Choose one thing you will do this week to care for your diabetes.	Close the session by asking participants to identify one action step they will take this week.

SKILLS CHECKLIST

Each participant will be able to:

1. draw up or dial the correct amount of medication;

2. inject the medication; and

3. rotate injection sites.

EVALUATION PLAN

Knowledge will be evaluated by achievement of learning objectives and by responses to questions during the session; skills will be evaluated by observing demonstration of techniques. The ability to apply knowledge will be evaluated by the recognition of feelings about diabetes, the development of personal self-care goals, the development and implementation of a plan to achieve those goals, and through program outcome measures.

DOCUMENTATION PLAN

Record class attendance and achieved objectives as appropriate using the Diabetes Self-Management Record, the Participant Follow-Up Record, or another form.

SUGGESTED READINGS

American Diabetes Association: Resource Guide 2009. Insulin. *Diabetes Forecast* 62(1):41–48, 2009

American Diabetes Association: Resource Guide 2009. Insulin pumps. *Diabetes Forecast.* 62(1):49–52, 2009

American Diabetes Association: *Practical Insulin,* 2nd edition. Alexandria, VA: American Diabetes Association, 2004

American Diabetes Association: *Intensive Diabetes Management,* 4th Edition. Alexandria, VA: American Diabetes Association, 2009

American Diabetes Association: Position statement: insulin administration. *Diabetes Care* 27(Suppl 1):S107–S109, 2004

Bergenstal RM, Johnson M, Powers MA, Wynne A, et al.: Adjust to target in type 2 diabetes. *Diabetes Care* 31:1305–1310, 2008

Blevins T, Schwartz SL, Bode B, Aronoff S, et al.: A study assessing an injection port for administration of insulin. *Diabetes Spectrum* 21:197–202, 2008

Blonde L, Merilainen M, Karwe V, and Raskin P for the TITRATE Study Group: Patient-directed titration for achieving glycemic goals using one-daily basil insulin analogue: an assessment or two different fasting plasma glucose targets—the TITRATE study. *Diabetes, Obesity, and Metabolism* 11:623–631, 2009

Brown AW: Clinicians guide to diabetes gadgets and gizmos. *Clinical Diabetes* 26:66–72, 2008

Carver C: Insulin treatment and the problem of weight gain in type 2 diabetes. *The Diabetes Educator* 32:910–917, 2006

Clark W: The benefits of tight control. *Diabetes Self-Management* 27(3):29–35, 2006

D'Arrigo T: A matter of balance: insulin and weight gain. *Diabetes Forecast* 61(5):16, 2007

Edelman SV: Internsive therapy in type 2 diabetes. *Insulin* (Suppl B):S34–S40, 2007

Fowler MJ: Diabetes devices. *Clinical Diabetes* 26:130–133, 2008

Funnell MM, Kruger DF, Spencer M: Self-management support for insulin therapy in type 2 diabetes. *The Diabetes Educator* 30:274–280, 2004

Funnell MM, Kruger DF: Type 2 diabetes: treating to target. *The Nurse Practitioner* 29:11–25, 2004

Funnell MM: Insulin detemir: a new option for the treatment of diabetes. *Journal of the American Academy of Nurse Practitioners* 19:508–515, 2007

Funnell MM: Overcoming barriers to the initiation of insulin therapy. *Clinical Diabetes* 25:36–38, 2007

Funnell MM: Quality of life and insulin therapy. *Insulin* 3:31–36, 2008

Gavin JR, Peragallo-Dittko V: The why and how of early intervention with insulin analogs. *The Diabetes Educator* 33(Suppl 3):52S–75S, 2007

Gebel E: Embracing insulin. *Diabetes Forecast* 61(6):45–47, 2008

Hamilton D, Hendricks S, Walsh B, Wilhelm K: Benefits of pramlintide for insulin using patients. *Practical Diabetology* 26(4):6–13, 2007

Henske JA, Griffith ML, Fowler MJ: Initiating and titrating insulin in patients with type 2 diabetes. *Clinical Diabetes* 27:72–75, 2009

Holman RR, Thorne KI, Farmer AJ, Davies MJ, Keenan JF, Paul S, Levy JC: 4-T study group addition of biphasic, prandial, or basal insulin to oral therapy in type 2 diabetes. *New England Journal of Medicine* 257:1716–1730, 2007

Iltz JL, Odegard PS, Setter SM, Campbell RK: Update on the pharmacologic treatment of diabetes. *The Diabetes Educator* 33:215–253, 2007

Kruger D: Symlin and byetta. *Practical Diabetology* 25(1):49–52, 2006

SUGGESTED READINGS *continued*

Larkin ME, Capasso VA, Chen, C-L, Mahoney, et al.: Measuring psychological insulin resistance. *The Diabetes Educator* 34:511–518, 2008

LaSalle JR: New insulin analogs: insulin detemir and insulin glulisine. *Practical Diabetology* 25(3):34–43, 2006

Lebovitz HE: *Therapy for Diabetes Mellitus and Related Disorders,* 5th Edition. Alexandria, VA: American Diabetes Association, 2009

Lush CW, Darsow T, Zhang B, Lorenzi G, Frias JP: Pramlintide as an adjunct to basal insulin: effects on glycemic control and weight in patients with type 2 diabetes. *Insulin* 2:166–172, 2007

Marrero DG, Crean J, Zhang B, Kellmeyher T, et al.: Effect of adjunctive pramlintide treatment on treatment satisfaction in patients with type 1 diabetes. *Diabetes Care* 30:210–216, 2007

McCarren M: *Guide to Insulin and Type 2 Diabetes.* Alexandria, VA: American Diabetes Association, 2007

Peyrot M, Rubin RR, Lauritzen T, Skovlund SE, Snoek FJ, Matthews DR, Landgraf R, Kleinebreil, DAWN Advisory Panel: Resistance to insulin therapy among patients and providers: results of the cross-national Diabetes Attitudes, Wishes and Needs (DAWN) study. *Diabetes Care* 28:2673–2679, 2005

Reid TS: Insulin for type 2 diabetes mellitus: separating the myths from the facts. *Insulin* 2:182–189, 2007

Rizvi AA, Ligthelm RJ: The use of premixed insulin analogues in the treatment of patients with type 2 diabetes mellitus: advantages and limitations. *Insulin* 2:68–78, 2007

Roberts SS: Insulin and type 2. *Diabetes Forecast* 60(5):25–27, 2007

Roberts SS: Insulin shots: choosing the right spot. *Diabetes Forecast* 60(7):43–44, 2007

Roberts SS: Symlin and Byetta. *Diabetes Forecast* 60(7):23–25, 2007

Robertson C: Physiologic insulin replacement in type 2 diabetes. *The Diabetes Educator* 32:423–432, 2006

Rowler MJ: Insulin and incretins. *Clinical Diabetes* 26:35–39, 2008

Rubin RR, Peyrot M: Factors affecting use of insulin pens by patients with type 2 diabetes. *Diabetes Care* 31:430–431, 2008

Spake A: Symlin up close. *Diabetes Forecast* 61(3):50–51, 2008

Yki-Jarvinen H, Juurinen L, Alvarsson M, et al.: Initiate insulin by aggressive titration and education (INITIATE). *Diabetes Care* 30:1364–1369, 2007

⮞ Normal Blood Glucose and Insulin Levels

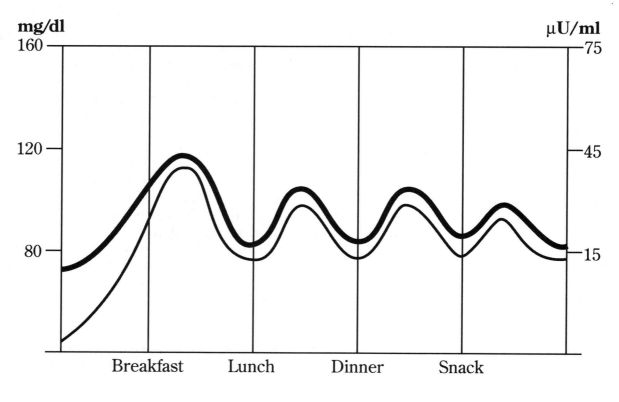

Breakfast	Lunch	Dinner	Snack	

━━━ Blood Glucose Level

─── Plasma Insulin Level

Insulin Action Times

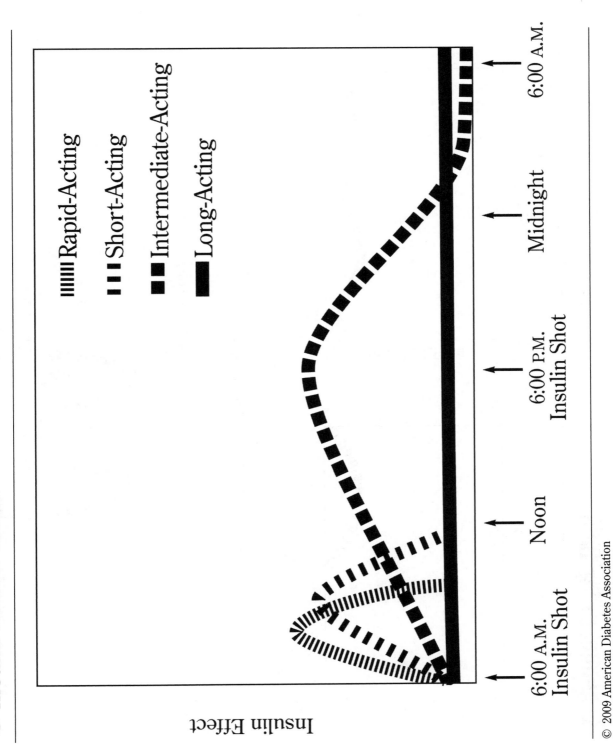

Insulin Programs

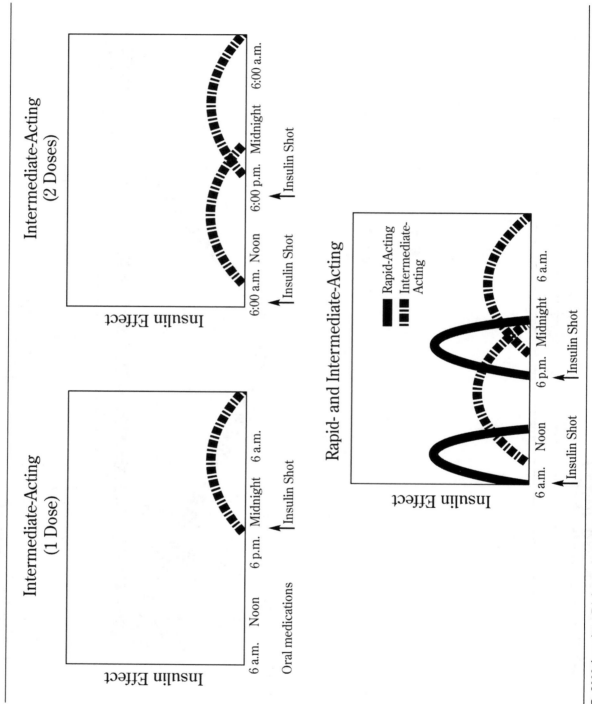

Intermediate-Acting
(1 Dose)

Intermediate-Acting
(2 Doses)

Rapid- and Intermediate-Acting

Insulin Effect

6 a.m.   Noon   6 p.m.   Midnight   6 a.m.

Oral medications   ↑ Insulin Shot

6:00 a.m.   Noon   6:00 p.m.   Midnight   6:00 a.m.

↑ Insulin Shot   ↑ Insulin Shot

■ Rapid-Acting
▦ Intermediate-Acting

6 a.m.   Noon   6 p.m.   Midnight   6 a.m.

↑ Insulin Shot   ↑ Insulin Shot

INSULIN PROGRAMS *continued*

➊ Insulin Programs

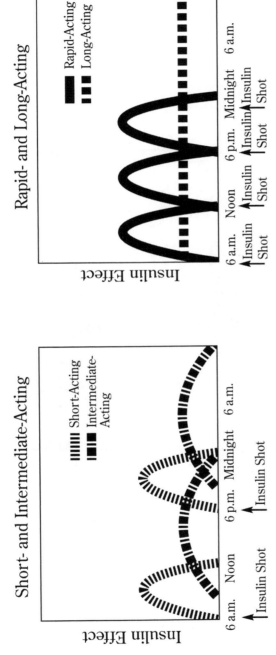

Short- and Intermediate-Acting

Short-Acting
Intermediate-Acting

Insulin Effect

6 a.m.   Noon   6 p.m.   Midnight   6 a.m.

↑Insulin Shot   ↑Insulin Shot

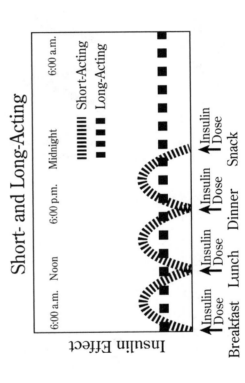

Rapid- and Long-Acting

Rapid-Acting
Long-Acting

Insulin Effect

6 a.m.   Noon   6 p.m.   Midnight   6 a.m.

↑Insulin Shot   ↑Insulin Shot   ↑Insulin Shot   ↑Insulin Shot

Short- and Long-Acting

Short-Acting
Long-Acting

Insulin Effect

6:00 a.m.   Noon   6:00 p.m.   Midnight   6:00 a.m.

↑Insulin Dose   ↑Insulin Dose   ↑Insulin Dose   ↑Insulin Dose

Breakfast   Lunch   Dinner   Snack

INSULIN PROGRAMS *continued*

Insulin Programs

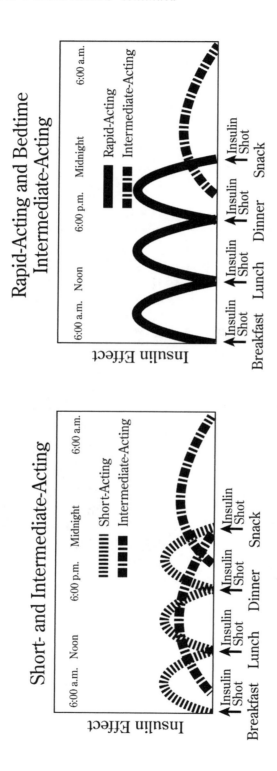

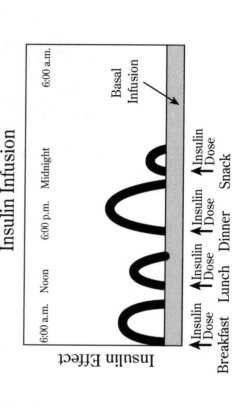

⬆ Timing of Regular Insulin and Meals

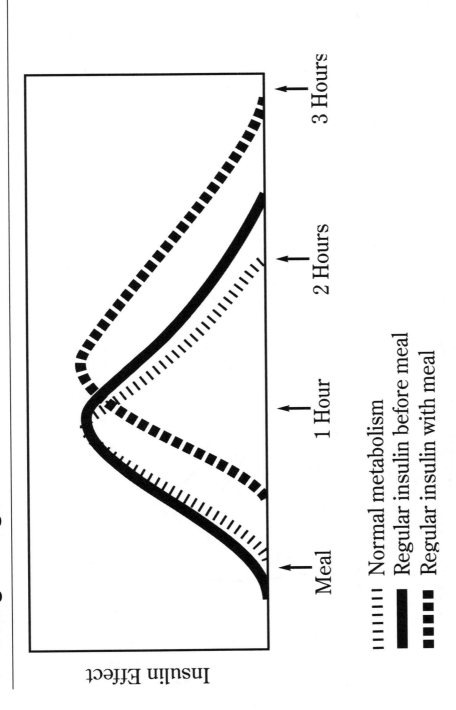

Insulin Effect

Meal 1 Hour 2 Hours 3 Hours

|||||| Normal metabolism

▬▬ Regular insulin before meal

▪▪▪▪ Regular insulin with meal

⬤ Injection Sites

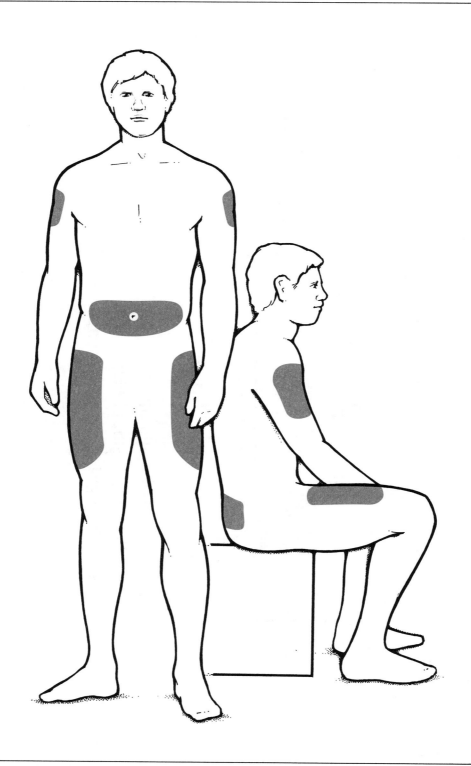

☞ Comparison of Insulins

Type	Source	Color	Approximate Length of Action (Hours)		
			Onset	**Peak**	**End**
Rapid-acting Lispro Aspart Glulisine	Analog	Clear	<15 minutes	30 min –1 hr	1–5
Short-acting Regular	Human	Clear	1/2–1	2–5	3–12
Intermediate-acting NPH	Human	Milky-white when mixed	1–4	4–10	12–18
Long-acting Detemir	Analog	Clear	1–2	—	24+
Glargine	Analog	Clear	2–4	—	24+
Mixtures NPL 75: L 25	Analog	Milky-white when mixed	15 min	1/2–4	24
Aprotamine 70: A 30	Analog	Milky-white when mixed	15 min	1–4	15–18
NPH 70: R 30	Human	Milky-white when mixed	1/2	2–12	24
NPL 50: L 50	Analog	Milky-white when mixed	15 min	1–2	24

H, human; R, regular; L, lispro; A, aspart.

⬆ Insulin Programs

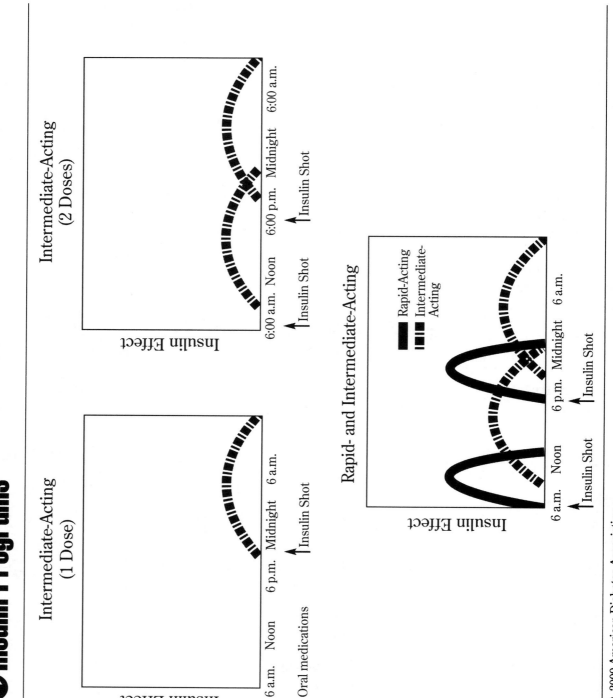

Intermediate-Acting
(2 Doses)

Insulin Effect

6:00 a.m. Noon 6:00 p.m. Midnight 6:00 a.m.

↑Insulin Shot ↑Insulin Shot

Intermediate-Acting
(1 Dose)

Insulin Effect

6 a.m. Noon 6 p.m. Midnight 6 a.m.

Oral medications ↑Insulin Shot

Rapid- and Intermediate-Acting

▮ Rapid-Acting
▮▮▮ Intermediate-Acting

Insulin Effect

6 a.m. Noon 6 p.m. Midnight 6 a.m.

↑Insulin Shot ↑Insulin Shot

194

INSULIN PROGRAMS *continued*

⬆ Insulin Programs

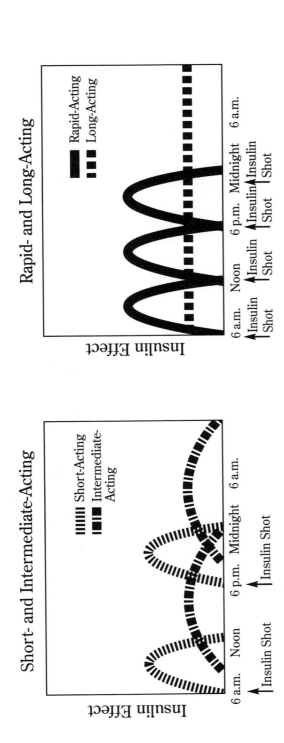

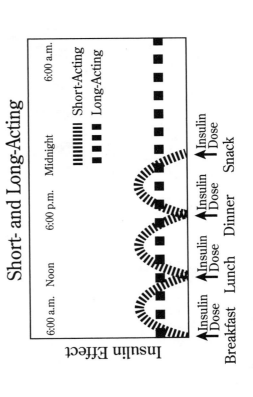

INSULIN PROGRAMS *continued*

Insulin Programs

Short- and Intermediate-Acting

6:00 a.m.	Noon	6:00 p.m.	Midnight	6:00 a.m.

Short-Acting
Intermediate-Acting

Insulin Effect

Insulin Shot — Breakfast
Insulin Shot — Lunch — Dinner
Insulin Shot — Snack

Rapid-Acting and Bedtime Intermediate-Acting

6:00 a.m.	Noon	6:00 p.m.	Midnight	6:00 a.m.

Rapid-Acting
Intermediate-Acting

Insulin Effect

Insulin Shot — Breakfast
Insulin Shot — Lunch — Dinner
Insulin Shot — Snack

Continuous Subcutaneous Insulin Infusion

6:00 a.m.	Noon	6:00 p.m.	Midnight	6:00 a.m.

Basal Infusion

Insulin Effect

Insulin Dose — Breakfast
Insulin Dose — Lunch — Dinner
Insulin Dose — Snack

Intensive Insulin Programs

Name _____ Date _____

BASAL INSULIN
The brand name and type of your basal insulin is:

_____

Please take the designated units of this insulin at the following times:

Breakfast	Lunch	Dinner	Bedtime

BOLUS INSULIN
The brand name of your bolus insulin is:

_____

Please take the designated units of this insulin at the following times:

Breakfast	Lunch	Dinner	Bedtime

INTENSIVE INSULIN THERAPY PROGRAM *continued*

Blood Glucose Ranges (mg/dl)	Insulin dose Breakfast	Insulin dose Lunch	Insulin dose Dinner	Insulin dose Snack

Please use the scale below to give your premeal insulin, according to your blood glucose levels.

Carbohydrate:Insulin Ratio _____.

For each 15 grams carbohydrate eaten, add _____ unit(s) to the designated dose.

For each 15 grams of carbohydrate not eaten, subtract _____ unit(s) from the designated dose.

For exercise, subtract _____ unit(s) from the pre-exercise dose.

For stress, add _____ unit(s) to the designated dose.

Correction dose _____ .

➡Giving an Insulin Injection

ONE KIND OF INSULIN

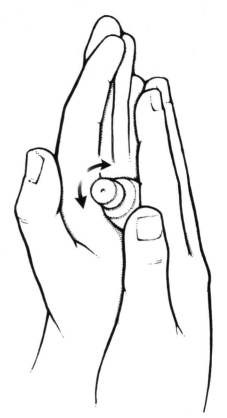

1. Gather your equipment:

   ■ syringe
   ■ insulin

2. Wash your hands.

3. Roll the bottle of insulin between the palms of your hands or shake gently to mix the insulin well. Do not shake vigorously. This can leave air bubbles that can get into the syringe.

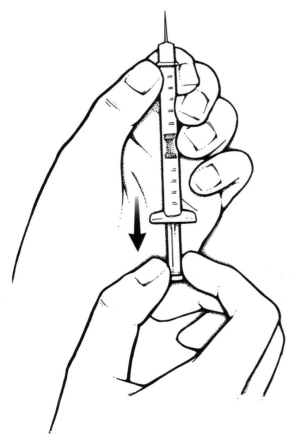

4. Take the needle cap off the syringe.

5. Hold the syringe with the needle pointing toward the ceiling. Keep the syringe at eye level, so you can easily see the markings on the barrel.

6. You must put air into the insulin bottle before you can get the insulin out of the bottle. First, pull the syringe plunger down until the top of the black tip crosses the mark of the dose to be taken. This draws air into the syringe.

   For example: If you take 40 units of insulin, draw about 40 units of air into the syringe.

GIVING AN INSULIN INJECTION *continued*

7. Now turn the syringe tip down. Put the
   needle through the rubber stopper of the
   insulin bottle. Push down all the way on the
   plunger, and hold the plunger in. This puts
   air into the bottle.

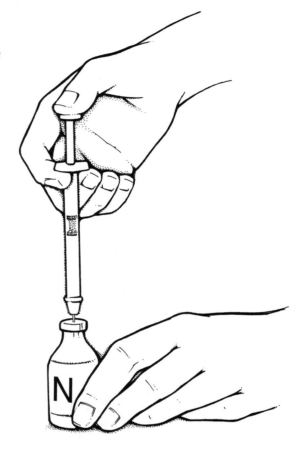

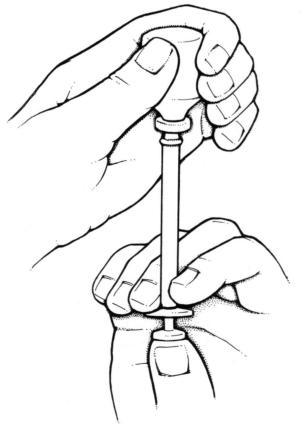

8. Turn the bottle and syringe upside down, so
   the bottle is on the top and the syringe is on
   the bottom. Leave the needle in the bottle
   with the plunger pushed all the way in.

GIVING AN INSULIN INJECTION *continued*

9. Make sure the tip of the needle is in the insulin. Pull down slowly on the plunger. This brings insulin into the syringe. Pull it down until the black tip is 2 or 3 units past your dose.

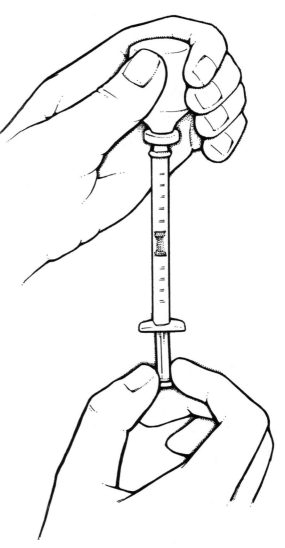

10. Push all of the insulin back into the bottle. This should get rid of any air bubbles.

11. Pull down slowly on the plunger to the exact line of your insulin dose. The right amount of insulin should now be in your syringe.

12. Look in the syringe for air bubbles. If you see air bubbles, push the insulin back into the bottle. Then pull the plunger back to the exact line of your insulin dose. If bubbles are still in the syringe, repeat the process until they are gone.

13. When all the bubbles are out and you have the right dose, pull the bottle straight up and off the needle. Put the needle cap back on the syringe over the needle. Put the syringe down. Check to be sure that you have the right dose. You'll know that it's right if the top of the plunger crosses the right mark on the syringe and there are no air bubbles.

14. Now you are ready to give yourself your shot. Take a deep breath and let it out slowly to help you relax.

GIVING AN INSULIN INJECTION *continued*

TWO KINDS OF INSULIN IN THE SAME SYRINGE

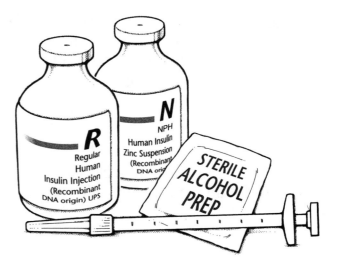

_____insulin (cloudy) _____ units

_____insulin (clear) _____ units

Total _____ units

1. Get your insulin bottles and syringe ready. Wash hands with soap and water.

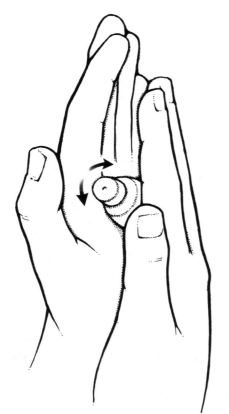

2. Roll _____ insulin between your hands or shake gently. This insulin looks cloudy.

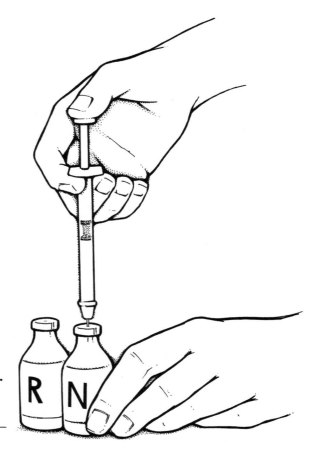

3. Take the needle cap off of the syringe.

4. Pull _____ units of air into the empty syringe. Put the needle through the rubber stopper of the bottle of cloudy insulin. Push air into the bottle. Remove the needle.

GIVING AN INSULIN INJECTION *continued*

5. Pull _____ units of air into the same empty syringe. Put the needle into your rapid- or short-acting insulin bottle. This insulin is clear. Push air into the bottle.

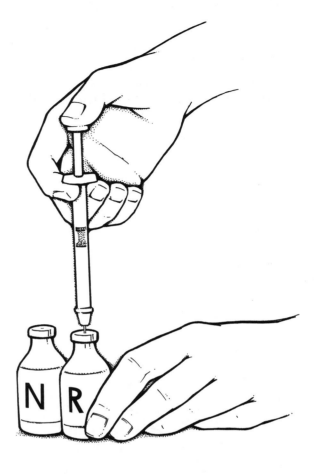

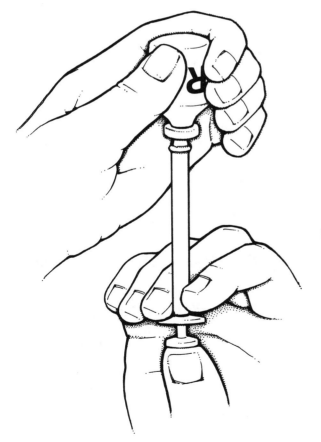

6. With the needle still in the regular insulin bottle, turn the bottle upside down. Pull the plunger halfway down the syringe. This brings insulin into the syringe. Push the insulin back into the bottle to get rid of the air bubbles. Now pull your dose of insulin into the syringe. Carefully measure _____ units of clear insulin. Pull the syringe out of the bottle.

GIVING AN INSULIN INJECTION *continued*

7. Turn the cloudy _____ insulin bottle upside down. Put the needle into the bottle. Pull the plunger back slowly to total _____ units. Pull the bottle off the needle.

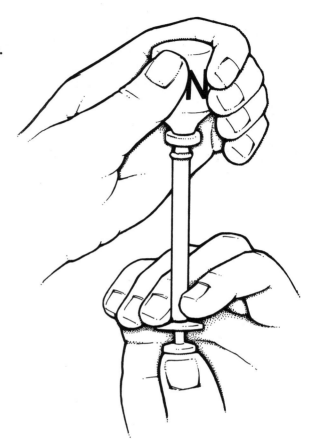

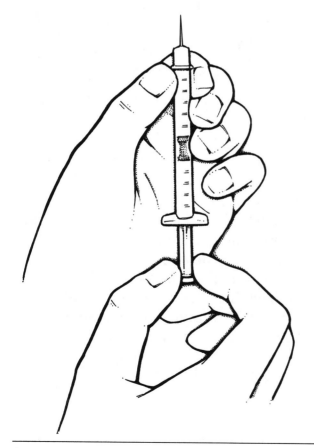

8. Check the total dosage. The dose should be:

_____ (cloudy) _____ units.

_____insulin (clear) _____ units.

Total of _____ units now in the syringe.

GIVING AN INSULIN INJECTION *continued*

GIVING THE INJECTION

1. You will inject yourself in your abdomen. Insulin is absorbed most evenly from this site. Your abdomen also has fewer nerves than other places and a pad of fat underneath. Pick a spot from the chart and then find this spot on yourself. Pick a spot at least 1 inch from the place you gave your last shot.

2. If desired, clean the spot with alcohol. Let dry.

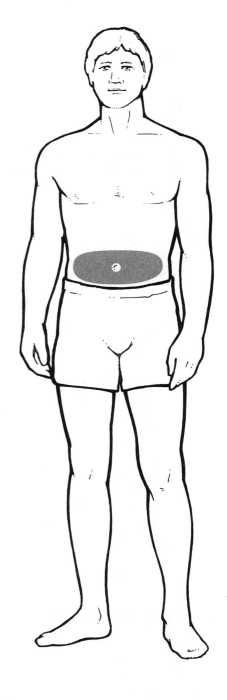

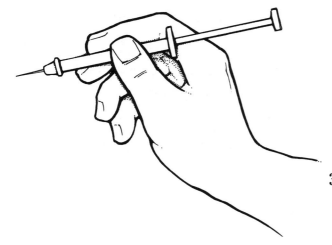

3. Remove the top from the needle. Hold the syringe in one hand as you would hold a pencil.

GIVING AN INSULIN INJECTION *continued*

4. With your other hand, pinch up a couple of inches of skin.

5. Stick the needle straight into the pinched skin. Put the needle all the way in through the skin with one smooth motion.

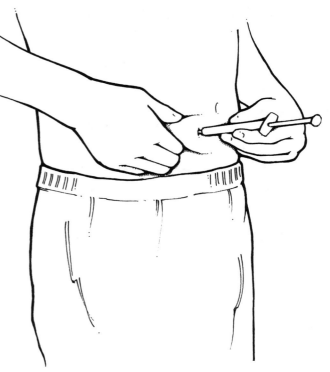

6. Slowly push the plunger all the way down and hold for 5 seconds. Be sure the insulin is in. Remove the needle.

7. Lightly press down on the site. Don't rub the spot. Don't worry if a drop of blood appears where the needle was.

8. When you are ready to discard your used needles and syringes, put them into a hard plastic or metal container with a screw-on lid. Label and discard according to local regulations.

9. Record the insulin dose you just gave yourself in your diabetes record.

It may be hard to give yourself a shot the first time, but with practice it will become much easier.

➥ Treatment of Low Blood Glucose

If your blood glucose test is:	The amount of food or drink to take is:
Between 50 and 69 mg/dl	15 g carbohydrate (1 carbohydrate serving **or** 1 cup fat-free [skim] milk)
Less than 50 mg/dl	30 g carbohydrate (2 carbohydrate servings)

You should feel better in 10–15 minutes after you treat yourself. If your blood glucose is still less than 70 mg/dl or you don't feel better 10–15 minutes after the treatment, take 1 more carbohydrate serving. Check your blood glucose an hour after the reaction to make sure that your blood glucose has gone above 70 mg/dl and stayed there.

▶ ▶ ▶ ▶ ▶

EXAMPLES OF TREATMENTS FOR LOW BLOOD GLUCOSE
(All equal about 15 gm carbohydrate or 1 fruit serving)

If your blood glucose is between 50 and 69 mg/dl, take the amount listed. If your blood glucose is less than 50 mg/dl, take twice the amount listed.

Foods	Amount
Orange or apple juice	1/2 cup
Grape or cranberry juice	1/3 cup
Non-diet soft drink	1/2 cup
Honey or corn syrup	1 Tbsp
Sugar packets	3
Life Savers	3–8 pieces
Glucose tablets	3–4 tablets

An additional carbohydrate snack may be needed at night or after exercise to keep your blood glucose above 70 mg/dl.

➲ How to Use Glucagon

Glucagon is an emergency drug that is given as a shot to raise the blood glucose level. It should be given when the person is not able to swallow or is at risk for choking, or in case of a severe insulin reaction or coma.

A prescription is needed to buy glucagon. It comes in two ways: in a kit or in a box to be mixed. If you use the kit, follow the package instructions.

To prepare glucagon for injection if you do not use a kit:

1. Remove the flip-off seals on bottles 1 and 2. Bottle 1 holds a diluting liquid and bottle 2 holds a white powder.

2. Draw the plunger of an insulin syringe (U-100) back to the 50-unit mark.

3. Steady the smaller bottle with the liquid in it (bottle 1) on the table. Push the needle through the stopper.

4. Inject the air from the syringe into the bottle and then turn the bottle upside down.

5. Withdraw as much of the liquid as possible into the syringe.

6. Remove the needle and syringe from bottle 1 and insert this same needle into bottle 2, the bottle with the powder. Inject all of the liquid from the syringe into bottle 2.

7. Remove the needle and syringe. Shake the bottle **gently** until the glucagon powder dissolves and the liquid becomes clear.

8. Withdraw the entire contents of bottle 2 (the mixed glucagon) into the syringe.

9. Inject the glucagon in the same way you would insulin, using the buttock, thigh, or arm.

10. Turn the person onto one side or stomach. (Vomiting is common after glucagon.)

11. As soon as the person is alert and not feeling sick, he or she should eat something, because glucagon acts for only a short period of time. First, give some juice or a non-diet soft drink, and then additional carbohydrate.

HOW TO USE GLUCAGON *continued*

12. If the person does not wake up within 15 minutes, the dose may be repeated. Call an ambulance.

13. Always call the doctor after an insulin reaction when coma or seizure occurs.

14. Check the package of glucagon periodically to be sure that it hasn't passed the expiration date. It's a good idea to keep an insulin syringe taped to the box so it will be ready.

#10   Monitoring Your Diabetes

▶ ▶ ▶ ▶ ▶

STATEMENT OF PURPOSE

This session is intended to provide information about the purpose of self blood glucose monitoring and how to record and use the results.

PREREQUISITES

It is recommended that participants bring their meters, as well as monitoring records.

OBJECTIVES

At the end of this session, participants will be able to:

1. explain that blood is tested to determine the actual level of glucose in the blood;

2. state the importance of A1C measurement;

3. state when to check blood glucose and urine ketones;

4. explain the importance of keeping a complete diabetes record;

5. interpret blood and urine tests and record results accurately;

6. define the usefulness of record keeping in blood glucose regulation;

7. list personal benefits and barriers of monitoring blood glucose levels;

8. identify strategies for monitoring routinely;

9. identify strategies for coping with feelings about monitoring results;

10. list at least four factors that can affect the results of blood tests;

11. name four factors that can affect monitoring results;

12. define personal glucose targets.

CONTENT

Monitoring blood glucose and other parameters, and interpreting and using the results for self-management decision making.

MATERIALS NEEDED

VISUALS PROVIDED	ADDITIONAL
1. Relationship of A1C to Risk of Complications 2. Normal Blood Glucose and Insulin Levels 3. Target Levels 4. Sample Diabetes Record	■ Chalkboard and chalk/Board and markers ■ Samples of blood glucose and ketone meters and test strips ■ Samples of lancets and lancet devices ■ Samples of records and log books ■ Samples of stickers to use for children

Handouts (one per participant)
1. Relationship of A1C Levels and Blood Glucose
2. Target Levels
3. Diabetes Record

METHOD OF PRESENTATION

Start by introducing yourself and telling what you do. Ask participants to introduce themselves. Explain that the purpose of this session is to provide information about the value and use of monitoring.

Begin by asking how they did with their short-term goal and what they learned from it. Present material in a question/discussion format, using the first question as a starting point. Provide appropriate content outlined below in response. Ask if there are additional questions, and respond, repeating the process for the entire session. Use the questions in the Instructor's Notes section to generate discussion if no questions are forthcoming after a period of silence. Keeping track of the content discussed in each session. Using the Diabetes Self-Management Record, the Participant Follow-up Record, or another form, helps you to evaluate if all needed content has been discussed.

Monitoring procedures are best taught on a one-on-one basis; however, you may want to demonstrate a blood glucose check to begin the session if any participants are unfamiliar with the procedure.

CONTENT OUTLINE

CONCEPT	DETAIL	INSTRUCTOR'S NOTES
1. Introduction	1.1 Monitoring your diabetes gives you information about your blood glucose level and the effects of meal timing, food intake, medication, activity, and stress.	Ask, "What questions do you have about blood glucose monitoring?" Ask participants how they currently monitor their diabetes. Many participants dislike the use of the word "test" and prefer "check" or "monitor." Ask, "What questions or concerns do you have about blood glucose monitoring?"
	1.2 Your diabetes record helps you keep track so you can use this information more easily.	Stress the importance of monitoring data for use by participants in daily self-care and

CONTENT OUTLINE

CONCEPT	DETAIL	INSTRUCTOR'S NOTES

decision making. Stress that they are monitoring for themselves, as well as their health care team.

2. Methods used to monitor blood glucose levels

2.1 Home blood glucose monitoring is a direct method that tells you what your blood glucose level is at that time.

Ask, "How can you find out your blood glucose level? Your blood glucose patterns?"

2.2 An additional measure is the A1C test. This is a measure of your blood glucose levels over the previous 6–12 weeks. It can be done in a laboratory or with a fingerstick drop of blood.

Ask, "Do you know your A1C? What does this number mean to you?" Distribute Handout #1, Relationship of A1C Levels and Blood Glucose. Fructosamine is a less frequently used measure of short-term control, generally a 2 to 3 week average.

2.3 Your red blood cells carry the memory of all your blood glucose levels. Glucose attaches itself to the hemoglobin in the red blood cell, forming glycated hemoglobin. (This is different from the test done for iron or anemia and used to be glycosylated hemoglobin or hemoglobin A1C.)

Less than 6% is generally considered the normal value. Use Handout #1, Relationship of A1C Levels and Blood Glucose. A1C results are not directly affected by food or activity on the day of the test. Remind participants to request this test if not done at least every 3–6 months.

2.4 Measuring A1C gives you the big picture of your glucose level, while a blood glucose check gives you a snapshot of that moment.

Remind participants that blood glucose levels change frequently during the day. Use Visual #2, Normal Blood Glucose and Insulin Levels.

2.5 If your readings and your A1C levels don't match, it may mean that your blood glucose levels are high or low at times when you are not checking— for example, after meals. Your A1C levels are not your grade on a report card, but data to help you and your provider make informed decisions.

Ask, "Have you ever been disappointed with your A1C level? How did you handle your disappointment?" Point out that your results are not a judgment of your efforts, but they provide information about whether changes are needed in how your diabetes is managed.

2.6 Your A1C reading is not a simple average, but a weighted average. You never have a complete turnover of red blood cells all at once. About half were

CONTENT OUTLINE

CONCEPT	DETAIL	INSTRUCTOR'S NOTES

formed within the last month. So your glucose levels in the last month count for about half of your A1C level, and cells from the previous 2–3 months make up the other half of the measure.

2.7 This number tells you about your risk for complications. Research has shown that keeping A1C levels at 7% or lower helps to prevent or delay the long-term complications of diabetes. Every time you lower your A1C level, you lower your risk.

Use Visual #1, Relationship of A1C to Risk of Complications. Ask, "Where is your A1C level now? Where would you like your A1C to be?" Stress the importance of this number for their long-term outcomes.

2.8 A1C results may also be reported as estimated average blood glucose levels (eAG). This average may be different than the average from your monitor.

Ask, "How does your average blood glucose level compare with your monitoring records?" Refer to Handout #1, Relationship of A1C Levels and Blood Glucose.

2.9 Your A1C is important for you because it helps you know how your blood glucose levels are affecting your body and how your treatment plan and hard work are paying off. Strategies to lower A1C levels are the same as strategies for lowering your blood glucose level. When your A1C is high, lowering your fasting blood glucose levels will have the most effect. As you get closer to normal, your post-meal blood glucose levels have the most effect on your A1C level.

Use Visual #1 to illustrate that every decrease in A1C helps lower their risk for complications. Ask, "What are strategies you could use to lower your A1C?" List these on the board. Examples include: change in medication type or dose; stress management; change in food choices or amounts; and increase activity level.

2.10 The Diabetes Control and Complications Trial (DCCT) was a large study of people with type 1 diabetes that showed that people in the group using intensive insulin therapy significantly reduced their risks for some of the long-term complications of diabetes compared with people using standard therapy. Participants in the intensive group had significantly lower blood glucose and A1C levels than those in the standard group.

Participants in the study are still being followed. Even though the two groups now have similar A1C values, the intensive group continues to have fewer complications.

CONTENT OUTLINE

CONCEPT	DETAIL	INSTRUCTOR'S NOTES
	2.11 The risk for diabetic retinopathy was decreased by 76%, neuropathy by 60%, and nephropathy by 35–56%.	Retinopathy = eye disease. Neuropathy = nerve disease. Nephropathy = kidney disease.
	2.12 The United Kingdom Prospective Diabetes Study (UKPDS) was a large study conducted among people with type 2 diabetes. The results showed that the risk for retinopathy, nephropathy, and perhaps neuropathy was reduced by lowering glucose levels. The overall complication rate was reduced by 25%. For every percentage point decrease in A1C, there was a 35% decrease in risk of complications.	This study was conducted among 5,102 patients with newly diagnosed type 2 diabetes. Participants were followed for an average of 10 years. There is no evidence for reduced risk at below-normal levels (<6.2%).
	2.13 The UKPDS also showed that reducing blood pressure significantly reduced strokes, diabetes-related deaths, heart failure, microvascular complications, and visual loss.	
3. Home blood glucose monitoring	3.1 Level of glucose in the blood results from interaction of: ■ meal plan ■ medicines for diabetes ■ exercise ■ stress.	Ask, "What questions or concerns do you have about home blood glucose monitoring? What have your experiences been with monitoring? How do you use the information?" Write the list on the board.
	3.2 Glucose levels change throughout the day and night.	Refer to the list on the board. Use Visual #2, Normal Blood Glucose and Insulin Levels. Ask, "What would you expect your glucose to do 2 hours after you eat? When your insulin is peaking?"
4. Blood glucose monitoring methods	4.1 All blood glucose meters require a drop of blood. Some meters require a larger drop of blood than others.	Ask, "What ways have you found to make testing less painful?" Examples: Use sides of fingers, use lancet devices, wash with warm, soapy water, and use a

CONTENT OUTLINE

CONCEPT	DETAIL	INSTRUCTOR'S NOTES
		different finger for each test. Show examples of various lancets and lancet devices. Review disposal procedure.
	4.2 The meter reads the blood glucose value from a test strip. The different meters vary in features, readability, portability, site of testing, and cost.	Show examples of various meters. Specific techniques for the chosen method will be taught on a one-on-one basis by the health care team.
	4.3 Choice of meter is based on personal preference, cost, features (e.g., memory), insurance coverage, and ease of use.	Demonstrate alternative site meters, if available, and visual strips if appropriate.
	4.4 Continuous glucose monitors (CGM) give a reading every few minutes. The information allows you to better understand trends, highs and lows; identify problems; and adjust insulin doses. These monitors also have alarms that alert you to dangerous levels.	Ask, "Have any of you tried CGM? What did you learn?" Provide information about CGM if requested. Women who are pregnant or planning to become pregnant and people who use an insulin pump are often candidates for CGM.
	4.5 With CGM, a tiny catheter is inserted subcutaneously. The catheter has a sensor which measures blood glucose in the interstitial fluid and sends the information to the meter or an insulin pump. These meters require calibration with SMBG.	Some people use CGM all the time while others use it occasionally to track trends and solve problems. Determining insurance coverage is a critical part of the decision-making process for CGM.
	4.6 Computer programs are available to you and your health care team that can download the results from your meter's memory.	Point out that this does not replace recording the numbers for pattern management.
5. When to check your blood	5.1 When to check is based on the information you need, your blood glucose goals, and your treatment plan.	Ask, "How often do you monitor?" Schools and workplaces may have policies about blood glucose monitoring.
	5.2 Checking blood glucose at various times of the day gives a better picture of your blood glucose patterns than checking at the same time every day.	

CONTENT OUTLINE

CONCEPT	DETAIL	INSTRUCTOR'S NOTES

Some options are:
- 1–8 times per day
- before each meal and at bedtime
- fasting and 2 hours after the start of each meal
- before and after each meal
- once a day, but at different times each day (e.g., Monday before breakfast, Tuesday before lunch)
- fasting and once more at different times of the day (as above)
- each day before breakfast.

Ask, "How often do you need to check to get the information you need?" Postprandial testing is especially useful for people using rapid-acting insulins or glucose dependent medications, people who are counting carbohydrates, people with disparate A1C and blood glucose levels, and people with type 2 diabetes or IGT.

5.3 Monitor every 2–4 hours when ill.

Ask, "How do you handle monitoring at work? At school? Away from home? How do you respond to people who ask about it?"

6. Factors that affect blood glucose test results

6.1 Factors that affect your blood glucose level:
- food and beverages
- medicine for diabetes
- other medicines
- exercise
- stress
- timing of food and diabetes medication
- time of day the test is performed.

Ask, "What have you noticed that affects your blood glucose level?" List these on the board and discuss. Point out that at times they may have unexplained glucose levels or levels that do not reflect their efforts. While frustrating, it is what your glucose level is most of the time that counts. Ask, "How do you handle your frustration over unexpected blood glucose results?" Having a strategy will diminish the chances of simply giving up on monitoring.

6.2 Outdated strips: check expiration date.

Ask, "What other factors can affect your test results?"

6.3 Technique errors:
- collection methods (e.g., inadequate blood sample)
- meter not correctly calibrated to strips
- meter needs to be cleaned.

Almost all meters are now calibrated to plasma glucose values. Plasma values are 10–15% higher than whole blood values. Some new meters do not require "coding" of strips.

6.4 Spoiled materials: do not use test materials if there is a color change on the test strip.

Store in a cool, dry place. Do not store test materials in direct sunlight, or on or near a stove, radiator, or window sill. Heat,

CONTENT OUTLINE

CONCEPT	DETAIL	INSTRUCTOR'S NOTES
		dampness, and altitude can affect your results.
	6.5 Meter malfunction.	Check the directions for the meter. If it still doesn't work, contact the manufacturer's toll-free hotline or your health care team.
	6.6 If your blood glucose results do not seem right to you, ask yourself if any of these factors might have caused the problem.	Multiple factors affect blood glucose values and participants do not have control over many of them.
7. Use of monitoring information	7.1 Monitoring gives you the information you need to make decisions as you care for your diabetes each day. Without this information, you aren't able to make informed decisions.	Ask, "What do you learn by monitoring?" Point out that blood glucose results are "just a number," not a judgment. They aren't a test that you pass or fail.
	7.2 You can determine if you are hypoglycemic by testing your blood glucose. Sometimes you feel as if you are having a reaction, but you are not certain.	A blood glucose level below 70 mg/dl generally indicates hypoglycemia.
	7.3 You can help detect and prevent nighttime hypoglycemic reactions by checking your blood glucose before bedtime. This is especially important if your blood glucose was lower than usual or you exercised more than usual that day.	If your blood glucose is low, eat a larger-than-usual bedtime snack. A change in your insulin dose is needed if the finding is consistent.
	7.4 You can determine the effects of a particular activity, food, or a stressful event on your blood glucose by doing "before and after" checks.	Monitoring can provide flexibility by increasing the ability to make adjustments and decisions.
	7.5 You can determine if your insulin dose was adequate for the amount of carbohydrate eaten or if your dose adjustments were effective.	
	7.6 In summary, anytime you want to know your blood glucose level, you can do a check.	
8. Blood glucose goals	8.1 Selecting your personal blood glucose targets is one of the most important decisions you can make	Stress the importance of setting blood glucose targets as a needed first step in choosing

CONTENT OUTLINE

CONCEPT	DETAIL	INSTRUCTOR'S NOTES

about your health. It is the basis for your treatment plan and for developing a collaborative relationship with your health care team.

treatment options. Clarity in goals helps establish a collaborative relationship with providers and decreases frustration on both sides.

8.2 It helps to know where you want your glucose levels to be most of the time as you set your personal blood glucose targets. Setting a range rather than an exact number is more realistic. These targets may change from time to time. You'll use these targets as a guide for using your monitoring data.

Ask, "What is normal blood glucose?" Use Visual #3, Target Levels. These goals are based on whole blood values. Plasma values and goals are 10–15% higher than whole blood values.

	People Without Diabetes (mg/dl)	**People With Diabetes (mg/dl)**
Before meals	80–125	70–130
After meals	80–130	<180

Remind participants that multiple factors affect blood glucose levels. Because they do not have control over many of these, it is often unrealistic to expect (and to set as a goal) blood glucose levels to always be in the normal or even the target range.

8.3 Fasting blood glucose tells what your blood glucose is before breakfast. The other levels take into account the effect of food. Blood glucose levels are highest just after a meal.

Point out that if participants have a lower fasting blood glucose level, blood glucose levels are generally lower for the rest of the day.

8.4 These are suggested blood glucose levels; however, you need to choose personal blood glucose goals based on your health, lifestyle, diabetes care goals, and other events in your life. Talk with your health care team about these targets, so you can work together to achieve them.

Ask, "Where would you like your blood glucose to be most of the time? How often do you need to check so that you have the information you need to help keep your blood glucose there? How confident are you that you can reach and maintain those targets?"

8.5 Some people find that their mood changes as their blood glucose levels change. They often notice this more when their levels are changing often.

"How do you feel emotionally when your results are in range? Out of range? How does this affect how you manage your diabetes? What are some ideas for ways to handle these times?"

CONTENT OUTLINE

CONCEPT	DETAIL	INSTRUCTOR'S NOTES
	8.6 Costs and barriers for optimizing glucose levels may include increased risk for low blood glucose, weight gain, expense, and effort involved.	Ask, "What costs and barriers do you see for yourself?" The meal plan may need to be changed to prevent weight gain with improved glucose control. ask, "What benefits do you see?" Listing these on a board can help participants consider their options (see Outline #15, *Changing Behavior,* p. 315).
	8.7 Benefits may include prevention of complications, feeling more energetic, and decreased symptoms.	
	8.8 If your blood glucose levels aren't in your target range, think about what may have caused the problem, such as ■ more (or less) food, activity, or medicine ■ illness ■ stress.	Ask, "What is it like for you when your blood glucose is out of range? How do you handle your feelings? How does it affect how you care for yourself?"
	8.9 Try not to get discouraged or dwell on what went wrong. Think about what you can do differently tomorrow. Many people find it more helpful to look for patterns in their blood glucose levels. Look at your record for the past 1–2 weeks. Were there times of the day when your blood glucose levels were too high or too low most days? If so, you may need a change in your medicines or meal plan.	Review participants' records for patterns, use Visual #4, Sample Diabetes Record, or develop an example with the group. Point out that it's often less frustrating to look at patterns. It is where the blood glucose level is most of the time that matters.
9. Tips for blood glucose monitoring	9.1 Blood glucose monitoring may be hard to do at first. As you learn to use the results to understand your body better and manage your treatment, it will become easier.	Ask, "What barriers have you encountered to monitoring? What strategies have you used to overcome the barriers?" Brainstorm a list of ideas.
	9.2 Getting the support of your family and friends can help you monitor more faithfully. Although they may be concerned, asking about your blood glucose levels each time you check may feel intrusive.	Ask, "How do your family and friends respond? How would you like them to respond? What are strategies you can use so that their response is helpful to you?"

CONTENT OUTLINE

CONCEPT	DETAIL	INSTRUCTOR'S NOTES
	9.3 Before you do a check, gather all monitoring materials and get them in order. You may want to keep your equipment in a small box or bag so that all materials are stored together.	Keeping all materials in a pouch or bag helps you be ready to take them with you.
	9.4 Keep your equipment near the place you usually check so it will take less time. Keep your diabetes record and a pen in the same place.	Some people own more than one meter to keep in different places. Humidity in a bathroom may damage strips.
	9.5 If you have trouble remembering, put a reminder where you'll be sure to see it (if you check in the morning, put your equipment by your alarm clock). Plan ways to make monitoring part of your daily routine.	
	9.6 To obtain an adequate drop of blood: ■ wash your hands in warm water before the finger prick ■ dangle fingers at your side for a few seconds before the finger prick ■ squeeze below the place on your finger you are going to prick until it turns red ■ prick the sides of your fingertips, not the fatty middle part or the fatty part of your palm just below your thumb. ■ keep your hand below the level of your heart while you wait for the drop to reach an adequate size ■ gently milk your finger ■ try your thumb or fourth finger—they have a rich blood supply.	Laser lancet devices are now on the market, as are devices that allow you to obtain blood from areas other than the fingertips.
	9.7 Do not use monitoring equipment that belongs to another person, and avoid sharing your equipment with others.	Point out the need for precautions to prevent blood-borne infections.
	9.8 Learn to use the results to adjust your medications, diet, or activity.	Teach pattern management here, if appropriate. Refer to Outline #19, *Carbohydrate Counting* (p. 399), and Outline #9, *All About Insulin* (p. 165).

CONTENT OUTLINE

CONCEPT	DETAIL	INSTRUCTOR'S NOTES
10. Recording and use of test results	10.1 Write down your results and bring to your appointments. Bring your meter also, so it can be downloaded.	Use Visual #4, Sample Diabetes Record. Be sure to include comments on the record—note any symptoms or deviations from your usual program.
	10.2 Monitoring alone will not lower your blood glucose. You can learn to **use** the results of your tests to adjust your diet, medicine, and exercise.	Ask, "What do you need to be able to do with the results to make monitoring worthwhile for you?" List on the board.
	10.3 Look for patterns in your blood glucose levels. Think about possible causes for your blood glucose patterns or changes from your usual pattern. This is the first step in using the results.	Ask, "Is your blood glucose often high or low at a certain time of day?" Put sample situations on a record form or use participant results and discuss. Distribute Handout #3, Diabetes Record, if desired.
	10.4 Call your doctor or nurse if any problems arise between visits or if there are major changes in your results. Also call if you have low blood glucose reactions for reasons you don't understand, or if your blood glucose levels change suddenly and you don't know why or what to do.	All participants should have individual blood glucose parameters and know when to contact their health care teams. Remind participants to ask for these parameters.
	10.5 Choose one thing you will do this week to care for your diabetes.	Close the session by asking participants to identify one step they will take this week.

SKILLS CHECKLIST

Each participant will be able to do a blood glucose check using the appropriate technique and record the results. Select participants will be able to do a urine ketone test using the appropriate technique and record the results.

EVALUATION PLAN

Knowledge will be evaluated by achievement of learning objectives and by responses to questions during the session. Skills will be evaluated by observing a return demonstration of techniques. The ability to apply knowledge will be evaluated by development and implementation of a personal monitoring plan and through program outcome measures.

DOCUMENTATION PLAN

Record class attendance and achieved objectives as appropriate using the Diabetes Self-Management Record, the Participant Follow-up Record, or another form.

SUGGESTED READINGS

American Diabetes Association: Bedside blood glucose monitoring in hospitals. *Diabetes Care* 27(Suppl 1):S104, 2004

American Diabetes Association: Resource guide. Blood glucose monitors and data management systems. *Diabetes Forecast* 62(1):53–66, 2009

American Diabetes Association: Tests of glycemia in diabetes. *Diabetes Care* 27(Suppl 1):S91–S93, 2004

Austin MM, Haas L, Johnson T, Parkin CG, Parkin CL, Spollett G, Volpone MT: AADE Position Statement: Self-monitoring of blood glucose: benefits and utilization. *The Diabetes Educator* 32:835–847, 2006

Bloomgarden DK, Feeman J, DeRobertis E: Early patient and clinician experiences with continuous glucose monitoring. *Diabetes Spectrum* 21:128–133, 2008

Bloomgarden ZT: Type 1 diabetes and glucose monitoring. *Diabetes Care* 30:2965–2971, 2007

Bode BW: Incorporating postprandial and fasting plasma glucose into clinical management strategies. Insulin 2:17–29, 2007

Brown AW: Clinicians guide to diabetes gadgets and gizmos. *Clinical Diabetes* 66–72, 2008

Dale L: Make a point about alternate site blood glucose sampling. *Nursing* 36(2):52–53, 2006

Fowler MJ: Diabetes devices. *Clinical Diabetes* 26:130–133, 2008

Freeman J, Lyons L: The use of continuous glucose monitoring to evaluate the glycemic response to food. *Diabetes Spectrum* 21:134–136, 2008

Garg SK, Kelly WC, Voelmle MK, Ritchie PJ, Gottlief PA, McFann KK, Ellis SL: Continuous home monitoring of glucose. *Diabetes Care* 30:3023–3025, 2007

Gebel E: Checking your blood glucose. *Diabetes Forecast* 62(4):32–34, 2009

Horner B, Chase HP: Continuous glucose monitoring. *Practical Diabetology* 26(1):26–42, 2007

International Expert Committee: International Expert Committee report on the role of the A1C assay in the diagnosis of diabetes. *Diabetes Care* 32:1327–1334, 2009

Kasturi KS, Petersen JR: Point-of-care glycosylated hemoglobin and its impact on diabetes care. *Practical Diabetology* 27(1):20–24, 2008

McAndrew L, Schneider Sh, Burns E, Levethal H: Does patient blood glucose monitoring improve diabetes control? *The Diabetes Educator* 33:991–1011, 2007

Nathan DM, Kuenen J, Borg R, Zheng J, et al.: Translating the A1C assay into estimated average glucose values. *Diabetes Care* 31:1473–1478, 2008

Perkins JM, Davis SN: The rationale for prandial glycemic control in diabetes mellitus. *Insulin* 2:52–56, 2007

Petersen JR, Finley JB, Okorodudu AO, et al.: Effect of point-of-care on maintenance of glycemic control as measured by A1C. *Diabetes Care* 30:713–715, 2007

Polonsky, WH: Ten good reasons to hate blood glucose monitoring. *Diabetes Self-Management* 17(3):24–30, 2000

Sheiner G: Continuous glucose monitoring. *Diabetes Self-Management* 25(3):42–50, 2008

Towfigh A, Romanova M, Weinreb JE, Munjas B, Suttorp MJ, Zhou A, Shekelle PG: Self-monitoring of blood glucose in patients with type 2 diabetes mellitus not taking insulin: a meta-analysis. *Am J Manag Care* 14(7): 468–475, 2008

Williams A: Talking meters. *Diabetes Self-Management* 24(3):6–18, 2007

➜ Relationship of A1C to Risk of Complications

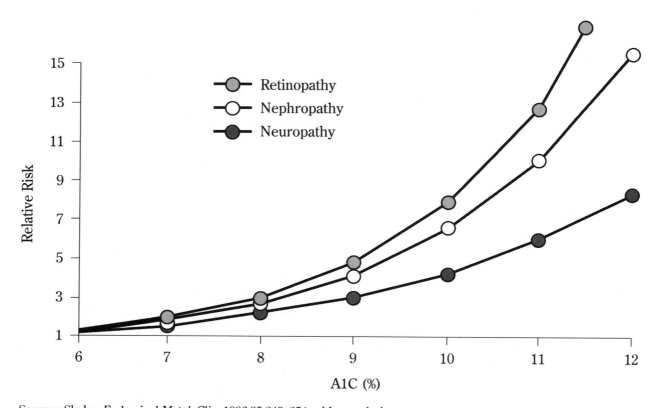

Source: Skyler. *Endocrinol Metab Clin.* 1996;25:243–254, with permission.

➲ Normal Blood Glucose and Insulin Levels

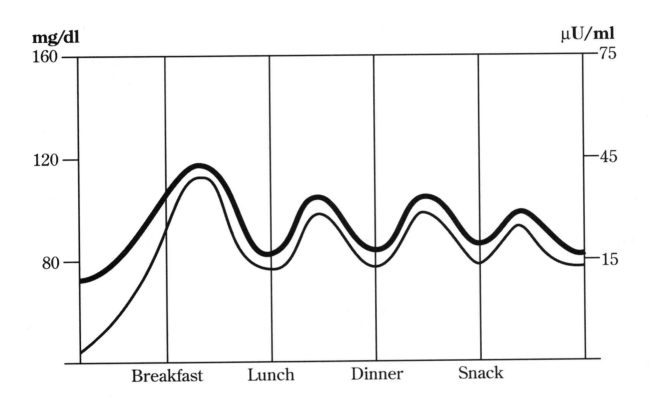

mg/dl   **μU/ml**

160   75

120   45

80   15

Breakfast   Lunch   Dinner   Snack

━━━ Blood Glucose Level

─── Plasma Insulin Level

➡ Target Levels

	People Without Diabetes	**People with Diabetes**
Blood glucose (plasma)		
Before meals	80–125 mg/dl	70–130 mg/dl
After meals*	80–130 mg/dl	Less than 180 mg/dl
A1C	Less than 6%	Less than 7%
Blood pressure	Less than 130/80	Less than 130/80

*Two hours after the first bite of food.

➡ Sample Diabetes Record

	Breakfast		Lunch		Supper		Bedtime		Other		Ketones	Comments
	Dose	Blood Glucose	Dose	Blood Glucose	Dose	Blood Glucose	Dose	Blood Glucose	Dose	Blood Glucose		
Sun	18L 6R	220			10L 4R			100			7 A.M. SM	Ate at 10 A.M.
Mon	18L 4R	80		120	12L 4R	170		140		30	7 A.M. Neg	Reaction 3 A.M.
Tues	18L 4R	240		180	12L 4R	240		110		70	7 A.M. SM	Walk 7-8 P.M.
Wed	18L 4R	90			10L 4R	120		80		90	10 P.M. Neg	Walk 7-8 P.M.
Thur	18L 4R	100			10L 4R	180					7 A.M. Neg	Walk 7-8 P.M.
Fri	18L 4R	120		150	10L 4R	160		120			6 P.M. Neg	
Sat	18L 4R	90		70	10L 4R	180		240			10 P.M. Neg	Ate 9 A.M. Tennis 10-12 Reaction 3 P.M.
Number of measurements		7		4		6		6		3		
Total of blood glucose values		940		520		1050		790		190		
Average of blood glucose values		134		130		175		132		64		

➲ Relationship of A1C Levels and Blood Glucose

The A1C blood test tells you your blood glucose levels over the past 3–4 months. This test, along with your home blood glucose checks, can give you a more complete picture of your blood glucose. It also helps you know your risk for long-term complications. The closer your A1C level is to normal, the lower your risk.

Hemoglobin is one part of a red blood cell. It carries oxygen throughout your body. The glucose (sugar) in your blood attaches to the hemoglobin, where it stays for the life of the red blood cell. The combined hemoglobin and glucose unit is called A1C. This test measures the percentage of total hemoglobin that has glucose attached to it. Because red blood cells live for about 120 days, these tests reflect your glucose levels for the previous 3–4 months. The results are not affected much by what you did the day before the test. This is not the same as the test for anemia or iron levels in your blood.

This chart shows how the A1C results compare with average blood glucose levels. The relationship between A1C and plasma glucose levels is shown.

A1C %	estimated Average Plasma Glucose eAg (mg/dl)
5	97
5.5	111
6	126
6.5	140
7	154
7.5	169
8	183
8.5	197
9	212
9.5	226
10	240
10.5	255
11	269
11.5	283
12	298

Your A1C level should be measured every 3–6 months so that you and your health care team can assess your overall diabetes care plan.

© 2009 American Diabetes Association

Target Levels

	People Without Diabetes	People with Diabetes
Blood glucose (plasma)		
Before meals	80–125 mg/dl	70–130 mg/dl
After meals*	80–130 mg/dl	Less than 180 mg/dl
A1C	Less than 6%	Less than 7%
Blood pressure	Less than 130/80	Less than 130/80

*Two hours after the first bite of food.

⬆ Diabetes Record

	Breakfast		Lunch		Supper		Bedtime		Other		Ketones	Comments
	Dose	Blood Glucose	Dose	Blood Glucose	Dose	Blood Glucose	Dose	Blood Glucose	Dose	Blood Glucose		
Sun												
Mon												
Tues												
Wed												
Thur												
Fri												
Sat												

Number of measurements _____ _____ _____ _____

Total of blood glucose values _____ _____ _____ _____

Average of blood glucose values _____ _____ _____ _____

▶ ▶ ▶ ▶ ▶

#11	**Managing Blood Glucose**

STATEMENT OF PURPOSE

This session is intended to identify and define the factors that influence blood glucose levels, show how these factors interrelate, and discuss the short-term complications of diabetes. Instructions for sick-day management and recognizing and treating hypoglycemia and hyperglycemia are included.

PREREQUISITES

It is recommended that participants have basic knowledge about the pathophysiology of diabetes. It is also suggested that participants bring their diabetes monitoring records.

OBJECTIVES

At the end of this session, participants will be able to:

1. define normal fasting blood glucose levels;

2. state personal benefits and barriers of near-normal blood glucose levels;

3. identify the three treatment components that affect regulation of blood glucose;

4. define hypoglycemia and hyperglycemia and list two causes of each;

5. define ketones and ketosis;

6. identify and discriminate between symptoms of hypoglycemia and hyperglycemia;

7. state actions to take that differ between hypoglycemia and hyperglycemia;

8. state action to treat hypoglycemia that is appropriate for the severity and the time of the reaction;

9. wear or carry diabetes identification;

10. state appropriate ways to manage blood glucose when ill, and state when to seek medical care;

11. identify personal food and drink choices to manage sick days.

CONTENT

Preventing, detecting, and treating acute complications.

MATERIALS NEEDED

VISUALS PROVIDED

1. Normal Blood Glucose and Insulin Levels
2. Insulin Action Times
3. Target Levels

Handouts (one per participant):
1. Treatment of Low Blood Glucose
2. How to Use Glucagon
3. Sick-Day Guidelines
4. Sick-Day Record

ADDITIONAL

- Chalkboard and chalk/Board and markers
- MedicAlert or other diabetes identification information
- Glucagon kit
- Samples of glucose products
- Ketone test strips

METHOD OF PRESENTATION

Start by introducing yourself and telling what you do. Ask participants to introduce themselves and say how long they have had diabetes and how it is being treated. Explain that the purposes of this session are to define factors that affect blood glucose levels and provide ways to use this information in the participants' own self-care. The first section is a review of factors that influence glucose levels. The second reviews acute problems related to blood glucose values.

Begin by asking how they did with their short-term goal and what they learned from it. Present material in a question/discussion format, using the first question as a starting point. Provide appropriate content outlined below in response. Ask if there are additional questions, and respond, repeating the process for the entire session. Use the questions in the Instructor's Notes section to generate discussion if no questions are forthcoming after a period of silence. You can also use participant monitoring records or develop examples that participants can use for problem solving.

Keeping track of the content discussed in each session, using the Diabetes Self-Management Record, the Participant Follow-up Record, or another form, helps you to evaluate if all needed content has been discussed.

CONTENT OUTLINE

CONCEPT	DETAIL	INSTRUCTOR'S NOTES
1. Managing blood glucose	1.1 This means keeping the factors that raise your blood glucose balanced with the factors that lower it. The body maintains this balance.	Ask, "What questions or concerns do you have about your blood glucose levels? What is your target blood glucose level? What is hardest for you in trying to keep your blood glucose in your target range?"
	1.2 Among people who don't have diabetes, blood glucose rises promptly after food is eaten, insulin is released	Use Visual #1, Normal Blood Glucose and Insulin Levels. Insulin production increases

CONTENT OUTLINE

CONCEPT	DETAIL	INSTRUCTOR'S NOTES
	by the pancreas in response to the increased blood glucose levels, and blood insulin levels rise. Usually, serum blood glucose goes no higher than 140 mg/dl and returns to the pre-meal level 2 hours after beginning to eat.	40 times within 5–15 minutes after starting a meal. Within 30 minutes, the pancreas releases a uniform stream of insulin for as long as it takes to digest the meal.
	1.3 Among people with diabetes, very little or no insulin is made, or the insulin doesn't work to lower blood glucose levels. You need to compensate for this lack of insulin action. You need to do what your body once did for you.	Ask, "How does glucose get into the blood? Where does it come from?" Injected insulin works more slowly than insulin made by the pancreas, and its effects last longer (even rapid-acting and short-acting insulins).
	1.4 Keeping the balance will help to prevent both the short-term (acute) and long-term (chronic) problems of diabetes.	Many people with diabetes object to the word "control" in relation to diabetes. Manage or regulate are more acceptable.
	1.5 The basic factors involved in blood glucose management are food, exercise, diabetes medicines (insulin or pills), and stress management. Meal planning and exercise are part of all diabetes treatment plans.	Ask, "What have you noticed about how different foods affect your blood glucose? Diabetes and other medicines? Exercise? Stress?"
	1.6 Knowing how these factors interact, your monitoring results, and your personal blood glucose targets are the basis for decisions you and your health care team make about your plan.	
	1.7 One of the most frustrating aspects of diabetes is the difficulty of keeping all of these factors in balance. Everyone's blood glucose goes off track now and then. There is no perfect treatment for diabetes. If you aim for perfection, you are setting yourself up for failure.	Ask, "What do you do when your blood glucose goes off track? How do you handle these feelings?" Acknowledge their frustration and the inadequacies of current therapy. Review the following material only if appropriate based on audience interest.
2. Meal plan	2.1 There are four basic purposes of a diabetes meal plan:	Ask, "What is your main purpose for using a meal plan?"

CONTENT OUTLINE

CONCEPT	DETAIL	INSTRUCTOR'S NOTES
	■ to provide appropriate food in amounts and at intervals that will balance with insulin or other medications to maintain target blood glucose levels ■ to achieve and maintain a reasonable body weight ■ to provide nutritional needs ■ to normalize blood fats, which minimizes risks for cardiovascular disease.	The insulin may be secreted by the individual's pancreas or administered by injection. Remind patients with type 2 diabetes that weight loss may increase the body's sensitivity to the insulin still being made by the pancreas, so they may not need to keep taking diabetes pills or insulin injections.
3. Physical activity	3.1 Exercise has the same beneficial effects for the person with diabetes as for those without diabetes.	Ask participants if they exercise and what their exercise program is, including type and schedule.
	3.2 Exercise usually will lower blood glucose in well-regulated diabetes.	Lower glucose levels can occur 24–48 hours after exercise.
	3.3 Consistent exercise at a comfortable level is the aim.	
	3.4 Aerobic exercise also helps reduce body fat.	
4. Medications to lower blood glucose	4.1 Oral agents stimulate the pancreas to produce more insulin, increase sensitivity to insulin, or alter your ability to absorb carbohydrates. Incretin mimetics help the insulin you make work more effectively.	See Outline #8, *Oral Medications and Incretin Mimetics* (p. 147).
	4.2 Insulin works to lower blood glucose. Combinations of insulins and other therapies are used to provide more even blood glucose levels throughout the day and to provide peak action when meals are eaten.	Ask, "What have your experiences been with taking multiple insulins and injections?" Use Visual #2, Insulin Action Times. See Outline #9, *All About Insulin* (p. 165).
5. Monitoring	5.1 Monitoring does not regulate your blood glucose. It gives you information about how well your meal plan, exercise, and medicines are balanced.	Ask, "What do you learn from monitoring? What are ways you use monitoring information?" See Outline #10, *Monitoring Your Diabetes* (p. 211).

CONTENT OUTLINE

CONCEPT	DETAIL	INSTRUCTOR'S NOTES
	5.2 Monitoring tells you if you are meeting the blood glucose targets you set for yourself.	Use Visual #3, Target Levels.
	5.3 You can learn to use the information from monitoring to make decisions throughout the day and adjust your blood glucose levels.	Stress the importance of their role in decision making.
	5.4 You can use the information to find your usual pattern of blood glucose.	
	5.5 You can use the information to determine how certain foods, activities, weight loss, or your emotions affect your blood glucose levels.	Problem-solve using participants' records or sample records.
	5.6 You can use the information to determine if your blood glucose is too high or too low.	Define these as the acute or short-term complications of diabetes.
6. Hypoglycemia	6.1 Regulating blood glucose helps to prevent the acute complications of diabetes. One of these is hypoglycemia or low blood glucose, sometimes called an insulin reaction.	Ask, "What questions or concerns do you have about hypoglycemia?" Hypo = low Glyc = glucose (sugar) Emia = blood
	6.2 Hypoglycemia is caused by too much effect of things that lower blood glucose (insulin, sulfonylureas, exercise) and/or too little food. Physical or emotional stress can also cause low blood glucose. Hypoglycemia is not likely to occur in diabetes managed with only diet and exercise.	For each type of insulin used by participants, ask if before-breakfast and/or evening doses would lower blood glucose levels the most. Alcohol can also lower blood glucose.
	6.3 The signs and symptoms of hypoglycemia are: blood glucose level below 70 mg/dl, sweating, weakness, hunger, anxiety, trembling, fast heartbeat, irritability, inability to think clearly, headache, drowsiness, numbness or tingling around lips, confusion, coma, and convulsions.	Ask, "What symptoms of hypoglycemia have you had?" Write these on the board. Nightmares or restlessness may be noted by others if hypoglycemia is nocturnal.
	6.4 Some people feel symptoms at higher levels and others cannot detect early symptoms at all. Some	If blood glucose levels have been elevated for some time, symptoms may occur at levels

CONTENT OUTLINE

CONCEPT	DETAIL	INSTRUCTOR'S NOTES
	people do not have any of the listed symptoms; however, most people have the same symptoms each time they are hypoglycemic.	above 70 mg/dl. If the blood glucose is 70 mg/dl or higher, advise patients to try to wait for symptoms to decrease or treat minimally. As blood glucose levels come into the target range, patients who have been hyperglycemic for some time and have felt low blood glucose symptoms at higher levels will notice that they don't feel symptoms until they drop close to 70 mg/dl.
	6.5 Hypoglycemia has a rapid onset (few minutes). The symptoms are often frightening and may be embarrassing as well.	Ask, "What is your biggest worry about going low?"
	6.6 Driving with low blood glucose levels is extremely dangerous. Always carry a source of glucose in your car. Have diabetes identification clearly visible. Keep a diabetes wallet card next to your driver's license.	Stress the need for those with hypoglycemia unawareness to check their blood before driving. A small card on the dashboard will inform helpers more quickly than a necklace or bracelet that may not be seen.
7. Treatment of hypoglycemia	7.1 Use a carbohydrate, such as sugar cubes, juice, or glucose tablets. You need to carry something with you to treat hypoglycemia at all times. Do not go off by yourself or lie down and wait for it to go away.	Distribute Handout #1, Treatment of Low Blood Glucose, and discuss. Show types of glucose products. Point out that participants who are lactose intolerant should not use milk for treatment.
	7.2 Use the rule of "15's." Treat the reaction with 15 grams of glucose. Wait 15 minutes. Check blood glucose again and repeat treatment if blood glucose remains below 70 mg/dl, or if there is no relief of symptoms.	Ask, "How do you treat your low blood glucose levels? How well does this work for you? What strategies do you use to keep from overtreating a reaction so that you are too high later?" Foods containing fat may retard the response to treatment.
	7.3 At night or after exercise, you may need to follow the initial treatment	Suggest that participants keep a box of juice near the bed for

CONTENT OUTLINE

CONCEPT	DETAIL	INSTRUCTOR'S NOTES

with a snack once the blood glucose level is above 70 mg/dl.

nighttime reactions as a way to prevent falls. There is no evidence that protein will maintain the blood glucose and prevent another reaction.

7.4 Glucagon is a hormone that helps the liver release its store of glucose into the bloodstream.

7.5 Glucagon can be given if a person is comatose or unable to eat. Call for emergency help if no glucagon is available. Glucagon may be less effective if administered in close succession, because the amount of stored glucose is less available.

Ask, "Do you have someone who knows what to do if you have a reaction?" Glucagon injection technique should only be taught to families of patients prone to severe hypoglycemia, who have asymptomatic hypoglycemia, or who are using intensive insulin therapy. Distribute Handout #2, How to Use Glucagon, if appropriate. Demonstrate kit.

7.6 Record the time of day, blood glucose level, and any precipitating causes.

Ask, "When do you tend to have low blood glucose reactions? What strategies do you use to prevent them?"

7.7 If you have more than one unexplained reaction a week, consult your health care team.

7.8 For your own safety, wear identification that states you have diabetes.

Distribute forms from the Medic Alert Foundation www.medicalert.com (888-633-4298) or others.

8. Hyperglycemia

8.1 Hyperglycemia (blood glucose levels above the normal range) is another acute complication.

Ask, "What questions or concerns do you have about hyperglycemia?"
Hyper = high
Glyc = glucose
Emia = blood

8.2 If your glucose reading is often higher than 130 mg/dl before meals and 180 mg/dl after meals or your A1C is higher than your target, it is too high and needs to be treated.

CONTENT OUTLINE

CONCEPT	DETAIL	INSTRUCTOR'S NOTES
	8.3 Hyperglycemia is caused by too little effect of things that lower blood glucose (insulin, other medications, exercise), and/or too much effect of things that raise blood glucose (insulin that has expired or "gone bad," eating more carbs than usual, weight gain, infection, or physical or emotional stress).	Hyperglycemia for no apparent reason may be caused by illness, infection, or emotional stress.
	8.4 The signs and symptoms of hyperglycemia are: higher blood glucose than usual, increased urine output, increased thirst, dry skin and mouth, fatigue and blurred vision, and, in the extreme, marked dehydration, lethargy, confusion, coma, and sometimes stroke. Hyperglycemia usually has a gradual onset.	Ask, "What symptoms of hyperglycemia have you had?" Write these on the board. Point out that you may not notice any symptoms.
9. Acute consequences of hyperglycemia	9.1 In type 1 diabetes during hyperglycemia, breakdown of fats caused by lack of insulin results in ketones appearing in the blood.	Discuss ketoacidosis only if appropriate for the audience. Mild ketosis can also occur during a weight-reduction diet.
	9.2 Ketones appear in the blood and urine when the body cells don't have enough glucose to use for energy because there is: ■ not enough insulin activity because of inadequate dose or illness ■ not enough carbohydrate, as in a weight loss diet or with hypoglycemia.	Blood glucose tests do not provide information about ketones. Urine or blood tests are needed for ketone results. Ask, "Do you check for ketones? Under what circumstances? How do you use this information?"
	9.3 The body burns fat and protein for energy when glucose is not available. Ketones are a waste product of this metabolism.	An analogy is ashes left in a fireplace when logs are burned.
	9.4 Ketones are acid. A buildup of ketones upsets the body's balance, and ketoacidosis results.	Ketoacidosis is acidosis due to ketones in the blood.

CONTENT OUTLINE

CONCEPT	DETAIL	INSTRUCTOR'S NOTES
	9.5 When hyperglycemia progresses, the excess ketones appear in the urine. This is a warning sign of impending ketoacidosis.	Blood or urine can be tested for ketones. Trace urinary ketones in the morning may indicate a nocturnal insulin reaction.
10. Ketone monitoring	10.1 Several products are on the market to check for urine ketones.	Show examples of various urine strips and meters that measure blood glucose and ketones.
	10.2 Urine checks reflect the amount of ketones in the blood during the time the urine was made by the kidneys. Blood tests show current levels.	Urine reflects ketones in the blood since the time of last voiding.
11. When to check for ketones	11.1 If you have type 1 diabetes: ■ check whenever your blood glucose is over 300 mg/dl ■ check whenever you feel ill ■ early-morning checks can tell you if you had a reaction during the night.	Present information specific for participants.
	11.2 If you have type 2 diabetes: ■ check whenever your blood glucose is over 300 or running high most of the time.	Ketoacidosis is rare in type 2 diabetes.
12. Results of ketone tests	12.1 If ketone results are positive, drink water or other sugar-free drinks. Extra insulin and fluids may help to prevent ketoacidosis.	This helps to flush ketones from the body. Provide information about insulin coverage, if appropriate.
	12.2 Check blood glucose and urine ketones every 2 hours until in the target range.	
	12.3 Call your health care team if levels remain elevated or you feel sick.	
	12.4 Symptoms of ketoacidosis are those of hyperglycemia (see 8.4) plus fruity breath; loss of appetite; nausea; vomiting; abdominal pain; faster, deeper breathing; confusion; and coma. If untreated, death may occur.	Encourage patients to seek help from their health care team or go to an emergency room. Drinking sugar-free fluids and taking rapid- or short-acting insulin may be used as an early treatment.

CONTENT OUTLINE

CONCEPT	DETAIL	INSTRUCTOR'S NOTES
	12.5 If you have stomach pain, nausea, vomiting, rapid breathing, or sweet, fruity-smelling breath, call your health care team or emergency room.	These are early signs of diabetic ketoacidosis (DKA).
	12.6 In type 2 diabetes, symptoms of severe fatigue, dehydration, abdominal pain, nausea, vomiting, and confusion without ketones are serious and should be reported right away. A coma can occur if these symptoms are not treated.	These are early symptoms of hyperglycemic hyperosmolar nonketotic syndrome. Encourage patients to seek help from their health care team or go to an emergency room.
13. Treatment of hyperglycemia	13.1 Treatment is based on cause.	Ask, "What has caused you to have high blood glucose levels? How did you manage it? Was the treatment effective?" Remind participants to try to determine possible causes.
	13.2 Take your usual medicines, eat planned meals, drink plenty of sugar-free fluids, and check your blood glucose and ketones (if >300 mg/dl) every four hours until back to your target range.	Fluids may help flush glucose and ketones from the body in early stages.
	13.3 Contact your health care team if you have any of the following: ■ blood glucose greater than 180 mg/dl for more than a week ■ any symptoms of hyperglycemia ■ presence of ketones ■ two consecutive blood glucose readings of more than 300 mg/dl ■ vomiting, confusion, or symptoms of severe dehydration.	Give appropriate guidelines for your setting or patient population. Check for moderate to large ketones in the urine.
14. Difference between hypo- and hyper- glycemia	14.1 Measure blood glucose as soon as either high or low blood glucose is suspected.	Generally, blood glucose must be 70 mg/dl or less to confirm hypoglycemia.

CONTENT OUTLINE

CONCEPT	DETAIL	INSTRUCTOR'S NOTES

14.2 Hypoglycemia occurs rapidly, within minutes. Hyperglycemia develops slowly, over hours or days.

14.3 If unable to check, treat with glucose as though hypoglycemia were present, and check blood glucose as soon as possible.

If symptoms are relieved by treatment with glucose, they were likely due to low blood glucose levels.

15. Sick-day management

15.1 An illness or infection can affect your blood glucose levels. Make a sick-day plan with your health care team before illness occurs.

Ask, "What questions or concerns do you have caring for diabetes when you are ill? What have your experiences been?" Distribute and review Handouts #3, Sick-Day Guidelines, and #4, Sick-Day Record.

15.2 Take your diabetes medicine as usual. Monitor your blood glucose at least every 4 hours. Check urine ketones every time you go to the bathroom if hyperglycemic.

Illness increases insulin resistance. More frequent monitoring is needed when blood glucose levels are elevated.

15.3 If possible, eat as usual. You may want to choose more soft or liquid foods. If you are unable to eat everything, try to have at least the carbohydrate foods. If you can't eat, drink high-carbohydrate liquids.

Ask, "What foods appeal to you when you are sick? What foods are you able to eat?"

See Handout #3, Sick-Day Guidelines, page 2. Make sure all participants have a plan that includes carbohydrate and medication adjustments, fever reduction information, monitoring information, and when to contact a health care professional.

15.4 If your blood glucose is high, (e.g., >250 mg/dl), you are vomiting, or you have urine ketones, call your health care team.

15.5 You need to tell all health professionals (doctors, podiatrists, and dentists) that you have diabetes.

This is particularly important before any type of surgery.

15.6 Prevention works better than trying to solve a problem. Annual flu shots are recommended for

Ask, "How do you remember to get your flu shot?" Pneumococcal revaccination is recommended

people with diabetes. Pneumococcal vaccine is also recommended.

for people over 65 if they were vaccinated before age 65 and the vaccine was more than 5 years ago.

16. Hints and tips

16.1 Everyone's blood glucose goes out of range now and then. This is often hard to cope with, especially when the results are unexpected.

Ask, "How do you handle these frustrations?" Some people have symptoms of low blood glucose as levels move nearer to the target range. If blood glucose is 70 mg/dl or higher, advise patients to try to wait for symptoms to decrease. If unable to tolerate symptoms, treat minimally (e.g., one saltine cracker).

16.2 Contact your health care team if your blood glucose is out of your target range nearly every day.

Close class by asking participants to identify their personal blood glucose goal (health outcome) and one step they will take this week to work toward this goal (behavior-change goal).

16.3 Choose one thing you will do this week to care for your diabetes.

Close the session by asking participants to identify one action step they will take this week to work toward their targets.

SKILLS CHECKLIST

Appropriate participants will be able to do a urine ketone check using the appropriate technique and record the results.

EVALUATION PLAN

Knowledge will be evaluated by achievement of learning objectives and by responses to questions during the session. Skills will be evaluated by observing a return demonstration of techniques. The ability to apply knowledge will be evaluated by development and implementation of a personal monitoring plan and through program outcome measures.

DOCUMENTATION PLAN

Record class attendance and achieved objectives as appropriate using the Diabetes Self-Management Record, the Participant Follow-up Record, or another form.

SUGGESTED READINGS

Hyperglycemia

American Diabetes Association: Hyperglycemic crisis in diabetes. *Diabetes Care* 27(Suppl 1): S94–S102, 2004

American Diabetes Association Resource Guide 2004: Urine ketone testing. *Diabetes Forecast* 57(1):69–70, 2009

D'Arrigo T: Rocky morning highs? *Diabetes Forecast* 61(7):41–44, 2008

Fowler M: Hyperglycemia crisis in adults: pathophysiology, presentation, pitfalls, and prevention. *Clinical Diabetes* 27:19–23, 2009

Kitabchi AE, Umpierrez GE, Miles JM, Fisher JN: Hyperglycemic crisis in adult patients with diabetes. *Diabetes Care* 32:1335–1343, 2009

Kitabchi AE, Umpierrez GE, Murphy MB, Kreisberg RA: Hyperglycemic crises in adult patients with diabetes. *Diabetes Care* 29:2739–2748, 2006

Kordella T: Diabetic ketoacidosis. *Diabetes Forecast* 58(3):40–43, 2005

Roberts SS: Ketones gone wild. *Diabetes Forecast* 59(12):23–25, 2006

Ruder K: The dawn phenomenon. *Diabetes Forecast* 59(7):63–64, 2006

Seley JJ: Inpatient management of hyperglycemia and diabetes. *Diabetes Spectrum* 21:230–272, 2008

University of New Mexico Diabetes Team: *101 Tips for Improving Your Blood Sugar,* 2nd Edition. Alexandria, VA: American Diabetes Association, 1999

Hypoglycemia

American Diabetes Association: Position statement: Hypoglycemia and employment/licensure. *Diabetes Care* 31(Suppl 1):S94, 2008

American Diabetes Association Resource Guide: Products for treating low blood glucose. *Diabetes Forecast* 81(1):RG50–RG53, 2008

American Diabetes Association Workgroup on hypoglycemia: Defining and reporting hypoglycemia in diabetes. *Diabetes Care* 28:1245–1249, 2005

Briscoe VJ, Davis SN: Hypoglycemia in type 1 and type 2 diabetes: physiology, pathophysiology, and management. *Clinical Diabetes* 24:115–121, 2006

Cryer PE: Insulin therapy and hypoglycemia in type 2 diabetes mellitus. *Insulin* 2:127–133, 2007

Fowler MJ: Hypoglycemia. *Clinical Diabetes* 26:170–173, 2008

Ginde AA, Pallin DJ, Camargo CA: Hospitalization and discharge education for emergency department patients with hypoglycemia. *The Diabetes Educator* 34(4): 683–692, 2008

Pearson T: Glucagon as a treatment of severe hypoglycemia. *The Diabetes Educator* 34:128–134, 2008

Raju B, Arbelaez AM, Brekenridge SM, Cryer PE: Nocturnal hypoglycemia in type 1 diabetes: an assessment of preventive bedtime treatments. *J Clin Endocrinol Metab* 91:2087–2092, 2006

White JR, Jr: The contribution of medications to hypoglycemia unawareness. *Diabetes Spectrum* 20:77–79, 2007

Sick Days/Surgery/Hospitalization

ACE/ADA Task Force on Inpatient Diabetes: American College of Endocrinology and American Diabetes Association consensus statement on inpatient diabetes and glycemic control. *Diabetes Care* 29:1955–1962, 2006

Baker St, Chiang CY, Azjac JD, Bach LA, Herums G, MacIsaac RJ: Outcomes for general medical inpatients with diabetes mellitus and new hyperglycemia. *Med J Aust* 188:340–343, 2008

Baldwin D, Villaneueva G, McNutt R, Bhatnagar S: Eliminating inpatient sliding-scale insulin. *Diabetes Care* 28;1008–1011, 2005

DiNardo M, Donihi AC, DeVita M, Siminerio L, Rao H, Korytkowski M: A nurse-directed protocol for recognition and treatment of hypoglycemia in hospitalized patients. *Practical Diabetology* 24(1):37–40, 2005

DiNardo M, Griffin C, Curll M: Outpatient surgery. *Diabetes Forecast* 58(5):50–54, 2005

SUGGESTED READINGS *continued*

DiNardo M, Weiss MA: Preparing your patients for hospitalization. *Practical Diabetology* 24(4):46–48, 2005

Donaldson S, Villanuueva G, Rondinelli L, Bladwin D: Rush University guidelines and protocols for the management of hyperglycemia in hospitalized patients. *The Diabetes Educator* 32:954–962, 2006

Gifford R, Childs BP: Diabetes care when you're sick. *Diabetes Forecast* 58(2):44–50, 2005

Miller C: Hyperglycemia in the critically ill—not so sweet. *Nursing* 36(10):cc1–cc4, 2006

Moghaissi ES, Korytkowski MT, DiNardo M, Einhorn D, et al.: American Association of Clinical Endocrinologists and American Diabetes Association consensus statement on inpatient glycemic control. *Diabetes Care* 32:1119–1131, 2009

Sadhu AR, Ang AC, Ingram-Drake LA, Martinez DS, et al.: Economic benefits of intensive insulin therapy in critically ill patients: the Targeted Insulin Therapy to Improve Hospital Outcomes (TRIUMPH) project. *Diabetes Care* 31:1556–1561, 2008

Smiley D, Umpierrez GE: Inpatient insulin therapy. *Insulin* 3:152–166, 2008

Spollett GR: Moving toward excellence in the care of hospitalized patients with diabetes. *Diabetes Spectrum*18:18–50, 2005

Spuhler VJ, Veale K: Tighten up glycemic control. *Nursing* 37(5):10–14, 2007

Wilson M, Weinreb J, Soo Hoo GW: Intensive insulin therapy in critical care. *Diabetes Care* 30:1005–1011, 2007

Normal Blood Glucose and Insulin Levels

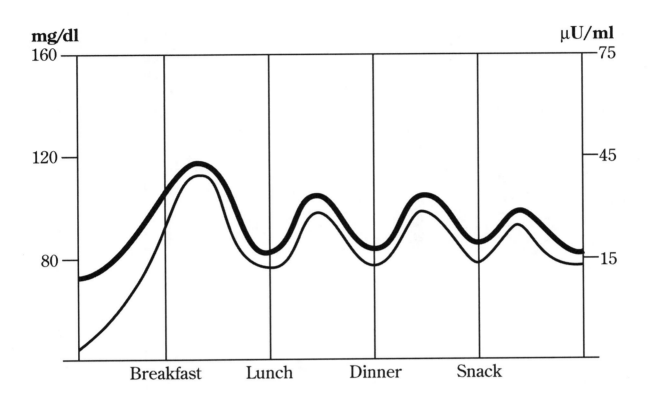

mg/dl   **µU/ml**

— Blood Glucose Level

— Plasma Insulin Level

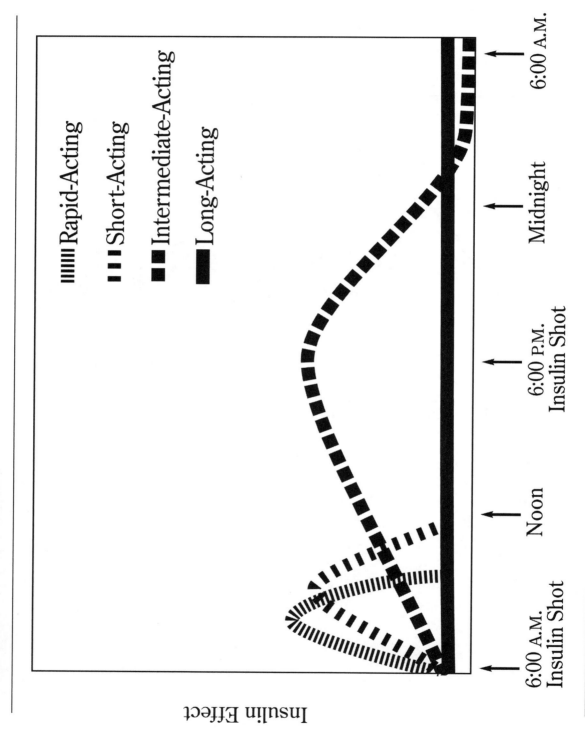

Insulin Action Times

Insulin Effect

IIIII Rapid-Acting
Short-Acting
Intermediate-Acting
Long-Acting

6:00 A.M. Insulin Shot

Noon

6:00 P.M. Insulin Shot

Midnight

6:00 A.M.

⬤ Target Levels

	People Without Diabetes	People with Diabetes
Blood glucose (plasma)		
Before meals	80–125 mg/dl	70–130 mg/dl
After meals*	80–130 mg/dl	Less than 180 mg/dl
A1C	Less than 6%	Less than 7%
Blood pressure	Less than 130/80	Less than 130/80

*2 hours after first bite of food.

➲ Treatment of Low Blood Glucose

If your blood glucose test is:	The amount of food or drink to take is:
Between 50 and 69 mg/dl	15 g carbohydrate (1 carbohydrate serving **or** 1 cup fat-free [skim] milk)
Less than 50 mg/dl	30 g carbohydrate (2 carbohydrate servings)

You should feel better in 10–15 minutes after you treat yourself. If your blood glucose is still less than 70 mg/dl or you don't feel better 10–15 minutes after the treatment, take 1 more carbohydrate serving. Check your blood glucose an hour after the reaction to make sure that your blood glucose has gone above 70 mg/dl and stayed there.

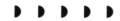

EXAMPLES OF TREATMENTS FOR LOW BLOOD GLUCOSE

(All equal about 15 g carbohydrate or 1 fruit serving)

If your blood glucose is between 50 and 69 mg/dl, take the amount listed. If your blood glucose is less than 50 mg/dl, take twice the amount listed.

Foods	Amount
Orange or apple juice	1/2 cup
Grape or cranberry juice	1/3 cup
Non-diet soft drink	1/2 cup
Honey or corn syrup	1 Tbsp
Sugar packets	3
Life Savers	3–8 pieces
Glucose tablets	3–4 tablets

An additional carbohydrate snack may be needed at night or after exercise to keep your blood glucose above 70 mg/dl.

➲ How to Use Glucagon

Glucagon is an emergency drug that is given as a shot to raise the blood glucose level. It should be given when someone is unable to swallow or is at risk for choking, or in case of a severe insulin reaction or coma.

A prescription is needed to buy glucagon. Glucagon needs to be stored in the refrigerator. Do not mix until you are ready to use it.

To prepare glucagon for injection if you do not use a kit:

1. Remove the flip-off seals from the vial and the syringe.

2. Push the needle of the syringe through the stopper of the vial.

3. Leave the syringe in place. Shake or swirl gently until the glucagon powder dissolves and the liquid becomes clear.

4. Turn the vial upside down and withdraw the entire contents of the mixed glucagon into the syringe.

5. Inject the glucagon in the same way you would insulin, using the buttock, thigh, or arm.

6. Turn the person onto one side or stomach. (Vomiting is common after glucagon.)

7. As soon as the person is alert and not feeling sick, he or she should eat something, because glucagon acts for only a short period of time. First, give some juice or a non-diet soft drink, and then additional carbohydrate.

8. If the person does not wake up within 15 minutes, the dose may be repeated. Call an ambulance.

9. Always call the doctor after an insulin reaction when coma or seizure occurs.

10. Check the package of glucagon periodically to be sure that it hasn't passed the expiration date. It's a good idea to keep an insuin syringe taped to the box so it will be ready.

⤭ Sick-Day Guidelines

These guidelines are for you to use when you have a minor illness, such as a cold, the flu, or an upset stomach. You may also use these guidelines when you have a dental procedure such as a tooth extraction and cannot chew. You will need to talk about sick days with your doctor, nurse, or dietitian—they may have specific guidelines for you.

You will need to check and keep a record of both your blood glucose every 2–4 hours and ketones every 4 hours. Take your temperature about every 4 hours, and keep a record of it, too. If you have a fever, drink some liquid at least once every half hour. If you notice any changes from your usual blood glucose pattern or changes in the way you feel, follow any special guidelines you may have been given.

Call your doctor if you have any of the following:

- rising ketone levels
- ketones for more than 12 hours
- blood glucose levels of greater than 250 mg/dl
- vomiting and/or other unusual symptoms
- high (101.5°F) or rising fever or fever for more than 24 hours

When you call your provider, have your sick-day record nearby so you can report your blood glucose and ketone levels, your insulin dose, and your temperature. (See Handout #4, Sick-Day Record.) If you are unable to reach your doctor quickly, go to the nearest emergency room. Call for help if you are alone and are unable to care for yourself.

If you take insulin, take your usual dose. **Do not omit your insulin.** The stress of being sick can raise your blood glucose level, even if you don't eat. If you take diabetes pills (oral hypoglycemic agents) to manage your blood glucose, take your usual dose.

When you are ill, it is important to eat the same amount of carbohydrate that you normally do. If possible, use your regular diet. If you are having a hard time swallowing, eat soft foods with the same amount of carbohydrate content as your regular diet (see list on page 3). If you can't eat everything, choose carbohydrate foods. If you are sick to your stomach or vomiting, take enough liquids to equal the amount of carbohydrates that you would normally eat. You can space the liquids out over the day. Taking a small sip every 10–15 minutes (for example, during every TV commercial) will help you keep the food or liquid down. The list of liquids and their carbohydrate content on page 3 can help you plan your sick-day diet.

© 2009 American Diabetes Association

SICK-DAY GUIDELINES *continued*

If your blood glucose is higher than 250 mg/dl, you need to drink sugar-free liquids, and you may need extra regular insulin. Your health care team will give you instructions when you call.

Even after you start to feel better, you will still need to check your blood glucose and ketones every 4 hours until you are back to your usual pattern. You may want to keep eating soft and liquid carbohydrates until your appetite is back to normal. If you've been very sick to your stomach, start by having clear liquids (things you can see through, such as broth, tea, regular soft drinks, Jell-O, apple or grape juice, and popsicles). When you can keep these down, move on to full liquids (orange or tomato juice, ice cream, and soup), and then to soft foods (oatmeal, toast, plain cooked vegetables, applesauce, rice, noodles, and crackers).

These guidelines are meant to give you the information you need to take care of yourself when you have a minor illness. Feel free to ask your nurse, doctor, or dietitian any questions you might have about this information.

CARBOHYDRATE CONTENT OF LIQUIDS AND SOFT FOODS

Food Item	Amount	Grams of Carbohydrate
Non-diet soft drink	1/2 cup	15
Orange juice	1/2 cup	15
Apple or pineapple juice	1/2 cup	15
Grape or prune juice	1/3 cup	15
Milk	1 cup	12
Ice cream, vanilla	1/2 cup	15
Cereal, cooked	1/2 cup	15
Gelatin, regular	1/2 cup	20
Sherbet	1/2 cup	30
Popsicle	1	24
Sugar	1 tsp	4
Coffee, tea, bouillon, broth	1 cup	0
Soup, thin creamy	1 cup	15
Soup, thick chunky	1 cup	20
Cream soup, made with water	1 cup	15
Cream soup, made with milk	1 cup	27
Pudding, regular	1/2 cup	30
Pudding, sugar-free	1/2 cup	15
Yogurt, plain or artificially sweetened	1 cup	17
Yogurt, fruit flavored	1 cup	40–60

EXAMPLE: LIQUID REPLACEMENT OF CARBOHYDRATES

Food Item	Amount	Grams of Carbohydrate
Broth	1 cup	0
Jell-O, regular	1/2 cup	20
7-Up, regular	1 cup (8 oz)	30
Ice cream	1/2 cup	10
Tea	1 cup	0
Total		**60**

⬆ Sick-Day Record

Physician Phone _____

Pharmacy Phone _____

Time	Food/Liquids	Insulin/ Medication	Blood Glucose	Urine Ketones	Symptoms (Fever, Nausea, Vomiting, Dizziness, etc.)

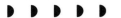

#12	**Stress and Coping**

STATEMENT OF PURPOSE

This session is intended to provide information about stress, how it affects glucose levels, and coping strategies. It is also intended to help participants recognize stressful situations in their lives and develop methods for coping with them.

PREREQUISITES

None.

OBJECTIVES

At the end of this session, participants will be able to:

1. define stress;

2. explain that what is stressful for one person may or may not be stressful for another;

3. explain the body's response to stress;

4. list the effects that stress may have on blood glucose;

5. identify and evaluate personally stressful situations;

6. list the ways in which they currently respond to stress;

7. identify one way to cope with a personally stressful situation.

CONTENT

Developing personal strategies to address psychosocial issues and concerns.

MATERIALS NEEDED

VISUALS PROVIDED	ADDITIONAL
None.	■ Chalkboard and chalk/Board and markers ■ Information about local diabetes and stress-management support groups and other local resources ■ Information about books on coping with diabetes or stress ■ DVD or audiotape about stress or relaxation techniques.

METHOD OF PRESENTATION

Start by introducing yourself and telling what you do. Ask participants to introduce themselves and say how long they have had diabetes. Explain that the purposes of this session are to encourage expression of feelings about stress, to provide information about stress and coping, and to practice relaxation techniques.

Begin by asking how they did with their short-term goal and what they learned from it. Present material in a question/discussion format, using the first question as a starting point. Provide appropriate content outlined below in response. Ask if there are additional questions, and respond, repeating the process for the entire session. Use the questions in the Instructor's Notes section to generate discussion if no questions are forthcoming after a period of silence.

Keeping track of the content discussed in each session, using the Diabetes Self-Management Record, the Participant Follow-up Record, or another form, helps you to evaluate if all needed content has been discussed.

A comfortable environment conducive to relaxation is recommended. Show a DVD, describe a stressful situation, or ask participants to describe stressful experiences to introduce the topic, if desired. End with one of the relaxation exercises or use a relaxation audiotape or DVD.

CONTENT OUTLINE

CONCEPT	DETAIL	INSTRUCTOR'S NOTES
1. Definition of stress	1.1 Stress can occur when: ■ an event produces a strain on a person ■ a person thinks of a situation as challenging or threatening, and physiological responses follow ("fight or flight").	Ask, "What is stress?" Using the board, list participants' definitions of stress. "What questions or concerns do you have regarding stress?"
	1.2 Stress is influenced by both the individual and the environment. Each of us defines what situations we see as stressful.	Ask, "What is stressful for you?" Stress is defined by our perceptions of a situation, not necessarily the reality.
	1.3 Positive as well as negative situations can be stressful, such as marriage, a new job, or retirement.	Point out that life would be pretty dull without stress. We all need challenges to keep life interesting. Ask, "Have you had situations that you viewed at the time as very stressful that you now see as valuable learning experiences?"

CONTENT OUTLINE

CONCEPT	DETAIL	INSTRUCTOR'S NOTES
	1.4 We all experience stress from time to time. Too many stresses or a long, intense, physical response to stress can lead to health problems and will affect both your blood glucose levels and your diabetes self-management efforts. Limiting stressful events or learning to cope with them is important for your health as well as management of your diabetes.	Ask, "What health problems are related to stress? How does feeling stressed affect your ability to manage your diabetes?"
2. Evaluating stressful situations	2.1 When something happens to people, they size up the situation and make a judgment about whether the situation could be good or harmful.	Ask, "How do you decide what is stressful to you?" Ask for examples of situations people may or may not perceive to be stressful (e.g., traffic jam, delayed flight).
	2.2 How stressful an event is depends on how good or harmful we think it is. Other things going on in our lives can change our perception of stress. A particular event may feel very stressful one day and not stressful another day.	
	2.3 Also, our beliefs, values, and goals affect the way we feel about events.	
	2.4 Change of any kind is almost always stressful.	
	2.5 Major life stresses (events such as illness or death in the family) are stressful for almost everyone. Some major life events, such as graduating from school, marriage, the birth of a child, a new job, or retirement, are positive and challenging situations that can cause a stress response.	Have participants identify major stressors in their lives.
	2.6 Minor life stresses are the irritating, frustrating, and distressing demands of daily life, such as being in a traffic jam, arguing with a coworker, tests, phone calls, or doctor visits. Events	Have participants list or name their minor stressors. Point out that what are major stressors for some, are minor for others.

CONTENT OUTLINE

CONCEPT	DETAIL	INSTRUCTOR'S NOTES
	such as holidays or vacations can also be stressful.	
3. How the body responds to stress	3.1 This is sometimes called the fight or flight response.	Ask, "How do you feel physically when you are in a stressful situation? (nervous, sweaty, pounding heart, or queasy stomach)." List on the board.
	3.2 The body prepares itself for stress by sending out stress hormones (catecholamines, glucagon, cortisol, and growth hormone). These hormones cause symptoms you can feel and changes in your behavior.	
	3.3 These stress hormones increase your heart rate and blood pressure, make your breathing rapid and shallow, and may cause your blood glucose to rise.	Ask, "How do you tell the difference between a response to stress and a low blood glucose reaction?" Sometimes the symptoms of stress and hypoglycemia are similar.
	3.4 The levels of glucose and ketones in the blood rise to provide the brain and muscles with important sources of energy. This energy is needed to either fight off stress or run away from it—the fight or flight response.	Ask, "Have you noticed that your blood glucose level is affected by stress?"
	3.5 If this extra energy is not used to fight or run away, it can leave you feeling tense and tired or cause a headache.	Use the list on the board to discuss.
4. Effects of stress on blood glucose	4.1 Stress makes managing diabetes more difficult. In an individual who does not have diabetes, insulin made by the pancreas prevents the blood glucose from rising too high in response to the stress hormones.	Point out that diabetes is both a physical and emotional stressor.
	4.2 In a person with diabetes, the pancreas may not make enough insulin to keep the blood glucose and ketone levels from going too high.	

CONTENT OUTLINE

CONCEPT	DETAIL	INSTRUCTOR'S NOTES
	4.3 In spite of this, research studies have shown that some individuals actually have a drop in blood glucose as an immediate response to stress.	
	4.4 High or fluctuating blood glucose levels may result. If stress is short-lived and repetitive, levels of blood glucose may "bounce" considerably.	
5. Effects of diabetes on stress	5.1 Some people find that they feel less able to deal with stress when they learn they have diabetes. Their energy for coping with other stressors is being used up on diabetes. They may also find that their moods change frequently as well.	Ask, "Have you noticed any changes in the way you handle stress since you learned you have diabetes?"
	5.2 Some people find that they feel less able to deal with stress when their blood glucose level is uneven or too high.	Ask, "Have you noticed any change in the way you handle stress when your blood glucose is high or low?"
6. Coping	6.1 One way to deal with a stressor is to eliminate it. If we can't eliminate the stress, we need to find a way to deal with it. This is called coping.	Ask, "What are ways you cope with stress?" List on the board. Diabetes is a stressor that we cannot eliminate so we need ways to cope with it.
	6.2 Everyone needs a variety of coping skills to use in different situations.	Remind participants of the many different styles and ways of coping using the list on the board.
	6.3 Each person deals with stress in his or her own way. We usually behave in ways that are familiar to us.	Ask, "How do you usually act before, during, and after a stressful situation?"
	6.4 Some of these strategies work and some leave us feeling tense, tired, angry, or sick. Some, such as smoking, drinking or eating too much, or drug abuse, cause other problems.	Many people eat more or differently when they feel stressed. There is nothing wrong with that as a strategy, except most of us make choices that have other negative consequences.
	6.5 Other techniques and ways of dealing with stress can help us to feel more	Many people find that prayer and meditation are helpful

CONTENT OUTLINE

CONCEPT	DETAIL	INSTRUCTOR'S NOTES
	in control, relaxed, and less tense after a stressful event.	strategies for dealing with stress.
	6.6 To determine if a strategy is effective, ask yourself, "Did it work? Did I feel better both temporarily and later? Is this an effective strategy to use in the future?"	People who learn to use varied coping skills and who are flexible in their approach to tough situations deal with stress more easily.
7. Tips for managing stress	7.1 There are three important factors in coping: ■ having enough information ■ feeling in control ■ having the support of others.	Ask, "What helps you cope with stress? What hinders you? What are ways other people help you? Hinder you?" Different coping strategies are effective in different situations.
	7.2 To evaluate your response to stress, you need to recognize your usual behavior in a stressful situation. Sometimes it helps to keep a stress diary for 3–4 days. Jot down stresses, how you react or cope, and how you feel during and after stressful situations. You may also want to write down your blood glucose level or use your monitoring record to note stress. This can help you predict or avoid stressful events, solve the problem causing the stress, or learn other ways to cope with things you can't change.	Encourage the group to brainstorm strategies for coping with stress. List them on the chalkboard. Ask, "Do you think any of these strategies you have not tried would work for you?"
	7.3 Do fewer things and do them better. One technique for managing stress is to reduce the demands on your time. Are you doing too much at work, at home, in the community, with friends? Carefully look at your typical day or week. Are there activities that you can give up? Set priorities for what you need to do. Save some time for yourself every day.	
	7.4 Identify your thoughts about your diabetes or other stress factors in your life. Thoughts can affect	Ask, "What are some thoughts you've had about diabetes? How did your thoughts affect your

CONTENT OUTLINE

CONCEPT	DETAIL	INSTRUCTOR'S NOTES

feelings and behavior. For example, some people view diabetes as a disaster, and some see it more as a challenge.

feelings or your behavior?"

7.5 Sometimes it is healthy to avoid stressful situations until you have time to think about how you might handle them positively.

7.6 Redirect your reaction to stress. Use the energy in some way. Exercise (walking, biking, jogging, or aerobics) is a way to release tension. During exercise, the body makes endorphins, the "feel good" hormones, which counteract the stress hormones.

Exercise is a form of controlled stress on the body. Exercise helps use up the stress hormones. With regular exercise, the body is better able to handle all types of stress. Exercise also increases overall stamina, which helps with long-term stress.

7.7 Many different relaxation techniques can be used to relieve stress: meditation, yoga, biofeedback, deep breathing, and visual imagery. They relieve tension by relaxing muscles. These techniques are usually done in a quiet, comfortable place where you will not be interrupted by the phone or other people. After you practice them there, you can use the same techniques anywhere you are experiencing stress.

7.8 Keep your sense of humor. Laughter releases endorphins and helps you decrease stress.

Ask, "Have you had experiences that were stressful at the time but were humorous later?"

7.9 Sometimes being with people who have similar problems helps to reduce stress. Talking about problems can help you solve them. It has been shown that people who get on-going support for managing diabetes do better in the long run.

Provide information about local support groups, stress management groups, or other local resources.

7.10 Spend your energy on hobbies, keeping a journal, or talking with friends.

CONTENT OUTLINE

CONCEPT	DETAIL	INSTRUCTOR'S NOTES
	7.11 Books are available that discuss coping with diabetes and other stresses.	Provide information about books or other resources that are available.
	7.12 If you want help to handle stress, or feel unable to cope, ask for professional help. Your health care team can help you find resources. It is helpful to find a mental health specialist (social worker, psychologist, psychiatrist, or nurse) who is experienced in working with people with diabetes.	
	7.13 Stress is something we all experience. Learning how to deal with stress effectively can help improve your quality of life and your ability to manage your diabetes.	
	7.14 Choose one thing you will do this week to care for your diabetes.	Close the session by asking participants to identify one action step they will take this week.
8. Relaxation techniques	8.1 Deep breathing, sometimes called diaphragmatic breathing, can be relaxing. When we are tense, we tend to breathe high in our chests in a rapid and shallow fashion. You can use the deep-breathing technique in a variety of stressful situations.	Practice deep breathing and relaxation for 5–10 minutes.

Deep Breathing Exercise

Have participants assume a comfortable position. Have the room quiet, without distractions.

Ask participants to breathe in slowly through the nose for 4 counts and breathe out slowly through the nose for 8 counts.

Ask participants to close their eyes and continue to breathe deeply and slowly.

Say the following in a clear, slow, calm voice: "Now relax all the muscles in your head and neck. You can feel all the tension leaving your face, neck, shoulders, arms, and hands. You are limp and relaxed like a rag doll. Continue to breathe deeply. Now relax your back, abdomen, buttocks, thighs, legs, feet, and toes. You are totally relaxed. Breathe deeply in for 4 counts and out for 8 counts."

8.2 Another method of handling stress is to use visual images to relax the mind and body. Sometimes called a "mental vacation," this technique can leave you refreshed and recharged.

Practice the visual imagery to end the session for 5–10 minutes. Speak slowly and in a relaxing manner as you go through the exercise, pausing between requests.

Visual Imagery Exercise

Ask participants to close their eyes and travel in their minds to a place in their lives that was beautiful and peaceful.

"It can be any place where you feel happy, relaxed, and at peace.

"What do you smell?
"What do you hear?
"What do you feel?
"What do you see?

"Continue relaxing for a few minutes. Let go of these images. Stretch. Open your eyes."

SKILLS CHECKLIST

None.

EVALUATION PLAN

Knowledge will be evaluated by achievement of learning objectives and by responses to questions during the session. Skills will be evaluated by observing a return demonstration of relaxation techniques. The ability to apply knowledge will be evaluated by development and implementation of a personal stress management plan and through program outcome measures.

DOCUMENTATION PLAN

Record class attendance and achieved objectives as appropriate using the Diabetes Self-Management Record, the Participant Follow-up Record, or another form.

SUGGESTED READINGS

D'Arrigo T: Taming the stress monster. *Diabetes Forecast* 59(12):81–85, 2006

Fisher L, Skaff MM, Mullen JT, et al.: Clinical depression versus distress among patients with type 2 diabetes. *Diabetes Care* 30:542–548, 2007

Hieronymus L, Geil P: Stress: finding peace amid the storm. *Diabetes Self-management* 22(2):15–20, 2005

Hill-Briggs F, Gemmell L: Problem solving in diabetes self-management and control: a systematic review of the literature. *The Diabetes Educator* 33:1032–1050, 2007

Lloyd C, Smith J, Weinger K: Stress and diabetes: a review of the links. *Diabetes Spectrum* 18:121–127, 2005

Polonsky WH, Fisher L, Earles J, Dudl RJ, Lees J, Mullan J, Jackson RA: Assessing psychosocial distress in diabetes. *Diabetes Care* 28:626–631, 2005

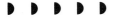

#13	**Personal Health Habits**

STATEMENT OF PURPOSE

This session is intended to provide information about personal health habits that are important for people with diabetes and to suggest ways to incorporate them into daily life. Foot care, skin care, recognizing and preventing infections, and dental care are included.

PREREQUISITES

None.

OBJECTIVES

At the end of this session, participants will be able to:

1. state why it is important for people with diabetes to be particularly attentive to their personal health habits;

2. recognize early signs and symptoms of infection;

3. list two components of dental care;

4. list four preventive foot care practices;

5. list three components of daily skin and foot care;

6. describe how to cut toenails safely;

7. state how to treat minor cuts and bruises;

8. state ways to improve circulation;

9. list symptoms of urogenital infections;

10. state reasons for need of increased frequency of health monitoring;

11. identify one health or complications screening they will do.

CONTENT

Developing personal strategies to promote health and behavior change. Preventing, detecting, and treating acute and chronic complications.

MATERIALS NEEDED

VISUALS PROVIDED

1. Foot Inspection
2. Cutting Your Toenails
3. Urogenital System

Handouts (one per participant)
1. Foot Care Guidelines

ADDITIONAL

■ Pencils for participants
■ Information about local resources for stopping smoking and foot and dental care
■ Mirror, samples of foot lotions, foot care instruments, wound care products, other foot care products
■ Monofilament to test sensation

METHOD OF PRESENTATION

Start by introducing yourself and telling what you do. Ask participants to introduce themselves. Explain that the purposes of this session are to provide information about health habits and to develop a personal foot care plan. One approach for teaching foot care is to have participants remove their shoes so that they can practice the skills they need to care for their feet.

Present material in a question/discussion format, using the first question as a starting point. Provide appropriate content outlined below in response. Ask if there are additional questions, and respond, repeating the process for the entire session. Use the questions in the Instructor's Notes section to generate discussion if no questions are forthcoming after a period of silence.

Keeping track of the content discussed in each session, using the Diabetes Self-Management Record, the Participant Follow-up Record, or another form, helps you to evaluate if all needed content has been discussed.

CONTENT OUTLINE

CONCEPT	DETAIL	INSTRUCTOR'S NOTES
1. Health habits	1.1 Health habits are very important for *everyone,* with or without diabetes.	Ask, "What questions or concerns do you have about your general health or health habits and diabetes?"
	1.2 Health habits include taking care of yourself physically and emotionally, such as getting adequate sleep, nutrition, and exercise. Other health habits include foot, skin, and	Ask, "What are some things you do to take care of your health?" List these on the board and discuss.

CONTENT OUTLINE

CONCEPT	DETAIL	INSTRUCTOR'S NOTES

	dental care, and screening for other health conditions.	
	1.3 It is important to obtain medical care at appropriate intervals. Don't neglect the other areas of your health.	Tell all health care providers that you have diabetes. Point out that certain cancers (e.g., colon and breast) occur more frequently among people with type 2 diabetes. These are highly treatable if found early and can be detected through routine screening.
2. Special care when you have diabetes	2.1 Having diabetes means paying special attention to some health habits.	
	2.2 Smoking is particularly harmful when you have diabetes. The combination of diabetes and smoking greatly increases the risk for cardiovascular disease and other problems.	Ask, "Is anyone interested in quitting at this time?" Provide a list of smoking cessation programs in your area and offer information on available over-the-counter or prescription aids.
	2.3 Alcohol can affect blood glucose and blood fat (triglyceride) levels.	Refer to Outline #5, *Planning Meals* (p.69), for more information.
3. Infections	3.1 Infections are more common and more serious in people who have diabetes.	Ask, "What questions or concerns do you have about infections?"
	3.2 The signs of infection are pain, redness, warmth of area, swelling, discharge, and fever.	Ask, "What signs would help you recognize an infection?"
	3.3 The first sign of infection may be elevated blood glucose levels.	Infections raise blood glucose levels; they also occur more often when blood glucose levels are high.
	3.4 Infections can occur without open cuts or injuries.	
	3.5 Call your health care team right away if you see any signs of infection.	

CONTENT OUTLINE

CONCEPT	DETAIL	INSTRUCTOR'S NOTES
4. Importance of dental care	4.1 People with diabetes are more prone to tooth decay and periodontal (gum) disease.	Ask, "What questions do you have about dental care? How do you care for your teeth?" Elevated glucose levels support bacterial growth.
	4.2 The bacteria that cause tooth decay have a higher chance of surviving when blood glucose levels are high. Having a dry mouth facilitates the build-up of plaque and bacteria.	
	4.3 Gum diseases include gingivitis and periodontis. Gingivitis is the mildest form and causes the gum to become red, swollen, and bleed easily.	The word periodontal means around the tooth. Both are related to plaque build-up. Brushing and flossing can help gingivitis.
	4.4 Over time, plaque may spread and grow under the gum line. Toxins released by the plaque cause the teeth and gums to become inflamed so that the tissues that support the teeth are broken down. The gums separate from the teeth forming pockets that can become infected. If untreated, the tissue and bones are destroyed and the teeth can become loose and may have to be pulled.	Antibiotics are often prescribed to treat periodontal disease. Treating periodontal disease can lower A1C levels.
	4.5 Periodontal disease can increase insulin resistance which results in high blood glucose levels. Over time, these high glucose levels increase your risk for long-term complications.	People with periodontal disease are two to four times more likely to have elevated glucose levels and have a three times greater risk for long-term complications.
	4.6 If you have periodontal disease, you may be referred to a periodontist, who specializes in gum disease.	More information is available as www.perio.org.
	4.7 Signs of gum disease are: ■ red, swollen, or tender gums or pain in your mouth ■ bleeding while brushing, flossing, or eating hard food ■ gums that are pulling away from	

CONTENT OUTLINE

CONCEPT	DETAIL	INSTRUCTOR'S NOTES

the teeth, causing the teeth to look longer
- loose or separating teeth
- pus between your gums and teeth
- sores in your mouth
- persistant bad breath or taste
- a change in the way your teeth or dentures fit together when you bite.

	4.8 Brush your teeth at least twice a day using a toothbrush and techniques that your dentist recommends. Note any bleeding or sores on gums.	Infected teeth can raise glucose levels. Dentures also need to be cleaned after every meal.
	4.9 Have regular dental exams. Be sure to tell your dentist that you have diabetes. Schedule your appointments after meals to decrease the risk of an insulin reaction.	See a dentist at least twice yearly or at recommended intervals.
	4.10 If you can't eat your regular meals because of dental work or tooth problems, use your sick-day plan for a soft or liquid diet.	
5. Importance of foot care	5.1 Decreased circulation causes slow healing of injuries.	Ask, "What questions or concerns do you have about caring for your feet? What do you do to take care of your feet?"
	5.2 Peripheral neuropathy (diabetic nerve disease in the leg and foot) causes decreased sensation and puts the foot at risk for undetected trauma.	Some people with diabetes have little or no feeling in their feet. They can injure or burn their feet without noticing it.
	5.3 Early discovery and treatment of foot injuries or other problems can prevent serious complications. Untreated problems may lead to infection and potentially to amputation. Most amputations from diabetes are preventable with early detection and treatment.	Two of the most important things participants can do are to get into the habit of looking at their feet each day and to seek prompt treatment for problems or changes.

CONTENT OUTLINE

CONCEPT	DETAIL	INSTRUCTOR'S NOTES
6. Prevention of foot problems	6.1 Wear shoes and socks that fit. Poorly fitting shoes are the most common cause of foot trauma. Socks made of a blend of fibers or wool allow feet to breathe. Change your shoes at least once during the day.	Ask, "What do you do to prevent foot problems? What questions do you have about choosing shoes and socks?" All-cotton socks retain moisture. Special "diabetic socks" are not necessary, but may offer a wider top to fit larger feet and legs.
	6.2 Shop for shoes in the afternoon when feet are larger. Buy shoes that have room for your toes to wiggle. Avoid shoes that are too tight. Try on both shoes and buy for the bigger foot. Shoes that don't fit well can lead to sores, blisters, and calluses. Break in new shoes slowly by wearing them for 1–2 hours a day at first.	If prescribed, special shoes are a covered benefit for participants with Medicare, as well as other insurance providers.
	6.3 When taking shoes off, look for areas of redness. These are most often caused by improper fit.	Ask participants to remove shoes and socks. The instructor should, even if participants do not.
	6.4 Shake out or feel inside your shoes for foreign objects before putting them on.	Demonstrate. Ask participants to check their shoes.
	6.5 Avoid heating pads, hot water bottles, and microwavable warmers. These can cause burns.	
	6.6 Avoid going barefoot indoors and outdoors.	Shoes help prevent injury. Hard-soled slippers are recommended.
	6.7 Wear wool socks to keep feet warm and waterproof shoes or boots for outdoor winter activities.	
	6.8 At the beach, avoid walking barefoot on hot sand or shells. Put sunscreen on tops of feet.	Beach sandals and swim shoes (e.g., Aquasocks) are available at stores that stock beach supplies.
	6.9 Take your shoes off when you see your provider as a reminder to check your feet.	Ask, "When did your provider last examine your feet?"

CONTENT OUTLINE

CONCEPT	DETAIL	INSTRUCTOR'S NOTES
	6.10 Your provider can test for sensation using a small device called a monofilament. This should be done at least once a year. You can also check at home. Ask your provider if there are any areas that are numb or to which you need to pay extra attention.	Encourage participants to ask for monofilament testing annually. Demonstrate the test with a monofilament. Monofilaments are available for home use from several sources.
7. Daily care of feet	7.1 Wash daily with mild soap and warm water and dry completely.	Ask, "What can you do to care for your feet each day?" Suggest times for foot care (during bath or dressing).
	7.2 Look at tops and bottoms of your feet for fissures, cracks, calluses, red spots, cuts, bruises, etc. Treat appropriately.	Demonstrate. Pass mirror for participants to use if they can't see bottoms of feet. Use Visual #1, Foot Inspection.
	7.3 If skin is dry, use lotion to keep feet soft. If feet sweat a lot, use powder. Lotions with a lot of perfume contain alcohol.	Show products. Care is particularly important if cracks or fissures are present. Soaking feet is drying for skin. Lanolin-based lotions are often recommended.
	7.4 Corns and calluses may be related to shoe fit. Remove calluses by gently rubbing with an emery board or pumice stone. Work on callused areas over time.	Point out corns, calluses, and other abnormalities during the demonstration.
	7.5 Treat corns or bunions by padding. Do not use caustic corn removers or sharp instruments.	These chemicals can burn your skin. Show appropriate products.
	7.6 Trim toenails to follow the curve of your toe and be even with the end of the toe. Nails are softer and easier to cut after a bath.	Show tools for cutting nails. Nails that have fungal infections or are ingrown should be cut by a professional. Use Visual #2, Cutting Your Toenails.
	7.7 If toes overlap, sheepskin or cotton placed between can prevent blisters.	
8. Other foot care	8.1 Treat small cuts by washing, rinsing well, drying, and covering	Show examples of tape, dressings, ointment, and antiseptics.

CONTENT OUTLINE

CONCEPT	DETAIL	INSTRUCTOR'S NOTES
	with sterile dressing held in place with nonallergenic tape.	
	8.2 Avoid iodine, merthiolate, mercurochrome, or liniment. These can burn skin, and their colors hide signs of infection.	
	8.3 If cuts do not show signs of healing within 2 days, contact your provider.	
	8.4 See a foot care specialist for continuing care of foot problems.	Refer as needed.
9. Decreased circulation to extremities	9.1 The signs and symptoms of decreased circulation are decreased hair growth, change in color (blue or red when standing, blanched when elevated), cold feet, and swollen feet and ankles.	
	9.2 Some clothing can further decrease circulation. Avoid tight clothing such as girdles. Make sure knee-high stockings do not cut off blood flow. The type with wide elastic tops generally allows more circulation. If you wear support stockings, make sure they fit without wrinkles.	Distribute Handout #1, Foot Care Guidelines. Help participants complete the Foot Care Plan portion. Ask, "When will you do your foot care?"
	9.3 Circulation (blood flow) can be improved (stop smoking or begin an exercise program including walking and foot exercises).	Demonstrate some foot exercises and have participants practice.
10. Urogenital infections	10.1 Symptoms include vulvovaginal itching and burning, urethral or penile discharge, frequent urination with urgency and pain, difficulty in initiating stream, fever, bloody urine, and suprapubic and back pain.	Use Visual #3, Urogenital System, to show the relationship between the kidneys, ureters, bladder, and urethra. Use words participants understand.
	10.2 Cultures of urine, discharge, and sometimes blood are needed to determine appropriate treatment.	
	10.3 Prevent bladder infections by urinating often, drinking fluids,	Empty the bladder every 2 hours while awake.

CONTENT OUTLINE

CONCEPT	DETAIL	INSTRUCTOR'S NOTES

| | and keeping blood glucose levels in your target range. | |

10.4 Do not ignore small problems; they may become big problems.

11. Regular examinations	11.1 Diabetes exams and tests: ■ every visit—foot and blood pressure check ■ every 3–6 months—A1C level ■ yearly—foot examination, tests for lipids, and microalbuminuria as appropriate.	Emphasize that a diabetes checkup may not assess total physical health. Participants still need routine screening for other health problems. Ask, "When did you last have these done?"
	11.2 Dilated eye exam: ■ adults and adolescents with type 1—within 3–5 years of diagnosis and annually thereafter ■ people with type 2—at diagnosis and annually thereafter	This can prevent blindness from retinopathy. Stress this point and that the pupils must be dilated by an eye specialist. It is not sufficient for your provider or an optician to examine the eyes during an office visit. Ask, "When was your last dilated eye examination?"
	11.3 **Before** becoming pregnant, have an exam by a diabetes doctor and obstetrician. Tight blood glucose management is necessary **before** and during pregnancy.	Close glucose regulation before conception and in early weeks of pregnancy will decrease risk of birth defects.
	11.4 Write down questions and problems before the visit, and bring the list with you.	
	11.5 Be sure to tell each of your providers that you have diabetes.	
12. Sleep	12.1 Sleep is an important part of good health. Having diabetes can affect your ability to sleep because of getting up to urinate or because of low blood glucose reactions.	Ask, "Do you ever have trouble getting enough sleep? What disturbs your sleep? What helps you sleep?" Write these on the board and discuss.
	12.2 Sleep apnea is a more serious problem. Your throat muscles relax and your airway closes. This wakes	Over a third of people with type 2 diabetes have sleep apnea. Sleep apnea increases the risk

CONTENT OUTLINE

CONCEPT	DETAIL	INSTRUCTOR'S NOTES
	you up briefly to take a breath, which disturbs your sleep pattern.	for heart attacks and mortality. For more information, go to www.sleepapnea.com.
	12.3 Some signs of sleep apnea are: ■ snoring loudly ■ kicking during sleep and other signs of restlessness ■ waking up choking and gasping ■ sleeping during the day, fatigued or lacking in energy ■ waking up not feeling rested, no matter how long you sleep.	This is not the same as Restless Leg Syndrome, which is also common among people with diabetes. Men who are over 45, obese, and have a neck circumference over 17 inches are at a higher risk for sleep apnea.
	12.4 Sleep apnea is diagnosed by a sleep study. Mild sleep apnea may be treated with decongestants or antihistamines and strategies to improve sleep patterns. Moderate or severe sleep apnea is treated with a CPAP device you wear while sleeping. This device uses pressure to keep your airway open.	CPAP stands for continuous positive airway pressure. Although it does take getting used to, most people say they feel better with improved sleep. Weight loss can also help with sleep apnea.
	12.5 Some ideas to improve sleep apnea are to: ■ go to bed and get up at about the same time every day ■ avoid getting overly tired ■ create a restful environment ■ use your bedroom only for sleeping and sex ■ avoid alcohol and stimulants ■ avoid naps during the day.	Refer to the list on the board.
	12.6 Choose one thing you will do this week to care for your diabetes.	Close the session by asking participants to identify one action step they will take this week.

SKILLS CHECKLIST

Each participant will be able to inspect feet, cut toenails safely, and treat small cuts and mild injuries.

EVALUATION PLAN

Knowledge will be evaluated by achievement of learning objectives and by responses to questions during the session. Skills will be evaluated by observing a demonstration of techniques. The ability to apply knowledge will be evaluated by the development and implementation of a personal foot care plan, through necessary screenings, and through program outcome measures.

DOCUMENTATION PLAN

Record class attendance and achieved objectives as appropriate using the Diabetes Self-Management Record, the Participant Follow-up Record, or another form.

SUGGESTED READINGS

Balay JL: Nutrition for dental health. *Diabetes Self-Management* 24(2):6–8, 2007

Bloomgarden ZT: The diabetic foot. *Diabetes Care* 21:372–376, 2008

Calianno C, Holton SJ: Fighting the triple threat of lower extremity ulcers. *Nursing* 37(3):57–63, 2007

Chasens ER: Obstructive sleep apnea, daytime sleepiness, and type 2 diabetes. *The Diabetes Educator* 33:475–482, 2007

Chasens ER: Understanding sleep in persons with diabetes. *The Diabetes Educator* 33:435–441, 2007

Christiana JR: Socks step out. *Diabetes Forecast* 59(9):66–68, 2006

Clayton W JR, Elasy TA: A review of the pathophysiology, classification, and treatment of foot ulcers in diabetic patients. *Clinical Diabetes* 27:52–57, 2009

D'Arrigo T: Beyond a great smile. *Diabetes Forecast* 60(13):60–62, 2007

Fain J: Understanding skin care. *The Diabetes Educator* 31:108–111, 2005

Kesselman P: Diabetic foot pathology. *Practical Diabetology* 25(2):41–43, 2006

Lasho DJ: Periodontal disease in the diabetic patient. *Practical Diabetology* 27(3):14–16, 2008

Neithercott T: The truth about pedicures. *Diabetes Forecast* 61(7):46–49, 2008

Reddy SG, Meffert JJ, Kraus EW, Becker LE: Dermatologic conditions in patients with diabetes. *Practical Diabetology* 27(2):6–10, 2008

Roberts SS: Foot care: what you need to know. *Diabetes Forecast* 58(5):35–37, 2005

Rudder K: A good night's sleep. *Diabetes Forecast* 59(10):56–59, 2006

Scheffler NM: All about wound care. *Diabetes Forecast* 59(5):48–51, 2006

Scheffler NM: Foot Surgery. *Diabetes Forecast* 58(12):52–54, 2005

Sieggreen MV: Stepping up care for diabetic foot ulcers. *Nursing* 35(10):36–43, 2005

Spollett GR, Crape CA: Dental issues in patients with diabetes. *Practical Diabetology* 60(2):28–31, 2007

Sweitzer SM, Fann SA, Borg TK, Buynes JW, Yost MJ: What is the future of diabetic wound care? *The Diabetes Educator* 32:197–212, 2006

⬤ Foot Inspection

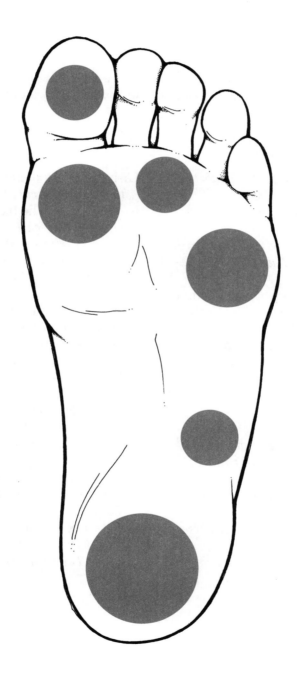

➲ Cutting Your Toenails

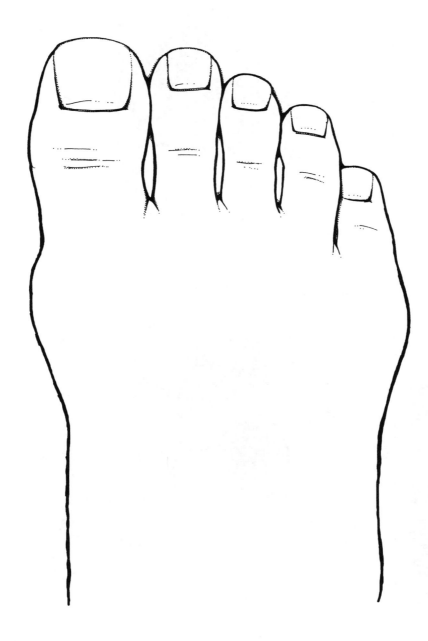

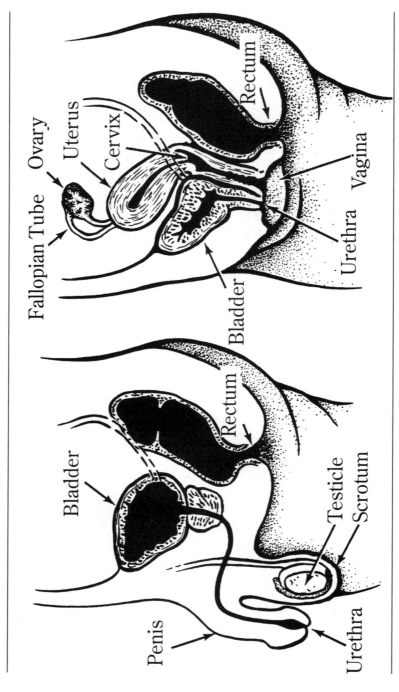

Urogenital System

Fallopian Tube
Ovary
Uterus
Cervix
Rectum
Vagina
Urethra
Bladder

Bladder
Rectum
Penis
Testicle
Scrotum
Urethra

© 2009 American Diabetes Association

➲ Foot Care Guidelines

INSPECTION

- ■ Look at your feet each day in a place with good light. Use a mirror if you can't bend over to see the bottoms of your feet. If looking at your feet is hard for you, ask a family member to help.
- ■ Look for dry places and cracks in the skin, especially between the toes and around the heel.
- ■ Check for ingrown toenails, corns, calluses, swelling, sores, or places that are red or pale. If corns, calluses, or other problems persist, see a foot doctor (podiatrist).

BATHING

- ■ Wash your feet daily in warm—not hot—water. Before you put your feet into the water, test the temperature with your wrist or elbow to prevent burning your feet.
- ■ Do not soak your feet, because soaking will dry your skin.
- ■ Use a mild soap and rinse well. Gently dry your feet with a soft towel, making sure to dry between the toes.
- ■ Cracks in the skin are places where infection can enter. To soften dry feet and keep the skin from cracking, use a mild cream or lotion, except between your toes where athlete's foot often occurs.
- ■ If your feet sweat a lot, lightly dust with foot powder. Wear socks that are mostly cotton, and change them if they become damp.

TOENAILS

- ■ Cut your toenails after bathing, when they are soft and easy to trim.
- ■ Cut or file nails to follow the natural curve of your toe. Avoid cutting nails shorter than the ends of your toes. File sharp corners and rough edges of toenails with an emery board so they don't cut the toes next to them.
- ■ Don't use sharp objects to poke or dig under the toenail or around the cuticle.
- ■ Ingrown toenails or nails that are thick or tend to split when cut need to be cared for by a foot care specialist.

FOOT CARE GUIDELINES *continued*

CORNS AND CALLUSES

■ After washing your feet, **gently** rub any corns and callused areas with an emery board or pumice stone to control buildup.

■ Avoid using do-it-yourself corn or callus removers. These can cause burns and may harm healthy skin around the problem area.

■ Never cut your corns and calluses with a razor blade. This can lead to infections.

■ Use pads on corns to reduce pressure.

SOCKS

■ Socks should fit well and be free of seams and darns that might reduce the blood supply.

■ Wear socks that are a blend of natural fibers to allow skin to breathe.

SHOES

■ Wear shoes or hard-soled slippers to cover and protect your feet. Avoid going barefoot, and use common sense about wearing sandals. Thong sandals can cause blisters between your toes, and you can step out of them and injure your feet.

■ At the beach, avoid walking barefoot on hot sand or shells, wear water shoes, and put sunscreen on the tops of your feet.

■ Choose the shoes that are most comfortable for your activities each day.

■ Before you put on your shoes, shake them out and then carefully feel inside for stones or rough spots that might hurt your feet.

■ The top part of the shoe should be soft and pliable. The lining should not have ridges, wrinkles, or seams. The toe area should be round and high to fit your toes. You may need to see an orthotic specialist for inserts, for special shoes, or to have your shoes adapted to your feet.

■ Shop for shoes in midafternoon when feet are larger. Buy shoes that feel good and have room for all the toes to wiggle and be in their natural place. Avoid shoes that are too tight or pinch. Try on both shoes, and if one of your feet is slightly larger than the other, buy for the bigger foot. Shoes that don't fit well can lead to sores, blisters, and calluses.

FOOT CARE GUIDELINES *continued*

- ■ If your feet are numb, you can't rely on how shoes feel to know if you have a good fit. Shop at a store where they fit your shoes or make an outline of each foot from stiff paper to insert in shoes when you are shopping.
- ■ Break in new shoes slowly by wearing them for 1–2 hours a day at first. Change your shoes at least once during the day.

CIRCULATION (BLOOD FLOW)

- ■ Exercise each day.
- ■ If you smoke, plan to quit or cut down.
- ■ Wear wool socks and warm, waterproof shoes or boots for outside winter activities.
- ■ Avoid heating pads, hot water bottles, or microwavable warmers. These can burn the skin. Instead, use wool socks to keep your feet warm.

TREATMENT OF INJURIES

- ■ Look at your feet if you stumble or bump a hard object to be sure that there is no damage.
- ■ If your foot is hurt, don't keep walking on it—that can cause more damage.
- ■ Treat blisters, cuts, and scratches right away. Wash with soap and water and apply a mild antiseptic. Never use strong chemicals such as boric acid, epsom salts, or any antiseptic that contains a dye. Remember, opening blisters yourself can lead to infections.
- ■ Cover all injuries with an adhesive bandage or dry sterile dressing.
- ■ If sores do not begin to heal within 2 days, or look worse after the first day, call your doctor.

FOOT CARE GUIDELINES *continued*

Foot Care Plan

_____ _____
Name   Date

It is especially important for me to:

_____

_____

_____

_____

_____

_____

Referral

Podiatrist:

Other:

Reason for referral:

Signature _____

Phone _____ Hours _____

| #14 | Long-Term Complications |

▶ ▶ ▶ ▶ ▶

STATEMENT OF PURPOSE

This session is intended to provide information about the chronic complications that can occur with diabetes.

PREREQUISITES

It is recommended that each participant have basic knowledge about diabetes and self-care, from either personal experience or from attending previous sessions. Readiness to learn about complications should be carefully assessed before this content is presented.

OBJECTIVES

At the end of this session, participants will be able to:

1. state that blood glucose and blood pressure control reduces risks for complications;

2. describe the major consequences of small blood vessel disease;

3. describe the symptoms that may occur with diabetic retinopathy and with diabetic nephropathy;

4. list treatments for diabetic retinopathy and diabetic nephropathy;

5. state the value of annual ophthalmologic and renal function examinations;

6. describe what happens to large blood vessels in arteriosclerosis;

7. list the risk factors and ways to decrease the risk for developing arteriosclerosis;

8. list consequences and symptoms of diabetic neuropathy;

9. list one treatment for neuropathy;

10. state that research into treatment for complications continues;

11. identify fears and concerns about the long-term complications;

12. identify strategies to reduce personal risk factors;

13. schedule screening for complications as recommended.

CONTENT

Preventing, detecting, and treating chronic complications.

MATERIALS NEEDED

VISUALS PROVIDED   **ADDITIONAL**

1. Relationship of A1C to Risk of Complications
2. Circulatory System
3. Normal Eye
4. Microaneurysms
5. Proliferative Retinopathy
6. Retinal Detachment
7. Normal Kidney
8. Large-Vessel Disease
9. Nervous System
10. Wound Healing

■ Information about local support groups and local resources for those with complications
■ Information about local smoking cessation, weight loss, and exercise programs

Handouts (one per participant)
1. Resources for Diabetes Complications

METHOD OF PRESENTATION

Start by introducing yourself and telling what you do. Ask participants to introduce themselves. Explain that the purpose of this session is to provide an overview of the long-term complications of diabetes so participants can identify symptoms early and seek treatment if complications occur.

Begin by asking participants how they did with their short-term goal and what they learned from it. Present material in a question/discussion format, using the first question as a starting point. Provide appropriate content outlined below in response. Ask if there are additional questions, and respond, repeating the process for the entire session. Use the questions in the Instructor's Notes section to generate discussion if no questions are forthcoming after a period of silence. Keeping track of the content discussed in one session, using the Diabetes Self-Management Record, the Participant Follow-up Record, or another form, helps you to evaluate if all needed content has been discussed.

When presenting this material, it is important to be sensitive to the participants' readiness to hear about complications and to their emotional responses to this difficult topic.

CONTENT OUTLINE

CONCEPT	DETAIL	INSTRUCTOR'S NOTES
1. Occurrence of long-term complications	1.1 In this session, you will learn some of the long-term problems people with diabetes can face, and you will	State that you understand this is a difficult topic to talk about, but it is needed so that they can

CONTENT OUTLINE

CONCEPT	DETAIL	INSTRUCTOR'S NOTES
	be given information about prevention, symptoms, and treatment options.	identify symptoms early and get treatment. Ask, "What questions or concerns do you have about complications?"
	1.2 Even though it may be hard to hear this information, you need to know for three reasons: ■ to make informed decisions about your blood glucose and other targets ■ to do all you can to prevent the complications ■ to recognize early signs or obtain screening for complications so they can be treated early.	Emphasize that causes for the development of complications are unclear, but are related to: ■ duration of diabetes ■ persistant hyperglycemia and hypertension ■ type of diabetes (to some extent).
	1.3 People with both type 1 and type 2 diabetes are at risk for all of the long-term complications.	Ask, "What experiences have you had? Have you known people with complications? What was their experience?"
	1.4 Some people get none of the complications, while others get one or more than one.	
	1.5 Evidence shows that some of the problems can be delayed or prevented with improved glucose and blood pressure levels. You are giving yourself the best chance for a long, healthy life by keeping these levels as close to the normal range as is safe for you. There are no guarantees, but you are greatly increasing your chances to prevent or delay these complications.	Review results of the Diabetes Control and Complications Trial (DCCT) and the United Kingdom Prospective Diabetes Study (UKPDS) from Outline #11, *Managing Blood Glucose* (p. 231). Show Visual #1, Relationship of A1C to Risk of Complications.
	1.6 Some of the problems are reversible or their progress can be slowed, if they are found and treated early.	The experiences of others with complications don't have to happen to you.
	1.7 There is good news: more and better treatments are now available. This is also an area of great research interest.	
2. Systems affected	2.1 Complications affect various systems of your body.	

CONTENT OUTLINE

CONCEPT	DETAIL	INSTRUCTOR'S NOTES
	2.2 In the large-vessel circulatory system, the heart, legs, feet, and brain are affected.	
	2.3 In the small-vessel circulatory system, the kidneys and eyes are affected.	
	2.4 In both the peripheral and autonomic nervous systems, many functions are affected.	This does not mean that you feel nervous.
3. Circulatory system	3.1 You have large and small blood vessels in your body. Small blood vessels are called capillaries. Veins and arteries are large blood vessels.	Use Visual #2, Circulatory System. Arteries carry blood and oxygen from your heart and lungs out to your cells. Veins then bring the blood back to get more oxygen and other needed nutrients.
	3.2 The large vessels move large amounts of blood into and out of your heart and lungs and supply blood to the arms, legs, and brain.	
	3.3 The small vessels provide blood to the eyes, kidneys, fingers, and toes.	
	3.4 In diabetes, both large and small vessels can be affected. Eye and kidney damage occur when the small vessels are affected. Heart and vascular damage occur when the large vessels are affected.	There are both macrovascular and microvascular complications of diabetes.
4. Eyes (diabetic retinopathy)	4.1 When you look at an object, the image is sent from the lens through the vitreous (area filled with clear gel-like fluid) to the retina.	Ask, "What questions/concerns do you have about diabetic eye disease?" Use Visual #3, Normal Eye. Point out that blurred vision is often a symptom of high blood glucose and that the vision will return to normal with lower blood glucose levels.
	4.2 The retina is a thin membrane at the back of the eye that receives the image.	Use the analogy of a camera: the retina is the film receiving the image from the lens.

CONTENT OUTLINE

CONCEPT	DETAIL	INSTRUCTOR'S NOTES

4.3 It is possible to look into the eye using an ophthalmoscope. The optic nerve, many small blood vessels, and the macula (the center of vision of the retina) can be seen.

Point out the blood vessels, optic nerve, and macula on Visual #3, Normal Eye.

4.4 In diabetes, weak spots develop in the walls of the smallest blood vessels. Balloon-like outpouchings occur (microaneurysms). This is *diabetic retinopathy.*

Use Visual #4, Microaneurysms. Blurred vision from elevated glucose levels is not the same as retinopathy.

4.5 These areas can leak, and fluid escapes. As these areas heal, scarring occurs. If the swelling occurs in the center of the retina, vision may be impaired. This is called macular edema.

This is nonproliferative retinopathy and may occur without any change in vision.

4.6 This interruption of the circulation causes formation of new, smaller blood vessels (neovascularization) in an attempt to provide blood flow to these areas.

This is called proliferative retinopathy. Use Visual #5, Proliferative Retinopathy.

4.7 These new vessels are very fragile and can easily break. When this happens, blood leaks into the space between the retina and the vitreous (the clear gel that fills the eyeball) and sometimes out into the vitreous itself.

4.8 When a hemorrhage occurs into the gel, it is like looking through a pool of blood or a spider web. This blood and the vision may eventually clear or partially clear. The scarring that results also causes some loss of vision. If bleeding occurs in or near the macula, visual loss can be severe; if untreated, total blindness may result.

The macula is the part of the eye you use to see things clearly. The other parts of the retina are used to see things around you and in the dark.

4.9 If scars develop, they may form fibrous attachments between the retina and vitreous. If these scars contract, the retina can be torn away from the back surface of the eye.

Use Visual #6, Retinal Detachment.

CONTENT OUTLINE

CONCEPT	DETAIL	INSTRUCTOR'S NOTES
	This is *retinal detachment*—if this happens, there is a rapidly developing partial or complete loss of vision. People have described this as being like a torn curtain in the eye, or dark streaks, or a black curtain coming across the eye. If this happens to you, SEE AN OPHTHALMOLOGIST OR GO TO THE EMERGENCY ROOM!	Blurred vision often occurs with high or low blood glucose levels. This is not related to detached retina. The areas where the retina pulls away cause blank spots in vision. *Immediate* care is necessary.
	4.10 Treatment for proliferative retinopathy consists of laser therapy to the retina. The laser produces a finely focused beam of light to cause microscopic-sized burns on the retina. This slows or prevents the development of abnormal new blood vessels or causes their disappearance. The laser can also be used to destroy nests of new blood vessels, which is especially important if they are bleeding. Freezing (cryotherapy) portions of the eye that the laser cannot reach can also stop new vessel growth and bleeding.	Point out that laser therapy is not painful, but it is uncomfortable. Laser therapy may need to be repeated at intervals throughout a lifetime with diabetes. Ask, "Have you had or known anyone who had laser therapy? What was your/their experience?"
	4.11 Glasses do not help to restore the vision lost in retinopathy. Glasses can only help when the problem is in the lens of the eye, and in retinopathy the problem is with the retina.	Use the analogy of the camera again; if the film is fogged, changing the lens won't help.
	4.12 There may be no symptoms at the time damage is occurring. The only way to find out is to have a dilated eye exam by an eye specialist who can look into the back of your eye and see very early changes.	Emphasize that this eye exam is more than just a refraction or glaucoma test. It must be done with the pupils dilated. Ask, "When did you last have a dilated eye exam?"
	4.13 Treatment at an early stage can often prevent severe visual loss and blindness. Regular eye exams are one of the most important things people with diabetes can do to protect their eyesight. Keeping	People with type 1 diabetes should get an exam within 5 years after diagnosis and yearly thereafter; people with type 2 diabetes should get an exam at diagnosis and yearly

CONTENT OUTLINE

CONCEPT	DETAIL	INSTRUCTOR'S NOTES
	your blood pressure within recommended targets is another way to help avoid retinopathy.	thereafter. Exams may be recommended less often (every 2 or 3 years) for those with no abnormalities. An exam is also needed as part of preconception care.
	4.14 Diabetes is the leading cause of new blindness in this country, but most of it is preventable. In the DCCT, risk for retinopathy was decreased by 76% with intensive therapy. The UKPDS demonstrated reductions in risk for visual loss with improved glucose and blood pressure levels.	Provide information about eye specialists in your area and/or encourage patients to seek a referral. Retinopathy is closely related to duration of diabetes.
5. Eyes (cataracts and glaucoma)	5.1 Another problem that can occur is cataracts. These have nothing to do with circulation, but are the result of the accumulation of sugars in the lens of the eye. This causes swelling and clouding.	There are two kinds of cataracts. Senile cataracts are not preventable and have a different cause. Metabolic cataracts are often seen in younger people (<40) with diabetes. Surgery is the main treatment.
	5.2 This is often an early complication of diabetes.	
	5.3 Glaucoma is a condition that leads to an increase in the pressure in the eye. This damages the optic nerve at the back of the eye. It can be treated with medications (eye drops). If not treated, it can cause a loss of vision. A person with diabetes is about twice as likely to develop glaucoma as a person without diabetes.	This type of glaucoma is called open-angle glaucoma. Ask, "Have you had the pressure in your eyes checked?" If the drops are not effective, a procedure called laser trabeculoplasty or surgery may be needed. Initially, there are no symptoms, but as the disease progresses, side vision may be affected, causing tunnel vision.
6. Kidneys (diabetic nephropathy)	6.1 Small blood vessels in the kidneys filter the blood; needed components are kept, and waste products including excess water are filtered out and disposed of as urine. About	Ask, "What questions/concerns do you have about diabetic kidney disease?" Use Visual #7, Normal Kidney.

CONTENT OUTLINE

CONCEPT	DETAIL	INSTRUCTOR'S NOTES
	200 quarts of blood are filtered each day.	
	6.2 Sometimes in diabetes, the small vessels thicken and the kidneys do not filter as they should. Necessary blood components, such as protein, are lost in the urine; waste products (e.g., creatinine, urea) are not adequately filtered out and eventually build up in the blood.	No symptoms are noticeable early in the development of diabetic kidney disease.
	6.3 To test kidney function, a spot, overnight, or 24-hour urine sample should be tested once a year for the presence of protein and for the amount of creatinine excreted. Blood tests for blood urea nitrogen (BUN) and creatinine can also be done.	Explain these tests and normal results. Ask, "When did you last have these tests done?" Encourage participants to ask for these tests and what the results mean. These tests should be done at diagnosis and annually for those with type 2 diabetes, and 5 years after diagnosis for those with type 1, and annually thereafter.
	6.4 The estimated rate of glomerular filtration (eGFR) can be calculated from the level of creatinine in the blood. It is the most accurate measure of the health of your kidneys.	These results are affected by age, race, diet, and body mass. The glomeruli act as filters. Creatinine should be checked annually for adults and the eGFR calculated, regardless of the albumin test results.
	6.5 The kidneys normally have a large reserve function. They can handle the needs of the body without causing any symptoms, until only 10% of the kidney function remains.	Ask, "Have you or anyone you know had kidney damage from diabetes? What was your/their experience?" Nephropathy occurs in 20–40% of patients with diabetes and is the leading cause of end-stage renal disease (ESRD).
	6.6 Two groups of medicines (called angiotensin-converting enzyme [ACE] inhibitors and angiotensin II receptor blockers [ARBs]) can delay the progression of diabetic nephropathy. In addition, keeping the blood pressure	Ask, "Are any of you taking ACE inhibitors or ARBs? What have been your experiences? Any side effects?" List drugs used on the board. Beta-blockers are effective for participants with

CONTENT OUTLINE

CONCEPT	DETAIL	INSTRUCTOR'S NOTES
	close to normal can slow the course of kidney damage.	uncomplicated hypertension, but their protective effect on the kidneys is not clear.
	6.7 Treatment for diagnosed nephropathy may include eating less protein. Some signs and symptoms (edema and hypertension) can be treated by improved glucose levels, eating less salt, and with medicines such as ACE inhibitors or ARBs.	By-products of protein metabolism are part of the waste products filtered by the kidneys. Protein levels of 0.8–10 g/kg/day are recommended in early stages of CKD, and 0.8 g/kg/day in later stages.
	6.8 Later symptoms are nausea, poor appetite, irregular heart action, fatigue, dry and itchy skin, slow thinking, confusion and memory failure, numbness and tingling in hands and feet, poor balance, depression, irritability, anemia, and bone loss.	These symptoms occur as harmful products build up in your bloodstream. Efforts to manage glucose, blood pressure, and cholesterol levels will continue.
	6.9 In the DCCT, intensive therapy decreased the risk for nephropathy by 35–56%. The UKPDS also demonstrated reductions in risk for nephropathy. You can help prevent or delay kidney failure by keeping your blood glucose and blood pressure close to normal and treating high blood pressure and bladder infections promptly.	Cautions: Untreated urinary tract infections can progress to kidney infection and damage; high blood pressure worsens diabetic kidney disease. Kidney damage is also related to diabetes duration.
	6.10 If kidney disease becomes worse, the kidneys may fail. The three treatment options are: ■ hemodialysis (a machine is used to filter the blood two to three times per week) ■ peritoneal dialysis (fluid flows into and out of the abdomen, and the peritoneum is used as a filter) ■ kidney transplantation.	These options are the same regardless of the cause of kidney failure.
7. Heart	7.1 Large-vessel problems in diabetes especially affect the heart, legs, and feet.	Ask, "What questions/concerns do you have about diabetes and heart disease?"
	7.2 Fats (cholesterol and triglycerides) are deposited along the walls of the	Use Visual #8, Large-Vessel Disease. Heart disease is the

CONTENT OUTLINE

CONCEPT	DETAIL	INSTRUCTOR'S NOTES
	vessels. This is called arteriosclerosis.	leading cause of death among people with diabetes.
	7.3 The vessels become stiff and less elastic, and the diameter of the vessel is smaller.	Ask, "Have you or anyone you know had heart disease and diabetes? What was your/their experience?"
	7.4 When this occurs in the coronary arteries, it can lead to heart attacks caused by not enough blood getting to the heart or to sections of the heart.	Arteriosclerosis is two to four times more common among men with diabetes and four to eight times more common among women with diabetes.
	7.5 When this occurs in cerebral arteries, it can lead to strokes.	Strokes are two to four times more common among people with diabetes.
	7.6 When this occurs in the large vessels of the general circulation, especially those leading to the legs and feet, many problems can result, such as calf pain (claudication), ulcers, and delayed healing of injuries.	These complications are four to forty times more common in people with diabetes.
	7.7 Hyperglycemia raises triglyceride levels.	Alcohol and high sugar intake can also raise triglycerides.
8. Risk factors for heart disease	8.1 The risk factors for heart disease are:	Ask, "What are risk factors for heart disease?"
	■ diabetes	Say, "You already have one of these risk factors that you can't change. But you can do things about some of the other risk factors to help delay or prevent problems."
	■ high blood fats (lipids)—your cholesterol level should be measured once a year	Ask, "Do you know your cholesterol level?" Review normal results. Encourage participants to request this test. Refer to Outline #18, *Eating for a Healthy Heart* (p. 379).
	■ high blood pressure (hypertension)—your blood pressure should be checked at every visit to your provider	Ask, "Do you know your blood pressure?" The goal in diabetes is <130/80 mmHg. Stress the importance of blood pressure management to protect heart,

CONTENT OUTLINE

CONCEPT	DETAIL	INSTRUCTOR'S NOTES

| | | kidneys, and eyes. Multiple medications are often needed. |

	■ smoking ■ heredity ■ gender	
		Males have higher risk for heart disease than females.
	■ stress ■ inactivity ■ obesity (more than 20% over ideal weight). }	These are contributing factors, although not proven to be direct causes of large-vessel disease.

9. Prevention, detection, and treatment of heart disease

9.1 Prevent heart disease by eliminating risk factors that are preventable. Smoking is one of the most important risk factors you can eliminate.

Ask, "Do you have any risk factors on which you would like to work?" Nicotine patches, gum, or medications may be helpful in smoking cessation. Provide information on smoking cessation programs in your area.

9.2 Lowering your cholesterol and blood glucose levels also decreases your risk. The UKPDS showed reductions of risk for heart failure and strokes with reductions in blood pressure. To lower your cholesterol, you can eat less saturated and trans fat (LDL) and more monosaturated fat (HDL), exercise more, and eat more soluble fiber and more cold-water fish.

Current cholesterol recommendations are:

HDL (men)	>40 mg/dl
HDL (women)	>50 mg/dl
LDL	<100 mg/dl
Triglycerides	<150 mg/dl

Encourage participants to ask for a cholesterol check, and what their results mean. Values for those with CHD may be different.

9.3 Heart problems can also be detected through electrocardiogram and Doppler studies.

9.4 The treatment is the same as people without diabetes. A daily aspirin and medications called statins are frequently used by people with diabetes.

Ask, "Do you take medication for your cholesterol? What have your experiences been?" List medications on the board.

10. Nervous system

10.1 Nerves conduct impulses (send messages) from one part of your body to another and back and forth to your brain.

Ask, "What questions or concerns do you have about nerve damage and diabetes?" Use Visual #9, Nervous System. Neuropathy is the most common complication of diabetes. Much

CONTENT OUTLINE

CONCEPT	DETAIL	INSTRUCTOR'S NOTES

research is currently being done in this area.

10.2 The peripheral nerves connect your brain and spinal cord to all other parts of your body, including the skin, muscles, and organs.

10.3 The names of the peripheral nerves are based on what they do. There are three types of these nerves.
- Sensory nerves send information to the brain about how things feel. For example, the sensory nerves tell the brain that the stove is hot when you touch it.
- Motor nerves send commands from the brain to the body about movements. For example, motor nerves cause you to take your hand off the hot stove.
- Autonomic nerves control the things your body does automatically. For example, autonomic nerves control digestion, heart rate and blood pressure, the bladder, and sexual function.

10.4 Diabetic neuropathy is classified by the type of nerves that are affected. Damage to the sensory nerves causes pain or a loss of feeling. Damage to the motor nerves causes muscle weakness. Damage to the autonomic nerves causes changes in the way your body controls certain functions.

Point out that having damage to one type of nerve doesn't mean that you will have other types of nerve damage; however, they often occur in combination.

10.5 Diabetes can affect all types of nerves. Why this happens is unclear, but the rate of conduction of impulses in the nerves is decreased, the nerve endings are damaged, and other disturbances occur.

Ask, "Do you have nerve damage or know someone who does? What is it like for you/them?"

CONTENT OUTLINE

CONCEPT	DETAIL	INSTRUCTOR'S NOTES
11. Feet, legs, and hands	11.1 Peripheral neuropathy (damage to the peripheral nerves) affects legs, feet, and, to a lesser extent, hands.	The longer nerves are affected first, in a stocking/glove/pattern.
	11.2 Symptoms are increased sensitivity with numbness or tingling, pain and burning, decreased sensation, and sometimes muscle weakness.	Symptoms depend on the type of nerves and the extent of the damage.
	11.3 Symptoms tend to come and go and may decrease with lower blood glucose levels.	
	11.4 If sensation is decreased, you can hurt yourself without realizing it because of an inability to sense heat or pain.	Pain is a protective mechanism.
	11.5 Another problem of the feet and legs involves large-vessel circulation. Decreased blood flow to the feet and legs means that wounds will not heal as quickly as they should.	Use Visual #10, Wound Healing. Point out the narrowed vessels with arteriosclerosis.
	11.6 The combination of circulatory and nerve problems in the legs can result in severe impairment. If you get a cut, you may not feel it. The decreased blood flow means that the wound will not heal quickly and may become infected.	Stress the importance of daily foot inspection and foot care to prevent amputations. Feet should be checked for sensation by your provider annually. Refer to Outline #13, *Personal Health Habits* (p. 265). Ask, "When did you last have your feet checked?"
	11.7 Increased sensitivity can lead to severe pain. While the pain may not completely go away with treatment, it should be eased with these therapies. It may take several trials with different medications and changes in dose to find the one that will work for you. It takes time and patience to find the right therapy.	Ask, "Do you have pain from neuropathy? How do you manage it?" Point out that if pain is not relieved with medication, to let their providers know.
	11.8 Treatment for pain includes: ■ medications	Narcotics are generally not used for long-term treatment. Medicine may include tramadol tricyclic antidepressants,

CONTENT OUTLINE

CONCEPT	DETAIL	INSTRUCTOR'S NOTES
		(e.g., amitriptyline [Elavil]) antiseizure medicines, (e.g., gabapentin duloxetine and pregablin), and OTC analgesics. There is insufficient evidence to determine if vitamin B is an effective therapy.
	■ walking to decrease leg pains ■ relaxation exercises, hypnosis, or biofeedback training ■ transcutaneous nerve stimulation (TENS) unit ■ acupressure and acupuncture. Pain clinics are also available in many cities.	A TENS unit is a battery-powered device that sends an electric current to the painful areas. The current blocks the pain message from going to the brain, which decreases the pain. These units are costly but may be covered by insurance.
	11.9 In the DCCT, risk for neuropathy was decreased by 60% with intensive therapy.	
12. Autonomic neuropathy	12.1 Damage to stomach nerves can cause delayed emptying, which causes nausea, stomach distention, and vomiting.	This is called *gastroparesis diabeticorum*. An early sign may be erratic blood glucose values.
	12.2 Damage to intestinal nerves leads to delayed emptying, causing a buildup of bacteria, constipation, and diarrhea.	Constipation and diarrhea may alternate, and nocturnal fecal incontinence may occur.
	12.3 Dizziness and unsteadiness on standing can occur as a result of a drop in blood pressure (postural hypotension).	
	12.4 Incontinence (leaking of urine) or retention and difficulty urinating may occur. This increases the risk for bladder infections.	Emphasize that frequent emptying of the bladder may help prevent urinary retention and stretching of the bladder.
	12.5 Damage to the nerves that control sexual function can also occur.	Ask, "Have you heard about this before? Do you have any questions/concerns?" Discuss according to the interest and

CONTENT OUTLINE

CONCEPT	DETAIL	INSTRUCTOR'S NOTES
		needs of the group. Refer to Outline #20, *Sexual Health and Diabetes* (p. 425).
	12.6 Men may experience erectile dysfunction. Treatments are available for ED. If this is a concern, bring this to the attention of your provider. Do not wait to be asked.	Of males who have had diabetes for 10+ years, 40–50% have impaired sexual function. Stress the importance of discussing this with your provider or other professional to get treatment.
	12.7 Women may have diminished orgasms or none at all. Sexual problems in women may be related to genital infections (vaginitis) or lack of lubrication (which can be hormonal after menopause).	Depression, fatigue, and not feeling desirable contribute to women's sexual dysfunction.
	12.8 Treatment is available for all aspects of neuropathy. Talk with your health care professional about your symptoms and concerns.	
13. What can you do?	13.1 There are things you can do to prevent or delay complications or to detect them and get early treatment.	Present this section as positive actions participants can take. Ask, "Are there actions you can take to prevent the complications? What barriers do you anticipate? What strategies can you use to overcome these barriers?"
	13.2 Keeping your blood glucose and blood pressure levels near normal will help prevent or delay eye, kidney, and nerve complications. Every improvement in blood glucose helps in preventing complications.	Review the results of the DCCT and UKPDS.
	13.3 Eliminate those risk factors that you can. Take care of yourself. Pay attention to little things, and treat them carefully.	Have information on smoking cessation, weight loss, and other programs in your area.
	13.4 Take care of your feet.	

CONTENT OUTLINE

CONCEPT	DETAIL	INSTRUCTOR'S NOTES
	13.5 See your eye specialist annually for a dilated eye exam.	
	13.6 Most of the complications can be treated more effectively if found early. Regular examinations are needed, especially of the eyes, kidneys, feet, and heart. Ask your provider for these exams and tests.	Review referrals and tests to request. Ask, "Does your provider review the results with you?" If not, ask for your results and what they mean.
	13.7 Research is being done on causes and treatment for complications that offers great hope for the future.	
	13.8 Living with the complications of diabetes—even with the *possibility* of complications—is very hard. If you find that you feel sad and depressed, find a health care provider or counselor you can talk to about your feelings. Help is available.	Have information available regarding local support groups. Distribute Handout #1, Resources for Diabetes Complications. End the session on a positive note or use one of the relaxation activities in Outline #12, *Stress and Coping* (p. 255).
	13.9 Choose one thing you will do this week to care for your diabetes.	Close the session by asking participants to identify one action step they will take this week.

SKILLS CHECKLIST

None.

EVALUATION PLAN

Knowledge will be evaluated by achievement of learning objectives and by responses to questions during the session. Skills will be evaluated by observing a return demonstration of techniques. The ability to apply knowledge will be evaluated by development and implementation of a personal monitoring plan and through program outcome measures.

DOCUMENTATION PLAN

Record class attendance and achieved objectives as appropriate using the Diabetes Self-Management Record, the Participant Follow-up Record, or another form.

SUGGESTED READINGS

Overview

Boren SA, Gunlock TL, Schaefer J, Albright A: Reducing risks in diabetes self-management: a systematic review of the literature. *The Diabetes Educator* 33:1053–1077, 2007

Brownlee M, Hirsch IB: Glycemic variability. *JAMA* 295:1707–1708, 2006

Cheung N, Wang JJ, Klein R, et al.: Diabetic retinopathy and the risk of coronary heart disease. *Diabetes Care* 30:1741–1746, 2007

Cusick M, Meleth AD, Agron E, Fisher MR, Reed GF, Knatterud GL, Barton FB, et al.: Associations of mortality and diabetes complications in patients with type 1 and type 2 diabetes. *Diabetes Care* 28:617–625, 2005

Fowler MJ: Microvascular and macrovascular complications of diabetes. *Clinical Diabetes* 26:77–82, 2008

Gebel E: Tension mounts. *Diabetes Forecast* 62(7):37–39, 2009

McEwen LN, Kim C, Karter AJ Haan MN, et al.: Risk factors for mortality among patients with diabetes. *Diabetes Care* 30:1736–1741, 2007

Retinopathy

Bartos BJ, Cleary ME, Kleinbeck C, Petzinger RA, et al.: Diabetes and disabilities: assistive tools, services and information. *The Diabetes Educator* 34:597–636, 2008

Bloomgarden ZT: Diabetic retinopathy. *Diabetes Care* 31:1080–1083, 2008

Clarke PM, Simon J, Cull CA, Holman RR: Assessing the impact of visual acuity on quality of life in individuals with type 2 diabetes using the short form-36. *Diabetes Care* 29:1506–1511, 2006

Cohen AS, Ayello EA: Diabetes has taken a toll on your patient's vision: how can you help? *Nursing* 35(5):44–47, 2005

Pettit DJ, Wollitzer Ao, Jovaovic L, He G, Ipp E: The California Medi-Cal Type 2 Diabetes Study Group. Decreasing the risk of diabetic retinopathy in a study of case management. *Diabetes Care* 28:2819–2822, 2005

Roberts SS: Eye disease, understanding retinopathy, part 2. *Diabetes Forecast* 59(2):25–26, 2006

Roberts SS: Eye disease, understanding retinopathy, part 1. *Diabetes Forecast* 58(12):25–26, 2005

Rogell GD: All about laser eye surgery. *Diabetes Forecast* 57(2):50–52, 2004

Simo R, Hernandez C: Advances in the medical treatment of diabetic retinopathy. *Diabetes Care* 31:1556–1561, 2009

Nephropathy

Castner D, Douglas C: Now onstage: chronic kidney disease. *Nursing* 35(12):58–63, 2005

Gross JL, De Azevedo MJ, Silveiro SP, Canani LH, Caramori ML, Zelmanovitz T: Diabetic nephropathy: diagnosis, prevention, and treatment. *Diabetes Care* 28:164–176, 2005

Roberts SS: Kidney tests: a crucial part of diabetes care. *Diabetes Forecast* 59(7):23–24, 2006

Roberts SS: Caring for kidneys. *Diabetes Forecast* 59(6):19–21, 2006

Wheeler ML: Dietary protein and its influence on diabetic nephropathy. *Practical Diabetology* 25(4):16–22, 2006

Yee J: Diabetic kidney disease: chronic kidney disease and diabetes. *Diabetes Spectrum* 21:8–38, 2008

SUGGESTED READINGS *continued*

Yu N, Milite CP, Inzucchi SE: Evidence-based treatment of diabetic nephropathy. *Practical Diabetology* 24(4):36–41, 2005

Cardiovascular

American Diabetes Association: Hypertension management in adults with diabetes. *Diabetes Care* 27(Suppl 1): S65–S67, 2004

Blaustein A: Mitigating cardiovascular risks in diabetes. *Practical Diabetology* 26(4):14–17, 2007

Bloomgarden ZT: Cardiovascular disease in diabetes. *Diabetes Care* 31:1260–1268, 2008

Boucher JL, Hurrell DG: Cardiovascular disease and diabetes. *Diabetes Spectrum* 21:154–193, 2008

Buse JB, Ginsberg HN, Bakris GL, Clark NG, et al.: Primary prevention of cardiovascular diseases in people with diabetes mellitus. *Diabetes Care* 30:162–167, 2007

Capuzzi DM, Freeman JS: C-reactive protein and cardiovascular risk in the metabolic syndrome and type 2 diabetes: controversy and challenge. *Clinical Diabetes* 25:16–22, 2007

D'Arrigo T: Padded footsteps. *Diabetes Forecast* 60(4):55–59, 2007

Gebel E: Meet LDL's partner in plaque. *Diabetes Forecast* 61(5):39–40, 2008

Gottleib SH: A good heart. *Diabetes Forecast* 60(3):43–44, 2007

Gottlieb SH: Stroke: feared but preventable. *Diabetes Forecast* 59(9):39–41, 2006

Gottlieb SH: A healing heart. *Diabetes Forecast* 58(4):29–31, 2005

Kordella T: The heart of a woman. *Diabetes Forecast* 58(7):42–47, 2005

Kordella T: C-reactive protein. *Diabetes Forecast* 56(6):51–54, 2004

Kruger DF, Cypress M, Maryniuk M, Childs BP, Tieking J: Pharmaceutical treatment of hypertension and dyslipidemia in people with diabetes: an educator's perspective, Part 2: dyslipidemia. *Diabetes Spectrum* 17:73–77, 2004

Mochari H: Lifestyle habits for a healthy heart. *Diabetes Self-Management* 27(3):46–51, 2006

Nesto RW: LDL cholesterol lowering in type 2 diabetes: what is the optimum approach? *Clinical Diabetes* 26:8–13, 2008

Peters AL: Clinical relevance of non-HDL cholesterol in patients with diabetes. *Clinical Diabetes* 26:3–7, 2008

Roberts SS: Cholesterol. *Diabetes Forecast* 58(3):33–35, 2005

Roberts SS: Back to basics: blood pressure. *Diabetes Forecast* 58(2):39–40, 2005

Skyler JS, Bergenstal R, Bonow RO, Buse J, et al.: Intensive glycemic control and the prevention of cardiovascular events: implications of the ACCORD, ADVANCE, and the VA diabetes trials. *Diabetes Care* 32:187–192, 2009

White JR Jr: Do people with diabetes need statins? *The Diabetes Educator* 34:664–673, 2008

Neuropathy

Bloomgarden ZT: Diabetic neuropathy. *Diabetes Care* 30:1027–1032, 2007

Boulton AJM, Armstrong DG, Albert SF, Frykberg RG, et al.: Comprehensive foot examination and risk assessment: a report of the Task Force of the Foot Care Interest Group of the American Diabetes Association, with endorsement by the American Association of Clinical Endocrinologists. *Diabetes Care* 31:1679–1685, 2008

Boulton AJM, Vinik AI, Arezzo JC, Bril V, et al.: Diabetic neuropathies: a statement by the American Diabetes Association. *Diabetes Care* 28:936–955, 2005

Boulton AJM, Vinik AI, Arezzo JC, Btril V, Feldman EL, Freeman R, Malik RA, Master RE, Sosenko JM, Ziegler D: Diabetic neuropathies. *Diabetes Care* 28:956–962, 2005

Boulton AJM: Management of diabetic peripheral neuropathy. *Clinical Diabetes* 3:9–15, 2005

Corbett CF: Practical management of patients with painful diabetic neuropathy. *The Diabetes Educator* 31:523–540, 2005

D'Arcy Y: Conquering pain. *Nursing* 35(3):36–41, 2005

SUGGESTED READINGS *continued*

Feigenbaum K: Treating gastroparesis. *Diabetes Self-Management* 23(5):24–33, 2006

Herzog RI, Chyun D, Young LH: Cardiac autonomic neuropathy. *Practical Diabetology* 25(1):34–38, 2006

Huizinga MM, Peltier A: Painful diabetic neuropathy: a management-centered review. *Clinical Diabetes* 25:6–15, 2007

Martin CL, Albers J, Herman WH, Cleary P, et al.: Neuropathy among the Diabetes Control and Complications Trial cohort 8 years after trial completion. *Diabetes Care* 29:340–344, 2006

Parrish CR, Pastors JG: Nutritional management of gastroparesis in people with diabetes. *Diabetes Spectrum* 20:231–238, 2007

Roberts SS: Gastroparesis. *Diabetes Forecast* 59(9):27–29, 2006

Roberts SS: Treat the tingling. *Diabetes Forecast* 59(8):24–27, 2006

Rushing J. Assessing for orthostatic hypotension. *Nursing* 35(1):30–32, 2005

Risk-Factor Reduction

Ford SK, Shilliday BB: Smoking and diabetes: helping patients quit. *Clinical Diabetes* 24:133–138, 2006

Hirat FE, Moss SE, Klein BEK, Klein R: Severe hypoglycemia and smoking in a long-term type 1 diabetic population. *Diabetes Care* 30:1437–1447, 2007

Levin ME, Pfiefer MA: *The Uncomplicated Guide to Diabetes Complications,* 2nd edition. Alexandria, VA: American Diabetes Association, 2009

Nursing 2007: Patient Education Series. Smoking cessation. *Nursing* 37(5):57–58, 2007

Rice VP, Stead LF: Nursing interventions for smoking cessation. *Cochrane Database of Syst Rev no.* CD001188, 2008

Stead L, Bergson G, Lancaster T: Physician advice for smoking cessation. *Cochrane Database Syst Rev no.* CD000165, 2008

Stead LF, Perera R, Bullen C, Mant D, Lancaster T: Nicotine replacement therapy for smoking cessation. *Cochrane Database Syst Rev* no. CD000146, 2008

University of New Mexico Diabetes Team: *101 Tips for Staying Healthy with Diabetes,* 2nd Edition. Alexandria, VA: American Diabetes Association, 1999

Willi C, Bodenmann P, Ghlai WA, Faris PD, Cornuz J: Active smoking and the risk of type 2 diabetes: A systematic review and meta-analyses. *JAMA* 298:2654CD0001462664, 2007

➲ Relationship of A1C to Risk of Complications

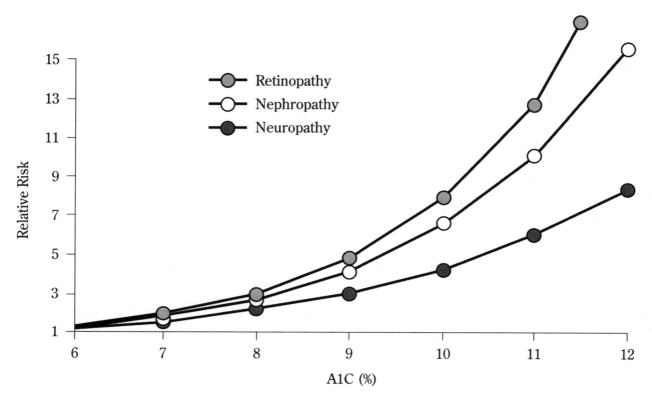

Source: Skyler. *Endocrinol Metab Clin*. 1996;25:243–254, with permission.

➲ Circulatory System

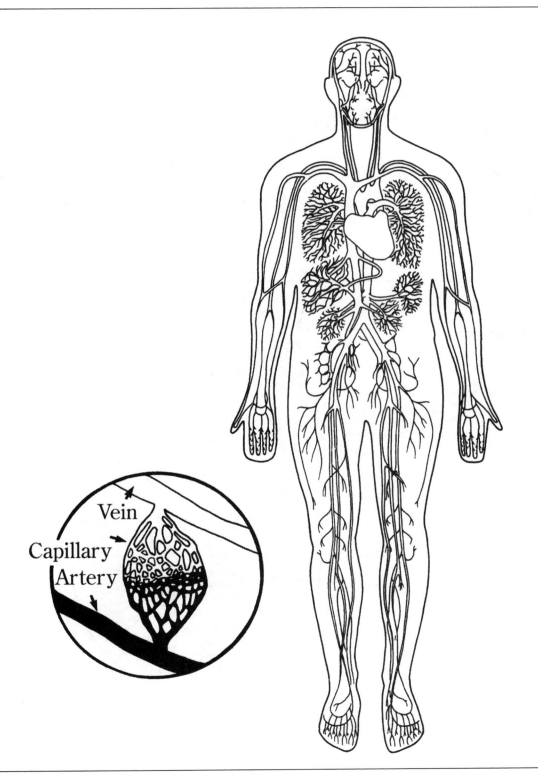

➲ Normal Eye

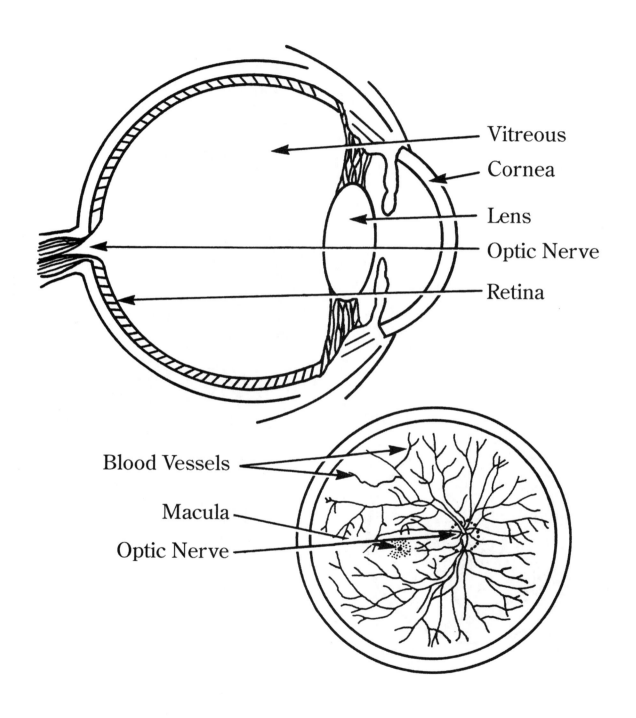

◑ Microaneurysms

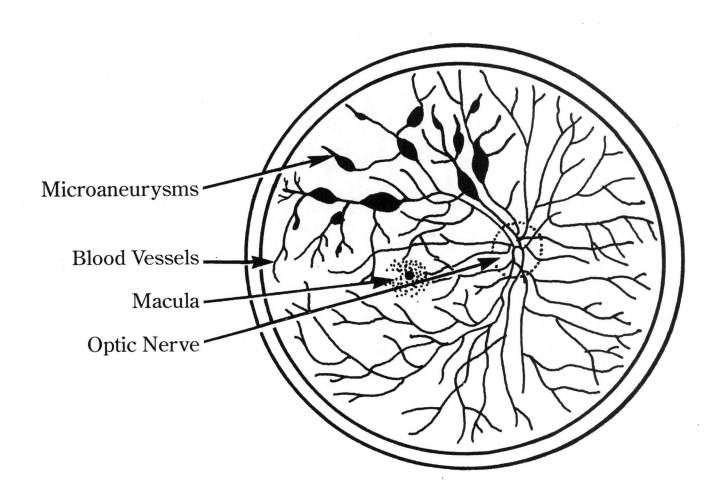

Microaneurysms

Blood Vessels

Macula

Optic Nerve

➲ Proliferative Retinopathy

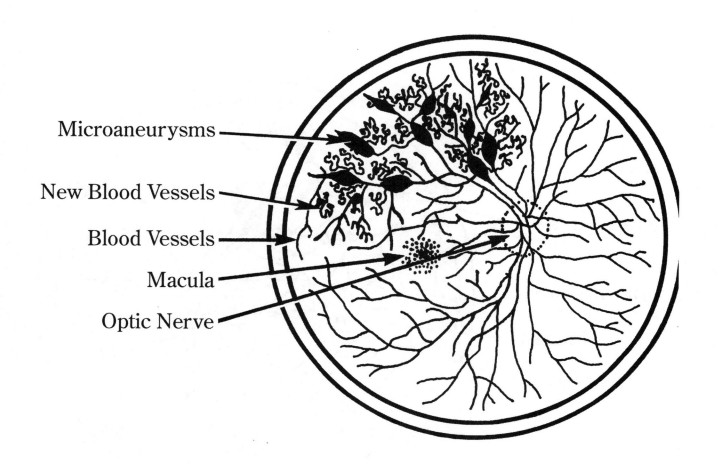

Microaneurysms

New Blood Vessels

Blood Vessels

Macula

Optic Nerve

➲ Retinal Detachment

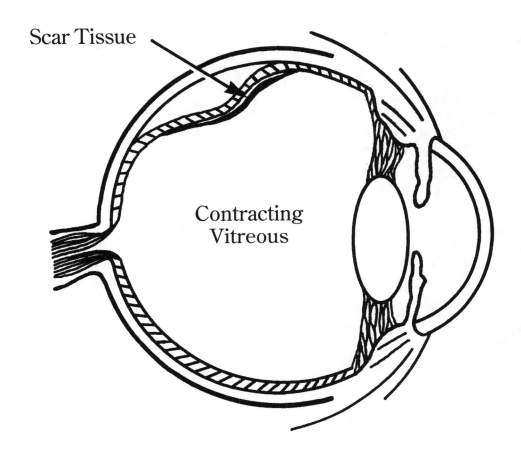

Scar Tissue

Contracting
Vitreous

⬤ **Normal Kidney**

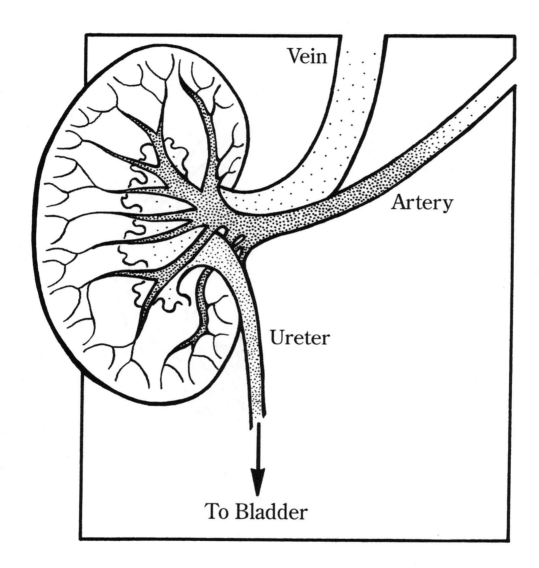

Vein

Artery

Ureter

To Bladder

➊ Large-Vessel Disease

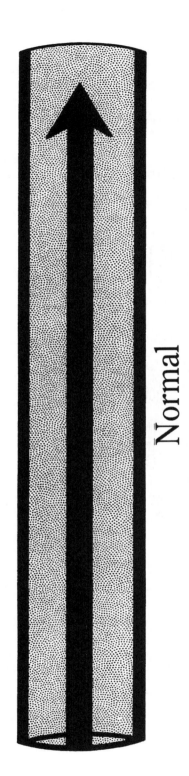

Normal

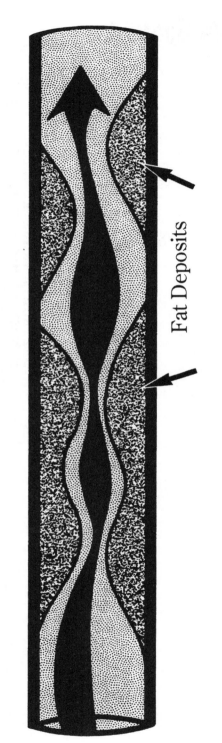

Fat Deposits

Arteriosclerosis

⬤ Nervous System

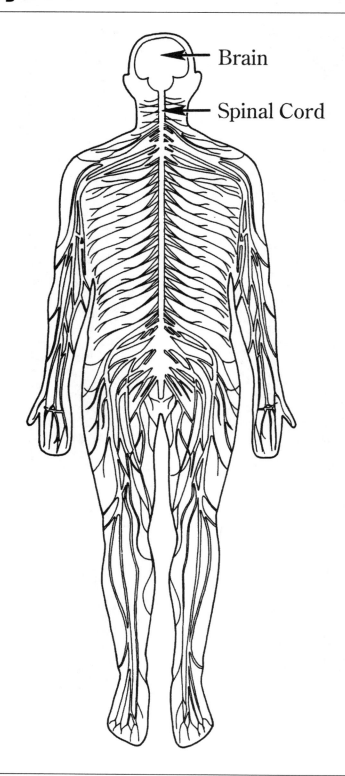

Brain

Spinal Cord

➤ Wound Healing

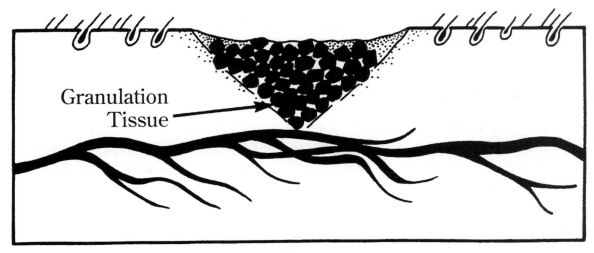

Granulation
Tissue

Normal Circulation

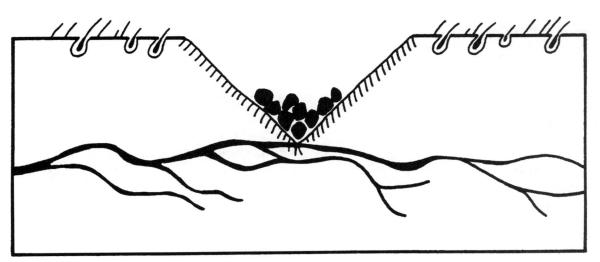

Arteriosclerosis

◐ Resources for Diabetes Complications

When people begin to experience the complications that can occur with diabetes, they often find that they need support and resources. There is help available. The following is a list of national organizations. Ask your health care team for more information about resources in your area.

VISION PROBLEMS

Services for the Blind is an agency that offers vocational or job training to legally blind persons. They can be contacted through the county Social Services Office (listed under "county government" in the white pages). They offer medical and surgical services and vocational training, including college, on-the-job, tutorial, and adjustment teaching.

Other service agencies

American Council of the Blind
1155 15th Street, NW
Suite 1004
Washington, DC 20005
800-424-8666
www.acb.org

Lions Club International
300 West 22nd Street
Oakbrook, IL 60523-8842
630-571-5466
www.lionsclubs.org

National Eye Institute
Information Specialist
Building 31, Room 6A32
Bethesda, MD 20892
301-496-5248
www.nei.nih.gov

National Federation of the Blind
1800 Johnson Street
Baltimore, MD 21230
410-659-9314
www.nfb.org

Sources for tapes or reading material

National Library Service for the Blind and Physically Handicapped
Library of Congress
1291 Taylor Street, NW
Washington, DC 20011
888-NLS-READ (657-7323)
www.loc.gov/nls/

Braille Exchange Lists
Braille Institute
741 N. Vermont Avenue
Los Angeles, CA 90029
323-663-1111
www.braillelibrary.org

American Printing House for the Blind
1839 Frankfort Avenue
Louisville, KY 40206
502-895-2405
www.aph.org

RESOURCES FOR DIABETES COMPLICATIONS *continued*

Correspondence course

Hadley School for the Blind
700 Elm Street
Winnetka, IL 60093
847-446-8111
www.hadley-school.org

Kidney disease

National Kidney Foundation
30 East 33rd Street
New York, NY 10016
800-622-9010
www.kidney.org

American Association of Kidney Patients
3505 E. Frontage Road
Suite 315
Tampa, FL 33607
800-749-2257
www.aakp.org

Kidney Directions
http://www.kidneydirections.com
Baxter health-care corporation online resource
for education materials.

Heart disease

American Heart Association
7272 Greenville Avenue
Dallas, TX 75231
800-242-8721
www.americanheart.org

Amputations

National Amputation Foundation
40 Church Street
Malverne, NY 11565
516-887-3600
www.nationalamputation.org

Neuropathy

The Neuropathy Association
60 East 42nd Street
Suite 942
New York, NY 10165
800-247-6968
www.neuropathy.org

| #15 | **Changing Behavior** |

▶ ▶ ▶ ▶ ▶

STATEMENT OF PURPOSE

This session is intended to present a problem-solving approach to diabetes self-management and health habits. Behavior change strategies and goal setting are included. This content is most useful if presented during the first or second session and participants are encouraged to choose a short-term behavioral goal as an experiment at each session. You can then use these experiences to generate discussion and involve the group in problem solving. The goal-setting form can be used during this or the last class as a way to help participants establish new goals or sustain the changes they made. It may be helpful to create a short version of the behavior change form for participants to use after this session, which would include questions 2, 9, 10, 11, 12, 13, and 14. You can also use the Participant Follow-up Visit form to record and track progress with participants.

PREREQUISITES

None.

OBJECTIVES

At the end of this session, participants will be able to:

1. state a specific strategy for making behavior changes;

2. create a LIFE plan;

3. identify a personal long-term goal related to diabetes;

4. make a behavior change plan;

5. set a behavior change goal;

6. make a commitment to carry out behavior change goals.

CONTENT

Developing personal strategies to promote health and behavior change.

MATERIALS NEEDED

VISUALS PROVIDED	ADDITIONAL
None.	■ Pencils for participants
	■ Chalkboard and chalk/Board and markers
Handout (one per participant)	
1. Behavior Change Plan	

METHOD OF PRESENTATION

Start by introducing yourself and telling what you do. Ask participants to introduce themselves and tell what they are currently doing to care for their diabetes. Explain that the purpose of this session is for participants to develop a clear plan for working on a problem they want to solve or a behavior they want to change.

Present material in a question/discussion format. Elicit and incorporate as many patient experiences and suggestions as possible into the discussion. The Behavior Change Plan handout can be used either as an in-class activity or at home by each participant. In either case, it is very important to review it with the participants so that they can choose a behavior change they believe will be meaningful to them. Help participants break down large goals into smaller, more achievable steps. Choosing one step will help them to feel that they can do it without being overwhelmed. End with the visualization, if desired.

Encourage family members and friends of participants to take part in the session, either by making a personal behavior change plan or by identifying how they will provide support.

CONTENT OUTLINE

CONCEPT	DETAIL	INSTRUCTOR'S NOTES
1. Health habits	1.1 The ways that you eat, sleep, exercise and take care of your health are habits, or behaviors. You have had these habits for many years, and they are rarely easy to change.	Ask, "How did you do with your short-term goal? What did you learn from it?"
	1.2 Taking care of diabetes may mean changes in your health habits.	Ask, "What changes have you made as a result of diabetes? What changes have been hard? Easy?"
	1.3 You will not be able to make a lot of changes overnight—no matter how much "willpower" you have. One definition of will power is importance + confidence.	Ask, "What questions or concerns do you have about making changes in your health habits?"

CONTENT OUTLINE

CONCEPT	DETAIL	INSTRUCTOR'S NOTES
	1.4 But you can make changes in your life. First you need to be ready, then learn how to make changes, then choose what you want to change, and then make a plan for change.	Emphasize that not being ready to change, not planning for change, not setting clear goals, setting a goal that's too hard, and lack of commitment are more likely reasons for not achieving goals than lack of "willpower."
2. Strategies for making changes	2.1 There are strategies that you can use in making behavior changes.	Ask, "What changes have you made in your habits in the past? What helped or hindered you in making these changes or reaching your goals? How did you overcome barriers you encountered?"
	2.2 Start with something you feel you can do and will be meaningful for you. Success will help you feel that you can make changes.	Ask, "What is hardest or the worst part for you about caring for your diabetes?" This is the level of importance.
	2.3 Start with something you feel ready to change.	Frustration or other negative feelings can serve as motivation for change.
	2.4 Because diabetes involves multiple changes in various aspects of your lifestyle, you may feel differently about different health habits. For example, you can be ready to exercise, but not ready to change your meal plan.	Ask, "On what areas do you feel ready to work?"
	2.5 Start by adding one new habit. It is easier to add a new habit than to give up one that you already have. For example, if you want to exercise, start with that behavior.	Ask, "How ready do you feel to make this change? How sure do you feel you can make this change?" This is the level of confidence or self-efficacy.
	2.6 Write down your new habits. Records, such as food diaries and exercise charts, can help you see how you are doing.	Point out that some people find weight charts frustrating, because things other than behavior can influence results.
	2.7 Make it easy to remember your new habits. For example, if it's hard for you to remember to take your pills before breakfast, put the bottle	Ask, "What other things have you done that serve as reminders to yourself to do things?"

CONTENT OUTLINE

CONCEPT	DETAIL	INSTRUCTOR'S NOTES
	on the kitchen table or by the alarm clock.	
	2.8 Get rid of reminders of habits you want to break. If you want to stop smoking, get rid of your ashtrays.	Ask, "Can you think of anything that reminds you of habits that you are trying to change?"
	2.9 Changing your daily routine may also help eliminate cues for certain behaviors or help you add a behavior.	Ask, "Are there ways to change your routine that will help?"
	2.10 Ask for help from your family and friends. Tell them how they can be most helpful to you. On-going support will help you stick with it over time.	Ask, "What kind of support from your family and friends is helpful to you?" Remember, if it does not help you, then it is not really supportive.
	2.11 Write a contract or agreement with your family or care team about the behavior changes you want to make.	
	2.12 Reward yourself when you make progress. Treat yourself to something when you reach each step toward your long-term goal. This isn't childish, but is a proven way to change habits.	A reward could be taking time to do something you enjoy, such as reading a book or doing a hobby.
3. Choices for behavior change	3.1 Before you can create a plan to make changes, it is helpful to have an overall roadmap.	Knowing where you are going helps create the best plan for how to get there.
	3.2 One approach is to create a LIFE plan for your overall diabetes care. LIFE = Learn all you can about diabetes and yourself; Identify your guiding principles: role, targets, flexibility; Formulate your plan; Experiment with and evaluate your plan.	Write the meaning of "LIFE" on the board. Discuss each area and invite participants to think about or write down their thoughts about each area.
	3.3 The purpose of this program is to help you learn about diabetes; however, it is just as important that you learn about yourself and your wants, needs, values, and capabilities. Knowing about yourself	Ask, "How would you describe yourself? Which of your cultural and religious beliefs affect how you care for your diabetes? What are the top 5 most important things in your life?

CONTENT OUTLINE

CONCEPT	DETAIL	INSTRUCTOR'S NOTES

helps you to better incorporate diabetes into your life.

How do these influence how you care for yourself?"

3.4 Identify your guiding principles. Three of these that affect how you will care for your diabetes are: your role, targets, and how much flexibility you need in your life.
Role: The reality is that you are in charge of your diabetes self-care; however, you can also choose to **take** charge. This is your role. You may choose to create all or part of your plan. There is no right way, just the one that will work best for you.
Targets: One of the ways to evalaute your plan is by knowing how it is helping you to reach your glucose, blood pressure, cholesterol, weight, and other targets.
Formulate your plan: This is **your** diabetes care plan.

Ask, "How much responsibility do you want for creating your plan of care?"

Ask, "What are your targets for blood glucose, A1C, blood pressure, weight, and cholesterol?" Some people find it helpful to set interim targets toward recommended targets.

Ask, "What strategies will you use to treat your diabetes? How likely is it that you will be able to carry out this plan?"

3.5 Experiment with and evaluate your plan. Because there is no "right" or "best" way to treat diabetes, most people try different ways to reach their goals. One way to think of this is as an experiment. A good thing about an experiment is that you cannot lose. No matter how it turns out, you learn from it.

The next step is to create an action plan.

Point out that some of life's most valuable lessons come from things that do not work well.

3.6 During the next part of the class, you can use some of these strategies to make a behavior change plan. The first step is deciding what you want to do. Think about your overall goals for caring for your diabetes. These are considered your long-term goals or outcomes. The targets you identified earlier are in this category.

Distribute Handout #1, Behavior Change Plan. Have each participant work through the steps as you review them, or work through the handout as a group on the board, then ask participants to develop a personal plan. Point out that they may not have responses in all categories.

CONTENT OUTLINE

CONCEPT	DETAIL	INSTRUCTOR'S NOTES
		If done in the group, ask the class to choose an area or situation that is relevant for most, such as blood glucose management or weight loss. Encourage participants to choose goals that are both meaningful and attainable. For example, maintaining normal blood glucose levels at all times in not realistic for most people with diabetes.
	3.7 Make a list of all your long-term goals related to diabetes.	Point out that a participant's goals may be different than those of the health care provider or their family members. It is critical that the goal be selected by the participant.
	3.8 What parts of living with diabetes are hardest for you? While it is tempting to choose a behavior, behaviors are reflections or symptoms of a problem. Changing the behavior without solving the problem or choosing a behavior that does not address a meaningful problem often means that the symptoms "pop up" elsewhere.	This helps participants focus on their concerns about living with and caring for diabetes. "Negative" feelings about a situation are often powerful motivators for change. Help participants identify and use the energy these emotions create.
	3.9 How does this issue make you feel? Keep in mind that there are no rules for managing diabetes. Just choices and consequences.	
	3.10 How does this need to change help you to reach your goals or feel better about it?	Ask, "What will happen if you don't do anything? How will you feel?"
	3.11 Where would you like to be in achieving this goal in a year? In six months from now? In three months?	Help participants evaluate appropriate time frames based on long-term goals.
	3.12 What would you like to accomplish in the next month? Week? This is your short-term goal.	Help participants set achievable short-term goals. For example, if the concern is a lack of exercise, and the long-term goal is to walk a mile every day, the

CONTENT OUTLINE

CONCEPT	DETAIL	INSTRUCTOR'S NOTES
		short-term goal may be to walk 1/4 mile three times a week by the end of the month, and two blocks by the end of the week.
	3.13 There are costs and benefits to any action or change that you want to make. Weighing the costs and benefits helps you decide how important this is to you.	
	3.14 What would be the costs to you for taking these actions or achieving this goal? For example, for weight loss, the costs may be giving up foods you enjoy, less flexibility, discomfort in social situations involving food, or changing the way you cook.	Do this with participants in an accepting, nonjudgemental way.
	3.15 What would be the benefits to you of taking action or achieving this goal? For example, if the goal is losing weight, the benefits may be that you will look better, feel better, or have better blood glucose control.	Point out that the benefits listed need to be personally meaningful. This provides the needed motivation for the long-term. Avoid pointing out benefits yourself.
	3.16 Think about the costs and benefits. Is it worth it to you to make this change? If the costs outweigh the benefits, you need to decide if you are still ready and willing to take action to improve this siuation or achieve this goal.	Ask, "On a scale of 1–10, how important is this goal to you?" Recognize that choosing to do nothing is an option. Only you can decide if the benefit is worth the cost. If the importance is less than 7, it is hard to stay motivated. In this case, ask, "What would it take to make this more important for you?"
	3.17 Make a commitment to yourself or another person.	
4. Making a plan	4.1 What are some steps you could take to improve this situation or move closer to your goal? Think of all the possible options you have and what you can do. In the weight	Options need to be generated by the participants to be meaningful. Encourage participants to choose behavior change strategies over which they have

CONTENT OUTLINE

CONCEPT	DETAIL	INSTRUCTOR'S NOTES
	loss example, options related to social situations may include saving meat and fat exchanges, not attending, meeting with the dietitian to discuss this topic, ignoring the meal plan on that occasion and monitoring more closely, taking extra insulin, or increasing activity that day.	control (e.g., skipping dessert three times a week rather than losing a specific number of pounds, or monitoring three times a day rather than achieving a certain blood glucose number).
	4.2 What are ways you can change your environment at home or work?	Ask, "Are there barriers to overcome?" Examples: Remove tempting foods from the house, place them out of sight, bring a lunch to work.
	4.3 What are ways you believe your family or friends can be most helpful to you? Think of how you will ask for help, and practice in your mind.	Ask, "Are there people who can help you?" Examples: Eat similar food, exercise with you, not eat tempting foods in front of you.
5. Setting behavior-change goals	5.1 Now, look at all the steps and options that you have identified and choose one to three steps that you will take toward achieving your short-term goal this week. These are your behavior-change goals.	These steps need to be readily achievable and specific. For example, if a morning exercise program is a goal, getting up half an hour earlier or buying comfortable shoes is an appropriate step.
	5.2 Feeling confident that you can carry out these behaviors increases the likelihood that you will start and continue with your plan.	Ask, "On a scale of 1–10, how confident do you feel that you can do what you have identified?" If less than 7, ask, "What would it take for you to feel more confident?"
	5.3 Set an I-SMART goal as your behavioral experiment. An I-SMART goal is: Important/Inspiring, Specific, Measurable, Actionable, Realistic, and Time-specific.	Remind participants that the advantage of an experiment is that it can always result in learning.
	5.4 Make a commitment that you will carry out this behavior change or step.	This can be verbal or written, with the educator, a partner, or significant other.

CONTENT OUTLINE

CONCEPT	DETAIL	INSTRUCTOR'S NOTES
	5.5 What is your time frame? Choose a deadline for starting or identify the number of times per week you will do the behavior.	Again, this needs to be realistic given the other demands and priorities that participants have. It may not be realistic to do something every day.
	5.6 How will you keep track of your new behavior?	Record keeping can be a very reinforcing part of behavior change. The system should be simple and easy to do, so that it is not a deterrent to change.
	5.7 Decide how you will reward yourself for achieving your long-term goal and short-term goal and for trying each behavior-change goal or step along the way.	This is a very important part of the behavior-change process that is often neglected. Having better health or preventing long-term complications is too elusive and futuristic to be rewarding for most people. Encourage patients to choose a reward that is meaningful enough so that it offers an incentive at times when the goal seems too hard to achieve, such as a reward for staying with behavior changes for 1 week.
6. Problem-solving	6.1 Are there any problems or issues that you can anticipate and plan for? For example, do you have a place to exercise in good and bad weather?	Ask, "Are there barriers that you can anticipate? What can you do to make a plan to overcome them?"
	6.2 If the plan doesn't work, think about what you learned from your experiments. The first step in solving problems is to identify the problem. Go back over the steps to see what you could do differently.	Encourage participants to think of these as problems to be solved, not failures. Point out that strategies they use to solve problems in other aspects of their lives are useful in diabetes as well.
	6.3 It could be that your goal is too big, you might be trying to do too much at one time, a different option will work better, the costs outweigh the	

CONTENT OUTLINE

CONCEPT	DETAIL	INSTRUCTOR'S NOTES
	benefits, or this goal isn't relevant for you at this time.	
	6.4 You may decide on a different long-term or short-term goal or choose a different option or behavior-change goal as your next experiment.	
	6.5 If you have a day when you don't meet your goals, try not to let it get you down. Think about what problems you encountered, what you learned, and what you might do differently the next time.	
7. Visualization	7.1 One technique that sometimes helps is visualization: imagining yourself as successful in meeting your goals. If you find this exercise helpful, you can do it yourself each day or when you feel discouraged.	After reviewing the plans, one way to end this session is by having the participants visualize themselves as successful at meeting their goals. Speak slowly and in a relaxing manner as you go through the exercise, pausing between requests.

Visualization Exercise

Ask participants to close their eyes and picture themselves in 3 months or a year when they have met their goal. Suggest that they picture:

- how they look
- how they feel physically
- how their family and friends feel about them
- how they feel about themselves

Ask that they keep their eyes closed for as long as they like and enjoy these feelings. Then, slowly open their eyes and come back into the present.

SKILLS CHECKLIST

Each participant will be able to identify a long-term diabetes-related goal and develop a behavior-change plan.

EVALUATION PLAN

Knowledge will be evaluated by achievement of learning and skill objectives and by responses to questions during the session. The ability to apply knowledge will be evaluated by development of personal long-term and behavior-change goals, by the development and implementation of a plan to achieve those goals, the ability to reflect on the outcome of the plan and solve problems that arise, and through program outcome measures.

DOCUMENTATION PLAN

Record class attendance, achieved objectives, and behavioral goals as appropriate using the Diabetes Self-Management Record, the Participant Follow-up Record, or another form.

SUGGESTED READINGS

Behavior Change

Aikens JE, Bingham R, Piette JD: Patient-provider communication and self-care behavior among type 2 diabetes patients. *The Diabetes Educator* 31:681–690, 2005

Anderson BJ, Rubin RR: *Practical Psychology for Diabetes Clinicians*, 2nd Edition. Alexandria, VA: American Diabetes Association, 2002

Anderson RM, Funnell MM, Burkhart N, Gillard ML, Nwankwo R: *101 Tips for Behavior Change in Diabetes*. Alexandria, VA: American Diabetes Association, 2002

Bodenheimer T, Davis C, Holman H: Helping patients adopt healthier behaviors. *Clinical Diabetes* 25:66–70, 2007

Bodenheimer T, MacGregor K, Sharifi C: *Helping Patients Manage Their Chronic Conditions*. Oakland, CA: California Healthcare Foundation, 2005

Eakin EG, Lawler SP, Vandelanotte C, Owen N: Telephone interventions for physical activity and dietary behavior change: a systematic review. *Am J Prev Med* 32(5):19–34, 2007

Green AJ, Bazata DD, Fox KM, Grandy S for the SHIELD Study Group: Health-related behaviors of people with diabetes and those with cardiometabolic risk factors: results from SHIELD. *Int J Clin Prac* 61:1791–1797, 2007

Heisler M, Resnicow K: Helping patients make and sustain healthy changes: a brief introduction to motivational interviewing in clinical diabetes care. *Clinical Diabetes* 26:161–166, 2008

Heisler M: Helping your patient with chronic disease: effective physician approaches to support self-management. *Semin Med Pract* 8:43–54, 2005

Kim S, Love F, Quistberg DA, Shea JA: Association of health literacy with self-mangement behavior in patients with diabetes. *Diabetes Care* 27:2980–2982, 2004

Neithercott T: 10 easy ways to get healthy right now. *Diabetes Forecast* 61(7):61–66, 2008

Peyrot M, Rubin RR: Behavioral and psychosocial interventions in diabetes: a conceptual review. *Diabetes Care* 30:2433–2440, 2007

Rhee MK, Slocum W, Ziemer DC, Cullen SD, et al.: Patient adherence improves glycemic control. *The Diabetes Educator* 31:240–250, 2005

Tomky D, Cypress M, Dang D, Maryniuk M, Peyrot M: AADE Position statement. AADE7 self-care behaviors. *The Diabetes Educator* 34:445–449, 2008

Turk PW, Mueller M, Egede LE: Estimating physician effects on glycemic control in the treatment of diabetes. *Diabetes Care* 31:869–873, 2008

Walker EA, Molitch M, Kramer MK, Kahn S, et al.: Adherence to preventive medications. *Diabetes Care* 29:1997–2002, 2006

SUGGESTED READINGS *continued*

Problem-Solving and Goal-Setting

Christian-Laygay J. Facilitating diabetes self-management goal setting in a real-world primary care center. *The Diabetes Educator* 33(Suppl 6):145S–150S, 2007

Estabrooks Pa, Nelson CC, Zu S, King D, et al.: The frequency and behavioral outcomes of goal choices in the self-management of diabetes. *The Diabetes Educator* 31:391–400, 2005

Funnell MM, Weiss MA: Patient empowerment: the LIFE approach. *Journal of European Diabetes Nursing* 5:75–78, 2008

Funnell MM, Anderson RM: Influencing self-management: from compliance to collaboration. In *Type 2 Diabetes Mellitus: An Evidence-based Approach to Practical Management.* Feinglos MN, Bethel MA, Eds. Secaucus, NJ: Human Press, 2008, p. 455–465

Gebel E: Hungry? *Diabetes Forecast* 62(3):37–41, 2009

Glasgow RE, Fisher L, Skaff M, Mullan J, Toobert DJ: Problem solving and diabetes self-management. *Diabetes Care* 30:33–37, 2007

Handley M, MacGregor K, Schillinger D, Sharifi C, Wong S, Bodenheimer T: Using action plans to help primary care patients adopt healthy behaviors: a descriptive study. *The Journal of the American Board of Family Medicine* 19:224–231, 2006

Hill-Briggs F, Gemmell L: Problem solving in diabetes self-management and control: a systematic review of the literature. *The Diabetes Educator* 33:1032–1050, 2007

Hochhauser M: Using technology to change diabetic patient behaviors. *Managed Care Quarterly* 13(4):18–21, 2005

Langford AT, Sawyer DR, Gioimo S, Brownson CA, O'Toole ML: Patient-centered goal setting as a tool to improve diabetes self-management. *The Diabetes Educator* 33(Suppl 6):139S–144S, 2007

Roberts SS: Setting goals the smart way. *Diabetes Forecast* 60(5)43–44, 2007

Weiss MA, Funnell MM: Your diabetes management plan: why it pays to have one. *Diabetes Self-management* 23(4):46–50, 2006

Weiss MA, Funnell MM: *The Little Diabetes Book You Need to Read.* Philadelphia: Running Press, 2007

⊝ Behavior Change Plan

1. What are all of your goals related to diabetes and its care?

2. What part of living with diabetes is hardest for you? How does that make you feel?

3. How does this situation need to change for you to reach your goals or feel better about it?

4. Where would you like to be regarding this situation or your goals a year from now?

   Six months from now?

   Three months from now?

   One month from now?

   Next week?

BEHAVIOR CHANGE PLAN *continued*

5. On a scale of 1–10, how important is this to you? (circle the number)

   1   2   3   4   5   6   7   8   9   10

   **Not at
   all important**

   **Extremely
   important**

6. What are some steps you could take to improve this situation or bring you closer to your goal?

7. In what ways can you change your environment (setting) at home or work (that is, eliminate negative triggers or change your routine)?

8. What are ways your family and friends can help you?

9. Write down one to three steps or behaviors that you will do when you leave here to change the situation or reach your goal.

10. How often will you do this behavior?

BEHAVIOR CHANGE PLAN *continued*

11. On a scale of 1–10, how confident do you feel that you can do this? (circle the number)

1   2   3   4   5   6   7   8   9   10

**Not at
all sure**   **Extremely
sure**

12. Write down how you will reward yourself for achieving this behavior.

13. Commitment:

I, _____ , will _____

_____

_____

_____

_____
Signature   Date

▶ ▶ ▶ ▶ ▶

| #16 | **Putting the Pieces Together** |

STATEMENT OF PURPOSE

This session is intended to help participants find and use information to deal with common situations, to provide information about resources available for people with diabetes, to obtain desired family support, and to obtain on-going support to sustain self-management of diabetes.

PREREQUISITES

It is recommended that each participant have basic knowledge about diabetes and self-care, from either personal experience or attending previous sessions.

OBJECTIVES

At the end of this session, participants will be able to:

1. identify strategies to cope with a variety of diabetes-related issues and situations;

2. find resources appropriate to particular situations;

3. state how to obtain a driver's license;

4. list strategies for dealing with possible problems associated with social activities and with traveling;

5. list strategies for obtaining desired family support;

6. create a disaster preparedness kit;

7. identify resources for obtaining desired on-going self-management support.

CONTENT

Developing personal strategies to address psychosocial issues and concerns.
Developing personal strategies to promote health and behavior change.

MATERIALS NEEDED

WORKSHEETS PROVIDED	ADDITIONAL
1–12. Problem Situations	• Membership brochures from the American Diabetes Association • Magazines and other information for people with diabetes • Information about local community resources • Information about obtaining a driver's license • Information about local syringe-disposal policies • Information about local resources for on-going self-management support

METHOD OF PRESENTATION

Start by introducing yourself and telling what you do. Ask participants to introduce themselves. Explain that the purposes of the class are to discuss a variety of issues that are common for people with diabetes and to provide information about social, vocational, medical, and financial resources that are available.

There are two options for this session. One option is to ask participants to describe situations or dilemmas they have encountered and use those for the group discussion. An alternative is to use the 12 situations included in this outline. These situations can also be used for discussion as part of other sessions. Choose only the situations and issues that are appropriate for the participants. You may choose to add a scenario that is relevant for your population. Begin by asking how they did with their short-term goal and what they learned from it.

Read each situation to the class, or ask each person in turn to read a situation aloud. Ask the participants to suggest ideas for dealing with the issue and resources that are available. Encourage participants to brainstorm ideas and discuss experiences. Point out that there are usually a variety of ways to deal with issues and problems and that no one way will work for everyone. Supply additional information from the instructor's resources sheets. Distribute pamphlets, membership forms, and so on, as indicated. Then move on to the next situation. End by asking participants to choose a short-term goal to try before the next session.

SKILLS CHECKLIST

Each participant will be able to suggest a strategy or resource for an issue or problem situation.

EVALUATION PLAN

Knowledge will be evaluated by achievement of learning objectives and by strategies and resources suggested during the session. The ability to apply knowledge will be evaluated by the ability to identify strategies for personal diabetes-related issues or problems, by the use of appropriate resources, and through program outcome measures.

DOCUMENTATION PLAN

Record class attendance and achieved objectives as appropriate using the Diabetes Self-Management Record, the Participant Follow-up Record, or another form.

SUGGESTED READINGS

American Diabetes Association: American Diabetes Association Resource Guide. *Diabetes Forecast* 62(1)33–93, 2009

American Diabetes Association: Position statement: Hypoglycemia and employment/licensure. *Diabetes Care* 31(Suppl 1):S97, 2008

Bourgeois P: Insurance: what our patients need to know. *Diabetes Spectrum* 18:62–64, 2005

Brubaker PL: Adventure travel and type 1 diabetes. *Diabetes Care* 28:2565–2572, 2005

Bunker K: Defeating discrimination. *Diabetes Forecast* 62(5):40–46, 2009

D'Arrugi T: The shift-work shuffle. *Diabetes Forecast* 60(7):50–52, 2007

D'Arrigo T: Disaster strikes. *Diabetes Forecast* 59(2):46–52, 2006

Funnell MM: Preparing for a disaster. *Practical Diabetetology* 24(3):31–33, 2005

Hernandez CL: Traveling with diabetes. *Diabetes Self-management* 20(6):118–122, 2004

Ruder K: Diabetes and your dollars. *Diabetes Forecast* 60(4):48–54, 2007

Stork ADM, van Haeften TW, Veneman T: Diabetes and driving. *Diabetes Care* 29:1942–1949, 2006

MEDICAL/COMMUNITY

You and your family have just moved to another state and you are unfamiliar with the town. You take two pills and long-acting insulin at bedtime for your diabetes. You realize that your medications are getting low. You don't have a local doctor. What might you do?

1. Brainstorm ideas such as calling your former health care team for written or telephone prescriptions, contacting local urgent or emergency care centers, or calling the local health department. If you use a chain pharmacy and have refills left, you can call a local branch for refills.

2. To find a new health care team:

   a. Have your current team refer you to one in your new community. If they can't do this, ask for a copy of your chart or a letter to introduce you to your new provider when you do locate one.

   b. Contact the American Diabetes Association (ADA), and request a list of health care professionals in your new location who are members of the ADA (www.diabetes.org).

   c. Contact the American Association of Diabetes Educators for an educator in your area who can refer you to a provider and help you find other needed resources (www.diabeteseducator.org).

   d. Look in the phone book to see if there is a diabetes clinic or other diabetes-related services nearby.

   e. Call the local hospital in the new community for names of providers.

   f. Write to the appropriate medical association or society in your new location for recommendations.

   g. When you get to your new town, ask friends or coworkers whose judgment you trust to recommend a care provider.

3. In some states, a prescription is not needed to buy syringes, needles, or monitoring equipment. Some health insurance plans have prescription coverage, and your diabetes supplies may be covered if they are ordered by prescription. Review local syringe disposal policies.

4. Laws that can affect people with diabetes include those regarding a driver's license, medical insurance, life insurance, and employment compensation. Review the specifics for your state. People with diabetes are protected under the Americans with Disabilities Act. For information about a driver's license, call the Bureau of Motor Vehicles or the Secretary of State in your new location. Some states put a notation on your driver's license to indicate that you have diabetes. Some reserve the right to deny or revoke licensure if an accident happens that is due to hypoglycemia.

SITUATION TWO

SOCIAL (FAMILY)

You are a 50-year-old woman with newly diagnosed type 2 diabetes. You have decided you want to lose one pound a week. You take insulin, but your provider says if you lose weight, there's a chance you may not need to stay on it.

Because you've always cooked all the meals for the family, your husband and sons expect you to keep doing so. Your teenage sons have already told you they do not want to eat "rabbit food." Your husband has kept on eating his snack foods in front of you. He makes a point of telling you that you shouldn't have "even a taste." How can you balance your needs with those of family members?

1. Lack of support may take the following forms:
   a. Trying to get the person with diabetes to indulge in food so other family members won't feel guilty
   b. Asking the person with diabetes to "try just a taste" of food because they feel sorry for the person
   c. Monitoring eating—being a "parent" to the adult person with diabetes
   d. Teasing about food or weight
   e. Refusing to make any changes in their eating habits.

2. Some possible ways to handle this lack of support are:
   a. Start with one area at a time and **ask** for support in each area.
   b. Have family members attend classes or talk with the health care team to gain a greater understanding of diabetes.
   c. Cook the same meals for all family members, and limit portion size for the person with diabetes.
   d. Ask family members to cook their own food.
   e. Work on assertiveness skills. Use "I" statements to ask for support ("I really need help staying with my diet," or, "It's really hard for me to avoid snack foods when they are around me," or, "I feel so much better when you are helping me").
   f. Join a diabetes support group in your area to get the help you need from others in similar situations.
   g. Remember, in most cases, family members are trying to be helpful. Try to provide your family with positive ways they can help you, such as:
      ■ notice weight loss
      ■ help plan menus
      ■ eat their snack foods away from you.
   h. Consider joining a weight loss group in your area or online.

SITUATION TWO *continued*

Weight Watchers International
The Jericho Atrium
175 Crossways Park West
Woodbury, NY 11797-2055
800-651-6000
www.weightwatchers.com

TOPS
4575 South Fifth Street
Milwaukee, WI 53207
414-482-4620
www.tops.org

Overeaters Anonymous
PO Box 44020
Rio Rancho, NM 87174
505-891-2664
www.oa.org

i. Purchase a diabetes cookbook that offers recipes the whole family can enjoy. Check your local bookstore, or contact the American Diabetes Association at 800-232-6733.

SITUATION THREE

SOCIAL

You are attending a family birthday dinner at your sister's house. Your sister, who takes pride in her cooking, has prepared a special meal with several courses. Most of the foods are combination dishes with sauces and gravies. After dinner, your sister personally hands you the dessert tray, insisting that you take some. She says, "I know several people with diabetes, and they eat anything." How can you handle this situation?

1. Some ways to handle this situation are:
   a. Eat smaller portions of the food that is served; don't take seconds.
   b. Avoid obviously sweet foods, high-fat foods, sauces, gravies, and alcohol.
   c. Take dessert, but eat none, eat only a small amount, or take it home and throw it away.
   d. Take a walk after eating.

2. Some ways to plan ahead are:
   a. Make a conscious decision before you go about what you will do. Weigh the costs, benefits, and barriers. If you decide to have dessert, think of it as a choice you have made, not as cheating. Realize that there is no right or wrong way to handle these situations, just choices and consequences.
   b. Remind your sister before you go that you have diabetes, and talk about the kinds of food you prefer to eat and those you'd rather avoid.
   c. Tell your sister how she can be of the most help to you. Do this at a time other than during the event.
   d. Offer to bring a dessert or other dish that fits your way of eating.
   e. Plan ahead for the special meal (for example, eat less fat that day). Don't take tempting leftovers home.
   f. Find out what the menu will be, then plan ahead what you will and will not eat. Reward yourself with something other than food for doing what you planned.

3. Other strategies for dealing with this type of situation are:
   a. Discuss assertiveness and how to develop it. Practice statements such as, "I appreciate the offer, but I can't possibly eat more," or, "I will feel better if I don't eat that."
   b. Talk about how to be appreciative without compromising health or diet, i.e., "Thank you for making this for me, I really appreciate your thoughtfulness, but. . . ."
   c. Discuss how personal attitude can influence a situation.
   d. Discuss the issue of "wasting" food versus "waisting" food.
   e. Be careful that these special days don't become a reason to overeat. On the other hand, don't let having diabetes keep you from being with your family.
   f. If one dinner doesn't go as you wanted, start over again tomorrow and think about ways to handle it differently the next time.

SICK DAYS

You wake up with the flu. Your body aches and you have a fever. You usually eat a hearty breakfast, but aren't sure you could keep any food down this morning.

1. Some ways to manage food intake when not feeling well are:

   a. Try to eat the same amount of carbohydrate as usual.

   b. Drink fluids in frequent sips. Try to drink at least once every 30 minutes or with every commercial break on TV.

   c. Clear liquids and soft foods may be appropriate. Consider what sounds good to you. Have the class brainstorm options.

2. Discuss changes needed in medicine or monitoring:

   a. Take your usual insulin dose even if you are unable to eat or are eating less.

   b. Check blood glucose every 2–4 hours.

   c. Check ketones every 4 hours or every time you go to the bathroom.

   d. Check fever and record every 4 hours. Take aspirin or acetaminophen as needed.

   e. You may need extra rapid- or short-acting insulin.

3. Talk about when to call the health care team:

   a. Call if ketones persist for more than 12 hours or are rising.

   b. Call if your blood glucose is higher than 250 mg/dl or you are vomiting persistently.

   c. Call if your fever is 101.5°F or higher, if your fever is rising, or if you have a fever for longer than 24 hours.

SITUATION FIVE

TRAVEL

You are flying to a tropical island for a vacation soon. At home, you take insulin injections twice a day, count carbohydrates, and walk 30 minutes every other day. How can you take care of your diabetes and enjoy your vacation?

1. Some ways to plan ahead are:
   a. Notify your health care team of your approaching trip. If possible, carry enough insulin and monitoring supplies with you. It is a good idea to pack extra in case of an emergency. Get a prescription for insulin and syringes before you leave. Get a letter from your provider about your diabetes, especially if you will be taking syringes through customs. Find out about the availability of insulin and monitoring supplies in the country where you will be traveling by calling the manufacturer, going online, or asking your pharmacist.
   b. An address for locating English-speaking physicians in foreign countries can be found in most travel books specific to the country you plan to visit. Bookstores or the local library may have books that provide this information.
   c. Airlines can provide special meals. You need to notify the airline 24 hours in advance if you would like a special meal. Many people find that they prefer the regular meal and eat only the foods that fit with their usual meal plan.
   d. Wear diabetes identification. Carry a telephone number and instructions to call that number if health care information about you is needed. Travel with someone, if possible.
   e. Take medication with you to control vomiting (especially if you get motion sickness) or diarrhea, and bring antacids to counteract new foods that might irritate your stomach.
   f. Write down the phrases for "Please get me a doctor," "Please get me some sugar or juice," "I have diabetes," "Where is a pharmacy?," "I need some insulin," and "I need to buy a syringe" in English and in the language of the country where you will be traveling. These can be found in a travel guidebook or dictionary of phrases.
   g. Carry your insulin and syringes with you. Do not pack them in your suitcase. Luggage compartments of airplanes are not insulated and the insulin may freeze. Take along more insulin than you will need, in case a bottle is lost or broken. You'll need to keep it cool (below 86°F) in your hotel room. Be sure to take along your monitoring supplies. Put your insulin in a small plastic bag (like other liquids) for security purposes.
   h. Find out what foods are available at your destination. Think through how your usual meal plan may have to be modified for these foods.
   i. Your diet and activity will be different, and your blood glucose can quickly get out of balance. You will probably want to check your blood glucose more often than at home. Take extra supplies so you can monitor as often as you need.
   j. Talk with your health care team to determine if immunizations or other special precautions are needed for the country or climate where you are going.
   k. Realize that with all of your efforts, things will probably not always go as planned. Do the best you can and enjoy the trip.

SITUATION FIVE *continued*

2. To make adjustments for time zone changes, ask your health care team about using multiple injections of rapid- or short-acting insulin before each meal while actually en route and converting back to the usual schedule when settled. Other options are to stay on your home schedule for short trips, or to gradually change to the new time zone before you go by changing your meal/insulin times by 30 minutes per day.

3. To handle delayed meals, carry some food in case of unexpected delays such as packaged peanut butter or cheese and crackers, juice boxes, and peanuts. If a meal is delayed and you have no emergency food, 1/2 cup of fruit juice or non-diet soft drink every 30 minutes until food is served should keep your blood glucose from going too low. Remember that fewer airlines provide food or snacks during the flight. Always carry some food with you as well as a way to treat a low blood glucose reaction.

SPECIAL EVENTS

You feel good about the way you have been caring for your diabetes. You want to keep doing well, but the holidays are coming. You know that both your schedule and usual meals will be different.

1. Strategies to manage diabetes during unusual or special times are:

   a. Set realistic blood glucose and exercise goals for the holidays and plan accordingly. Make conscious decisions about your self-care behaviors, weighing costs, benefits, and barriers.

   b. Decide how you will handle different situations. Remember that there is no right or best way. Decide what is going to work best for you for each particular occasion based on your past experiences and what you know about yourself.

   c. If you decide to stick as close to your plan as you can, write down what you are going to eat at the beginning of each day. You may want to share that plan with another person. Save fats and meats to "spend" at a special meal.

   d. If you choose to ignore your plan for one day, go back to it the next day.

   e. If you don't have time for your regular exercise program, try to increase your daily activity level.

   f. Limit alcohol.

   g. Check your blood glucose more often.

   h. Take extra insulin to cover additional food, or increase your activity level.

   i. Make a plan for meals at different times.

   j. If going to a gathering where a meal will be served, offer to contribute food that fits with your meal plan, such as vegetables, homemade bread, or diet soft drinks. Suggest a walk after the meal.

   k. If things don't go as you had hoped, plan how you will do better tomorrow.

FINANCIAL

Diabetes is expensive. You have figured out what you want to do to take care of your diabetes but are concerned about how you will be able to afford to pay for some of your medicines or monitoring supplies.

1. Ways to economize are:
   a. On diabetes supplies:
      - Shop wisely and compare prices. They can vary a great deal from store to store.
      - Check prices of mail-order pharmacies—they are sometimes less expensive.
   b. On food:
      - Shop wisely and plan ahead; use lists, coupons, and specials; buy fewer prepared or fast foods; or buy generic brands when possible.
      - Explore food cooperatives, community meal programs, low-cost meals through Meals-on-Wheels, and so on.
      - Grow a garden—some communities offer gardening plots if you don't have space.
2. Options for financial help are:
   a. Talk to someone in your hospital social services department about your financial problems (have the telephone number available).
   b. Contact the Department of Social Services, which is a state agency (have the telephone number available).
      - Apply for Medicaid. Financial eligibility requirements change, so you will need to check. The public library has copies of the eligibility manuals. Coverage varies greatly. If you are financially eligible and over 21 years old, you'll need to be medically approved by the Department of Social Services. If you are under 21, you just need to qualify financially.
      - Apply for food stamps. Eligibility is based on income and size of family. Generally, those who qualify for Medicaid also qualify for food stamps.
   c. Most pharmaceutical companies or service organizations may be able to offer help. A program called *Partnership for Prescription Assistance* provides access to over 600 public and private assistance programs. Contact them at 1-888-477-2669 or www.pparx.org.
   d. Apply for disability assistance.
      - Social Security disability benefits provide monthly checks to workers who are disabled. The amount paid is based on average earnings under Social Security over a period of years. Services offered are counseling, job retraining, and job placement. Call the Social Security office or your hospital social worker.
      - Supplemental Security Income (SSI) is provided to people in need who are over 65 years old or to blind and disabled people of any age. This is a supplement, an addition to your income, and is not meant to meet all of your living expenses. If you qualify for SSI payments, you can also usually qualify for Medicaid.

FINANCIAL (HEALTH INSURANCE/EMPLOYMENT POLICIES)

Your spouse has retired and you are moving. Your spouse is now eligible for Medicare, but you are not. Your group coverage at work has paid for your medical bills, diabetes medicines, and supplies, which have been quite expensive at times. You need to have health insurance coverage until you can find a new job. You are also concerned that you are less likely to be hired because of your diabetes.

1. **Health insurance.** The Health Insurance Portability and Accountability Act of 1996 helps people with chronic health conditions obtain and keep health insurance.

   a. Federal government.
      - *Medicare:* beneficiaries are retired or are disabled according to the Social Security Act. Medicare offers specific benefits for people with diabetes.
      - *Veterans Administration (VA):* payment for care within the VA Medical System only.
      - *Public Health Service and Indian Health Service:* federally funded care for specific small groups.
      - *Champus:* a program for reimbursing health care providers in the private sector for care of members of the armed forces and their dependents.

   b. State government.
      - *Medicaid:* criteria and coverage vary greatly.

   c. Fee-for-service insurance.
      - *Blue Cross/Blue Shield (BC/BS):* various plans with coverage for groups or individuals.
      - *Commercial Insurance Companies:* each makes its own decisions about coverage and to whom they will offer insurance.
      - *Self-Insuring Groups (e.g., companies and unions):* insure their members while employing BC/BS or commercial carriers as administrators.

   d. Prepaid health plans.
      - *Health Maintenance Organization (HMO):* a health care plan with its own coverage policy. There are a variety of HMOs with different provider models.

   e. Group coverage.
      - A group insurer may only refuse or limit coverage of a new enrollee with a health condition treated or diagnosed in the 6-month period before enrollment for a maximum of 12 months. Having once met the 12-month waiting period, a person cannot be denied coverage when changing jobs as long as he or she has had continuous coverage.

- Make the most of group coverage wherever you get it. See that all eligible family members are included in your plan so they can take advantage of the conversion privilege if you leave the plan. For them to exercise the privilege, you will probably have to convert as well.

- If you are covered on someone else's group plan, such as your spouse's, familiarize yourself with all conversion possibilities. This is critical if the person who has primary coverage is planning to leave the job.

f. Single policies.

- You may be able to purchase individual health insurance from the company that provided your group coverage at a reduced rate for a period of time (COBRA).

- You can convert from a group policy to an individual one, free from preexisting condition exclusions, if you have had continuous coverage for the previous 10 months, are not eligible for group coverage, and have exhausted your COBRA coverage.

- If you buy a policy on your own, look for one with guaranteed (not optional) renewability and unlimited or very high major medical benefits.

- Many states require companies to offer "pooled risk" policies for people with diabetes. This decreases the cost of premiums. Contact your State Insurance Commissioner.

g. If you cannot get regular health insurance.

- Look for policies that have liberal preexisting condition rules. Those are the clauses that exclude claims resulting from health problems that you were treated for before you took out the policy. Two years is a typical exclusion time, but some plans offer 1 year or less.

- Compare coverage, costs, and preexisting rules for several mail-order plans. These do not require a medical exam, but you may be asked specific questions about your health—whether you've been hospitalized recently and why—to exclude certain conditions.

- When you're between jobs, shop for interim health insurance for coverage. Typical interims are 30, 60, or 90 or more days. These are generally open enrollment plans (no medical exam) and have liberal preexisting condition clauses.

- Contact the American Diabetes Association for information about obtaining health insurance or other assistance.

2. Find out about the coverage for diabetes.

   a. Treatment: How often can I see my doctor? Can I see a dietitian and nurse educator?

   b. Education: Are diabetes education programs covered?

   c. Supplies: Are insulin, syringes, and diabetes pills covered? Monitoring supplies? Insulin pump? Supplies for the insulin pump?

   d. Complications: Are screening and treatments for complications covered?

   e. Specialty referral practices: Can I see an endocrinologist? An ophthalmologist? A podiatrist? A mental health specialist? An obstetrician who manages high-risk pregnancies? Other specialists as needed?

3. **Employment policies.** Americans with diabetes have been protected under the Americans with Disabilities Act since 1992. Changes in this Act in 2009 offer more protections for people with

SITUATION EIGHT *continued*

diabetes. A fact sheet is available from the Equal Employment Opportunity Commission (EEOC) (www.eeoc.gov) and from the American Diabetes Association.

a. The law guarantees equal opportunity for individuals with disabilities in employment, public accommodations, transportation, state and local government services, and telecommunications.

b. The law covers employment practices, including job application procedures, hiring, firing, advancement, compensation, training, and other terms, conditions, and privileges of employment (e.g., tenure, layoff, leave, fringe benefits, and so on).

c. During an interview, you cannot be asked if you are disabled. An employer can only ask if you can perform the particular job functions. This is also true if the employer already knows that you have diabetes.

d. Once you have been offered the job, you must disclose the fact of your diabetes to be protected under the Act. You need to explain that you need to do certain diabetes-related things during work hours. Then you need to negotiate with your new employer about how the job requirements and your diabetes management needs can both be "reasonably accommodated."

e. If you feel you are discriminated against because of your diabetes, you may be able to receive free counseling through a federally mandated program called the National Association of Protection and Advocacy Systems (NAPAS). Each state has a representative. For more information, go to www.napas.org or call 202-408-9514. You can also contact the American Diabetes Association for help with discrimination issues.

SITUATION NINE

FINANCIAL (LIFE INSURANCE)

*You never worried about life insurance before, but now you're getting married
and feel you should offer this security to your spouse. You call your friendly agent
to find out what life insurance is going to cost and learn that it
will cost almost 50% more than it costs a friend of yours who does not have
diabetes.*

1. To obtain life insurance at reasonable cost:

   a. Before you assume you're not insurable at reasonable cost, ask your agent or a company that offers this service to investigate.

   b. Group life insurance coverage is less expensive and often does not require a medical exam. Coverage is automatic after you join the group and meet certain time limits or employment standards.

      ■ If you're covered at work, you may be able to take on more insurance under the same plan, for a fee. It's usually the cheapest way available to get more insurance.

      ■ Seek out other groups, whether or not you have on-the-job coverage. Often unions, credit unions, fraternal societies, and the like offer group life insurance to members.

      ■ Convert your group coverage when you leave your job. Many employers offer up to 30 days to get a new, individual policy from the same company, with no medical exam required and no medical questions asked. You may have a choice of converting to a whole-life policy or to a less costly 1-year term policy that you could convert later into whole life. Either will cost you more than group coverage. The 30-day conversion is your best recourse if you fear a health problem will cause an insurer to turn you down or "rate" you for more expensive premiums than normal for your age. Compare the facts about other plans as soon as you know you'll be leaving your job.

   c. Buy insurance with a "waiver of premium" clause (cost: about 38–40¢ a year per $1000 face value for a 30-year-old man) so that your premiums will be paid and your insurance kept in force even if you become disabled and can no longer work.

   d. Some companies offer life insurance to people with diabetes at group rates providing they meet certain requirements. For example:

      John W. Hall & Assoc., Inc.   This policy is underwritten by the Sentry Life
      P.O. Box 14868   Insurance Company.
      Shawnee Mission, KS 66285-4868
      913-268-7878

   e. Look into policies that allow you to use the dividends to purchase additional insurance.

   f. Consider buying a "convertible term" that can be converted to permanent insurance without a physical exam. Rates are pegged to your age when you convert.

SITUATION NINE *continued*

    g. Investigate whole-life policies that will permit additional purchases up to set amounts in future years—again, without a medical exam.

2. "Graded death benefit" life insurance (sometimes called "modified" or "guaranteed issue life") is written by a few companies in most states. The key to this insurance is its terms: open enrollment with no medical exam required. Depending on the coverage and the company, premiums can run about 10–50% higher than regular policies—but the insurance may be your only protection. Terms and costs vary. Your best approach is to write several of these companies for more information.

FOR SPOUSES

Your spouse has diabetes and you want to show your support. You are also worried about your ability to handle the situation and about your own health.

1. It's not always easy to live with someone who has diabetes. It can be difficult to deal with the emotions and changing moods that many people with diabetes experience. The decisions your spouse makes will affect your future as well. Discuss some of the situations that class members describe. Ways that spouses and family members can be helpful are to:
   - Learn about diabetes.
   - Ask the person who has diabetes for ways you can be helpful. Let them know how they can be helpful to you as well.
   - Recognize positive changes.
   - Eat the same foods as your spouse.
   - Exercise with your spouse.
   - Avoid nagging, "policing," and taking over the responsibility.
   - Listen when your spouse needs to talk about his or her diabetes.
   - Attend diabetes classes and/or a support group with your spouse.
   - Be honest about your feelings.

2. Ways that spouses can get the support they need are:
   - Talk with friends or family.
   - Do what you need to take care of yourself and your health.
   - Consider joining a support group.

STAYING ON TRACK

Congratulations! You are a graduate of a diabetes education program, and you are ready to start doing the best you can to take care of yourself. However, you are concerned about staying up-to-date and motivated. You also know that people who get the support they need are better able to sustain the changes they made while attending diabetes education. How can you get the help you need?

1. Reassure participants that it is not always easy to make a lot of changes. It is also difficult to sustain these changes and maintain the motivation they need over a lifetime of diabetes. Along with their health care team, they may find it helpful to obtain on-going self-management support through a local or online support group, or to find a "diabetes buddy" for mutual support.

   a. Other suggestions may include:
   - Make a plan for change. Select a goal, then break it down into smaller steps.
   - Start by adding one new habit. It is easier to add a new habit than to break one that you already have.
   - Write down your new habits. Make them easy to remember by using reminders.
   - To change an old habit, choose the habit that is easiest for you to change. Success will help you feel that you *can* make changes.
   - Get rid of reminders of habits that you want to break and of tempting foods, too.
   - Join a diabetes support group. (Have information about local groups available.)
   - Ask for help from your family and friends. Tell them how they can be most helpful.
   - Write a contract or an agreement with a family member, friend, or health care giver about the changes you want to make.
   - Reward yourself when you make progress. Treat yourself to something you enjoy when you reach each step toward your larger goal.
   - Volunteer or find other ways to provide help to others. Serving as a support person for another person with diabetes is a way to sustain your own motivation.

   b. Motivation comes from commitment to goals. Reevaluate your goals and your treatment plan now and then, and reaffirm your commitment.

2. People can continue learning about diabetes in many ways. Some ideas are:

   a. Join the American Diabetes Association (ADA). Have membership forms and information about local activities and programs available. Many groups offer summer camping experiences for young people.

   b. Read periodicals. The ADA provides a subscription to *Diabetes Forecast* when you become a member. Other magazines are also available.

SITUATION ELEVEN *continued*

c. Use the Internet to get information from reputable websites.

d. Read books. Many books are available for people with diabetes at bookstores, online, or at your local library. For a current listing, contact:

American Diabetes Association
1701 N. Beauregard Street
Alexandria, VA 22311
800-ADA-ORDER (800-232-6733)
www.diabetes.org

National Diabetes Education Program
One Information Way
Bethesda, MD 20892-3560
888-693-NDEP (6337)
www.yourdiabetesinfo.org

e. Continue your diabetes education. Provide information about follow-up plans for your program or other local options.

DISASTER PREPAREDNESS

Because of recent news stories, one of the members of your diabetes support group wants to make sure that if a disaster occurred, she could manage her own diabetes. What advice would you give?

1. American Diabetes Association Standards of Care recommend that each person with diabetes have a disaster preparedness kit and plan that is updated annually.

2. Provide information about local resources for disaster preparedness.

3. Brainstorm with the group to develop a list of items to include in a "diabetes kit." Identify items needed based on likely possibilities for your area.

4. Ideas for items include:
   - List of medications and prescription numbers (using a national pharmacy is helpful);
   - Meeting point for all family members;
   - Meter and strips (unexpired);
   - Non-perishable food items and a 3-day supply of water;
   - Treatment for a low blood glucose level;
   - Syringes and other medication supplies;
   - Cash and telephone card;
   - List of critical record numbers (e.g., bank account, credit card, insurance);
   - Hand sterilizer;
   - Telephone numbers of your family members, physician, and pharmacy;
   - Flashlights, batteries, battery-operated radio and television, candles, and matches;
   - First aid kit.

5. Along with the American Diabetes Association, other resources include:

   American Red Cross
   www.redcross.org

   Emergency Preparedness and Response
   www.bt.cdc.gov

   Federal Emergency Management Agency
   www.fema.gov

   Prepare.org
   www.prepare.org

⊖ Situation One

MEDICAL/COMMUNITY

You and your family have just moved to another state, and you are unfamiliar with the town.

You take two pills and long-acting insulin at bedtime for your diabetes. You realize that your medications are getting low. You don't have a local doctor. What might you do?

1. How can you get a prescription?

2. How do you find a new health care team?

3. You realize that state laws can vary. What are your state's laws about purchasing syringes and insulin? About disposing of used syringes?

4. What other laws can affect you as a person with diabetes? What are your state's laws about people with diabetes having a driver's license?

➲ Situation Two

SOCIAL (FAMILY)

You are a 50-year-old woman with newly diagnosed type 2 diabetes. You have decided you want to lose one pound a week. You take insulin, but your provider says if you lose weight, there's a chance you may not need to stay on it.

Because you've always cooked all the meals for the family, your husband and sons expect you to keep doing so. Your sons have already told you they do not want to eat "rabbit food." Your husband has kept on eating his snack foods in front of you. He makes a point of telling you that you shouldn't have "even a taste." How can you balance your needs with those of your family members?

1. What problems might happen when you get home?

2. What are some ways to handle this situation?

⬤➤ Situation Three

SOCIAL

You are attending a family birthday dinner at your sister's house. Your sister, who takes pride in her cooking, has prepared a special meal with several courses. Most of the foods are combination dishes with sauces and gravies. After dinner, your sister personally hands you the dessert tray, insisting that you take some. She says, "I know several people with diabetes, and they eat anything." How can you handle this situation?

1. What are some ways to handle this situation?

2. What are some ways you can plan ahead for these special events?

3. What are other ideas for dealing with this type of situation?

⮕ Situation Four

SICK DAYS

You wake up with the flu. Your body aches and you have a fever. You usually eat a hearty breakfast, but aren't sure you could keep any food down this morning. What can you do?

1. What can you do to take care of yourself and your diabetes when you feel so awful?

2. When should you call your health care team?

➲ Situation Five

TRAVEL

You are flying to a tropical island for a vacation soon. At home, you take insulin twice a day, count carbohydrates, and walk 30 minutes every other day. How can you take care of your diabetes and enjoy your vacation?

1. What plans do you need to make for your diabetes care as you travel and once you arrive?

2. What adjustments will be necessary for time zone changes?

3. You have stopped over in Houston to refuel. It is your suppertime, but the plane is delayed by severe thunderstorms. The flight crew will not serve a meal until the plane is in flight. What can you do?

⬤➤ Situation Six

SPECIAL EVENTS

You feel good about the way you have been caring for your diabetes. You want to keep doing well, but the holidays are coming. You know that both your schedule and usual meals will be different. How can you have fun but not undo all of your hard work?

1. What are strategies you can use so that you stay on track?

You usually take your evening NPH and regular insulin at about 5:30, eat dinner at 6:00, and have a snack before bedtime at about 10:00 p.m. Today you have been invited to a dinner at a friend's home at 8:00 p.m.

1. How might you handle this change in your schedule?

➲ Situation Seven

FINANCIAL

Diabetes is expensive. You have figured out what you want to do to take care of your diabetes and are concerned about how you will be able to afford to pay for some of your medicines or monitoring supplies.

1. What can you do to economize?

2. Where can you go for help?

➡ Situation Eight

FINANCIAL (HEALTH INSURANCE/ EMPLOYMENT POLICIES)

Your spouse has retired and you are moving. Your spouse is now eligible for Medicare, but you are not. Your group coverage at work has paid for your medical bills, diabetes medicines, and supplies, which have been quite expensive at times. You need to have health insurance coverage until you can find a new job. You are also concerned that you are less likely to be hired because of your diabetes.

1. What options do you have to obtain health insurance?

2. What questions should you ask to get the best coverage?

3. During an interview for a new job, what are the employer's legal responsibilities related to your diabetes? What are your responsibilities?

⬇ Situation Nine

FINANCIAL (LIFE INSURANCE)

You never worried about life insurance before, but now you're getting married and feel you should offer this security to your spouse. You call your friendly agent to find out what life insurance is going to cost you and learn that it will cost almost 50% more than it costs a friend of yours who does not have diabetes.

1. How can you get life insurance without paying so much?

2. What can you do if your agent tells you that you can't get life insurance?

⊖ Situation Ten

FOR SPOUSES

Your spouse has diabetes and you want to show your support. You are also worried about your ability to handle the situation and about your own health.

1. What are some ways you can be helpful?

2. What are ways you can get the support that YOU need?

➔ Situation Eleven

STAYING ON TRACK

Congratulations! You are a graduate of a diabetes education program, and you are ready to start doing the best you can to take care of yourself. However, you are concerned about staying up-to-date and motivated. You also know that people who get the support they need are better able to sustain the changes they made while attending diabetes education. How can you get the help you need?

1. What are some ways you can include diabetes care in your daily routine?

2. You also want to keep learning about diabetes, new treatments, and new research. List some ways you can continue learning about diabetes.

⬤➡ Situation Twelve

DISASTER PREPAREDNESS

Because of recent news stories, one of the members of your diabetes support group wants to make sure that if a disaster occurred, she could manage her diabetes. What advice would you give?

1. What advice would you give?

'''''Supplementary Outlines

#17	Food and Weight

▷ ▷ ▷ ▷ ▷

STATEMENT OF PURPOSE

This session is intended to provide an understanding of how different foods affect body weight. Information about nutrients and food groups introduced in Outline #4, *Food and Blood Glucose* (p. 53), will be reviewed and expanded to predict the caloric density of foods. Weight reduction is one means to lower blood glucose levels and reduce cardiovascular risks (high LDL cholesterol and triglyceride levels and elevated blood pressure). The information may be appropriate for anyone interested in losing weight, in avoiding the weight gain that may occur with better blood glucose management and that is common with intensive insulin regimens, or in decreasing their cardiovascular disease risk factors. Understanding caloric density can also be applied to weight gain efforts or to maintaining calorie intake during periods of poor appetite. The focus in this session is on helping participants identify and develop strategies to change food behaviors to reach personal weight goals.

PREREQUISITES

It is recommended that participants have attended session #4, *Food and Blood Glucose* (p. 53), or have achieved those objectives. It is also helpful if participants bring a food diary.

OBJECTIVES

At the end of this session, participants will be able to:

1. name the six basic food groups and the nutrients in each group;

2. name the nutrient that supplies the most calories;

3. give examples of foods high in calories and low in calories;

4. identify triggers for emotional eating and strategies to address them;

5. identify one behavior change they could make to work toward achieving their weight goals.

CONTENT

Incorporating Nutritional Management into Lifestyle.

MATERIALS NEEDED

VISUALS PROVIDED	ADDITIONAL
None.	■ Chalkboard and chalk/Board and markers
	■ Food models or pictures of foods
Handouts (one per participant)	■ Commercial food product containers or labels that
1. Nutrients and Calories in Food Groups	show foods of various caloric densities
	■ *Choose Your Foods: Exchange Lists for Diabetes* (booklet available from the American Diabetes Association, 800-232-6733)
	■ *Choose Your Foods: Exchange Lists for Weight Management* (booklet available from the American Diabetes Association, 800-232-6733)

METHOD OF PRESENTATION

Start by introducing yourself and telling what you do. Ask participants to introduce themselves. Explain that the purpose of the session is to expand the information about different groups of foods and the nutrients in each group from session #4, *Food and Blood Glucose* (p. 53), to learn how different foods affect body weight and use their food diary from session #3, *The Basics of Eating* (p. 37), to identify their weight goals and behaviors to achieve these goals. This information can be used by participants to make food choices that help them reach their personal weight goals.

Present material in a question/discussion format, using the first question as a starting point. Provide appropriate content outlined below in response. Ask if there are additional questions and respond, repeating the process for the entire session. Use the questions in the Instructor's Notes section to generate discussion if no questions are forthcoming after a period of silence. You can also use participant monitoring records or develop examples that participants can use for problem solving. Keeping track of the content discussed in each session, using the Diabetes Self-Management Record, the Participant Follow-up Record, or another form helps you to evaluate if all needed content has been discussed.

CONTENT OUTLINE

CONCEPT	DETAIL	INSTRUCTOR'S NOTES
1. Diabetes and weight management	1.1 Weight loss is one way to lower blood glucose and to reduce risks for heart and blood vessel disease.	Ask, "What questions or concerns do you have about diabetes and weight?"
	1.2 For most people, weight loss is an on-going struggle. Losing 7–10% of your body weight can have a big impact on your blood glucose levels.	Ask, "Have you ever tried to lose weight? What worked or did not work for you? What did you learn?" Acknowledge any struggle implied in their comments. Most people feel self-conscious and guilty about their weight and weight loss attempts.

CONTENT OUTLINE

CONCEPT	DETAIL	INSTRUCTOR'S NOTES
	1.3 Keeping weight off once you lose it can also be difficult. If you lose weight too quickly, it often returns.	Ask, "Have you ever lost weight and then regained it? Why do you think that happened?"
	1.4 Studies show that people who are successful in maintaining weight loss regularly exercise, eat breakfast, weigh themselves often, and view paying attention to their weight as part of a routine.	
	1.5 Your weight is determined by: ■ food eaten ■ activity level ■ heredity and body build ■ body chemistry ■ medicines. Some things you can change and some things you cannot change.	Point out the benefits of healthy eating regardless of weight.
	1.6 Understanding yourself, what food means to you, and your triggers for overeating are critical for losing weight and keeping it off. If eating when stressed is an issue, learning and coping skills may be more helpful than "dieting."	Ask participants to reflect for a few minutes about these issues. At the end of the time, ask if anyone has any thoughts or insights they want to share. Be neutral in your response to issues raised and involve other participants. Asking if others have had similar experiences often helps to identify strategies for problem areas.
2. Calories	2.1 Eating fewer calories is one way to lose weight.	A calorie is a measure of stored energy.
	2.2 The minimum recommended calories to obtain needed vitamins and minerals is 1,200 for adult females and 1,500 for adult males. Fad diets and quick weight loss plans can harm health and interfere with diabetes management. Weight loss of no more than 1–2 lbs per week is safe and less likely to be regained.	Very-low-calorie diets are sometimes prescribed to improve pancreatic function in type 2 diabetes. They should be attempted only under medical supervision.

CONTENT OUTLINE

CONCEPT	DETAIL	INSTRUCTOR'S NOTES
	2.3 Awareness of the calorie content of food can help you choose foods to lose weight or to avoid weight gain. Because glucose calories are lost in the urine when blood glucose levels are high, it is easy to gain weight when you lower your blood glucose.	A decrease of 500 calories per day will result in about a 1 lb weight loss per week.
	2.4 Awareness of the calorie content of food can also help you choose foods to gain weight or avoid weight loss.	
3. Role of carbohydrate, protein, and fat in weight management	3.1 Carbohydrate, protein, and fat all contribute calories when digested.	Review information about nutrients and food groups in Outline #4, *Food and Blood Glucose,* (p. 53), as needed. Use Handout #1, Nutrients and Calories in Food Groups.
	3.2 Fat provides more calories per gram than carbohydrate or protein and is most easily changed into body fat. However, too much of any nutrient beyond your calorie requirements is stored as fat.	Counting fat grams is an effective way for some people to limit total calories.
	3.3 Excess fat intake leads to excess fat on our bodies. Fat can be stored almost directly on the body.	A total of 97% of excess dietary fat is converted to body fat.
	3.4 Foods high in water and/or fiber have fewer calories per bite. Fresh fruits, vegetables, and whole grains have the fewest calories per bite. These foods tend to require more chewing, take longer to eat, and help you feel full and satisfied without a lot of calories.	Ask, "What foods are low in calories?" Use food models or pictures of food to illustrate. See Outline #18, *Eating for a Healthy Heart* (p. 379), for more detailed information about fiber.
	3.5 Calories from high-fat foods, such as regular salad dressing and peanut butter, can add up quickly. Both approach 100 calories per tablespoon.	From a pitcher with 1/2 cup (8 Tbsp) salad dressing, pour dressing onto lettuce or crinkled-up paper. From a shallow container with 1/4 cup peanut butter, spread some on a piece of bread. Ask participants to estimate the amounts used. Measure the amount left in each

CONTENT OUTLINE

CONCEPT	DETAIL	INSTRUCTOR'S NOTES

container and calculate the calories in the portions used.

3.6 Meat, cheese, and milk contain valuable nutrients but can be high in fat (e.g., sausage, cheddar cheese, and whole milk). You can obtain the nutrients and limit fat and calories by choosing lean meat, fish, poultry without skin, low-fat cheese, and skim milk.

Compare the calorie level of equal amounts of high- and low-fat milk and meats. Refer to *Exchange Lists for Diabetes Management* or *Exchange Lists for Weight Loss* for lists of very lean, lean, medium-fat, and high-fat meats.

3.7 Fried chicken, french fries, cream sauce, some frozen dinners, and snack chips are examples of foods that are high in fat.

Ask participants to name other high-fat foods. Show food models or labels.

3.8 Foods with added sugar (e.g., cookies and candy) or compact foods (e.g., granola or dried fruit) are high in calories as well as carbohydrate per bite.

The makers of some low-fat dessert and snack items have replaced fat with extra sugar. The products tend to be high in carbohydrate and may have as many calories as the higher-fat versions.

3.9 Most dessert items are high in both sugar and fat. Examples are cake, cookies, pies, ice cream, chocolate, and candy.

Ask, "What foods are high in sugar and fat?" Research shows that people are born enjoying foods that combine sugar and fat.

3.10 In summary, to decrease calories without eating less total food:
- Eat more fresh fruits, vegetables, and whole grains.
- Choose measured amounts of lean meat, fish, poultry, and skim milk.
- Limit added-fat and high-fat foods.
- Limit calories from liquids.

Note that this is the recommended way of eating for everyone.

3.11 You don't have to give up your favorite foods. To decrease calories without eliminating types of food:
- Limit portion sizes.
- Choose a low-fat version of the food.
- Limit number of portions per day or week.
- Limit between-meal snacking.
- Eat high-calorie foods less often.

Ask, "What are strategies you use to include your favorite foods?" Write these on the board.
For example, if a participant likes a cheese and bologna sandwich for lunch each day, he or she could:
- have half a sandwich and a salad

CONTENT OUTLINE

CONCEPT	DETAIL	INSTRUCTOR'S NOTES
		■ use low-fat bologna, cheese, and/or mayonnaise ■ have it 1 or 2 days a week ■ trade one high-fat food for another item he or she likes less.
	3.12 A calculated meal plan can include all of these ways to limit calories.	
4. Tips for changing behaviors to eat fewer calories	4.1 Changing a series of behaviors is usually required before new food choices are habits. You can use several strategies to help.	Ask, "What has helped you to make changes in the past? What strategies have worked to help you lose weight?" Brainstorm a list of ideas for changing behavior and write on the board. Ask, "Would any of these work for you?" Offer information from sections 4 and 5 not included on the brainstorm list.
	4.2 Recording everything you eat or drink for a week can help you see patterns you want to change. Writing down the time, place, and your feelings can make you more aware of situations that affect your food choices.	Ask, "Do you know what you want to change?" Offer copies of Handout #2, Food Diary, from Outline #3, *The Basics of Eating*. (p. 37).
	4.3 Planning meals and snacks ahead may help avoid overeating (a bag lunch avoids temptation in the cafeteria, a snack after work may avoid nibbling through dinner preparations, and regular grocery shopping helps prevent fast food meals).	Different approaches to overall meal plans are covered in Outlines #5, *Planning Meals #19* (p. 69), and *Carbohydrate Counting* (p. 399).
	4.4 Water, coffee, tea, diet soda, sugar-free KoolAid, club soda, and flavored water may help you feel full and satisfied, but provide few (or no) calories. Because beverages can be quickly consumed, it is easy to "overeat" when drinking fruit juice, punch, and regular soft drinks.	
	4.5 Planning for small amounts of your favorite foods (even if they are high in carbohydrate, fat, and calories)	Ask, "Is there a food you crave? What approach would work best for you?" A dietitian can

CONTENT OUTLINE

CONCEPT	DETAIL	INSTRUCTOR'S NOTES
	helps some people stick with their overall meal plan. Others overeat sweets once they start and do better avoiding them. If you crave certain foods, you may be cutting back too much on a particular nutrient.	help find ways to include favorite foods and reduce cravings.
	4.6 Buy high-fat foods in single-portion sizes—"economy packs" can encourage overeating or eating when not hungry. There are many ways to eat less fat: ■ Choose high-fat foods less often. ■ Eat smaller amounts of the same foods you eat now. ■ Omit some high-fat foods. ■ Substitute a similar food with less fat per bite; many lower-fat and lower-calorie alternatives are now available at restaurants and in the grocery store.	Ask, "Do you think eating less fat would help you reach your goal(s)? What ways could you eat less fat?" Write on board and discuss. Examples: Eat peanuts once a week instead of every night; eat one slice of cheese instead of two; stop buying bacon. Examples: Substitute ground sirloin for hamburger; eat regular instead of premium ice cream; use lite instead of regular salad dressings; buy low-fat crackers; choose a grilled instead of a deep-fried chicken sandwich.
5. Other ways to help manage weight	5.1 Look for other things to do if you eat when you are not hungry. Examples: Go for a walk, call a friend, drink water or diet soft drinks, chew sugarless gum, or knit. Urges to eat do pass.	Ask, "Do you ever eat when you are not really hungry? Do you eat when you are stressed or at other times? Are there strategies you have used that help?" Write these on the board without making judgments.
	5.2 Figure out a strategy for when you are feeling deprived or have cravings.	Ask, "Do you ever feel deprived when you are trying to lose weight? What strategies have you found that are helpful?" Write these on the board and discuss. Refer individuals with eating disorders, anxiety, or depression to a mental health professional.
	5.3 Individual counseling from a dietitian or joining a support group may help you reach your goals.	Refer individuals with suspected eating disorders, anxiety, or depression to a mental health professional.

CONTENT OUTLINE

CONCEPT	DETAIL	INSTRUCTOR'S NOTES
	5.4 Check your blood glucose before treating symptoms of a reaction. Frequent eating to avoid or treat reactions is a common source of excess calories for persons treated with insulin.	Refer to Outline #11, *Managing Blood Glucose* (p. 231), for information about treatment for hypoglycemia.
	5.5 As you lose weight, you may notice that your blood glucose levels are lower. Talk with your provider if you think you need less insulin or oral medication.	Low blood glucose reactions are one sign less medication is needed. Review as needed, including nocturnal hypoglycemia.
	5.6 Exercise helps with weight management by burning calories, relieving stress, and maintaining muscle mass.	See Outline #7, *Physical Activity and Exercise* (p. 121).
	5.7 Exercise helps people with type 2 diabetes improve blood glucose levels by helping insulin to work better and decreasing glucose output from the liver. You may need less medication as you exercise more.	
	5.8 Medicines to help with weight loss are available. These may help people lose and maintain a modest weight loss when combined with a reduced-calorie diet. Consult your provider about the benefits and risks of these drugs.	One medication, Xenical (Orlistat), blocks absorption of fat. It prevents about 30% of dietary fat from being absorbed. Patients can expect a loss of about 10% of their body weight. The main side effects are cramping and diarrhea. A less potent form (Alli) is available over the counter. Sibutramine (Meridia) is an appetite suppressant. The average weight loss is 10–14 lb. Common side effects are dry mouth, constipation, and insomnia. Serotonin-uptake inhibitors can be used to promote weight loss. These are not stimulants, but help decrease appetite and improve insulin sensitivity. These may be recommended for people who are at least 20–30% over their desirable body

CONTENT OUTLINE

CONCEPT	DETAIL	INSTRUCTOR'S NOTES
		weight. Usually mild and short-term side effects include dry mouth, drowsiness, and diarrhea. An acute side effect is primary pulmonary hypertension. Neurotoxicity is another concern.
	5.9 Surgical options are becoming more widely available, but have risks as well as benefits.	A thorough physical and psychological assessment and extensive education is needed as part of the decision-making process.
6. Planning for change	6.1 There are many approaches to managing weight through your food choices: ■ Set a long-range goal that is important to you, is realistic, and is inspiring. ■ Assess the way you are eating now. Use your food diary to determine your current eating habits and whether there are foods you could easily eliminate of decrease. ■ Develop a plan on which you are willing and able to work. ■ Choose one behavior change you can do before the next class. ■ Start with a behavior that will be easy for you to change or one that worked for you in the past. ■ Commit to that behavior change for the next week.	Examples: In the next 4 months, lose 7 lbs or exercise 45 minutes daily. Use the food diary to help participants identify problem areas that can be used as the basis for action planning. See Outline #15, *Changing Behavior,* (p. 315). Choose a short-term goal to try before the next session. Examples: Try diet soft drinks; carry your lunch; measure amount of cereal eaten; and drink 2% instead of whole milk.

SKILLS CHECKLIST

None.

EVALUATION PLAN

Knowledge will be evaluated by achievement of learning objectives and by responses to questions during the session. The ability to apply knowledge will be evaluated by development of personal weight goals, by the development and implementation of a plan to achieve those goals, and through program outcome measures.

DOCUMENTATION PLAN

Record class attendance and achieved objectives as appropriate.

SUGGESTED READINGS

Bloomgarden ZT: Diabetes and obesity: part 1. *Diabetes Care* 30:3145–3151, 2007

Bloomgarden ZT: Diabetes and obesity: part 2. *Diabetes Care* 31:176–182, 2008

Bloomgarden ZT: Weight control in individuals with diabetes. *Diabetes Care* 29:2749–2754, 2006

Boucher JL, Benson GA, Kovarik S, Solem B, Vanwormer JJ: Current trends in weight management: what advice do we give to patients? *Clinical Diabetes* 26:100–114, 2008

Cheskin LJ, Mitchell AM, Jhaveri AD, Mitola, AH, et al.: Efficacy of meal replacements versus a standard food-based diet for weight loss in type 2 diabetes. *The Diabetes Educator* 34:118–127, 2008

Christian VJ, Polonsky WH: Overcoming the psychological challenges to weight loss. *Diabetes Forecast* 58(4):54–58, 2005

Craig J: How to maintain lost weight. *Diabetes Spectrum* 21:186–188, 2008

Ferrannini E, Mingrone G: Impact of different bariatric surgical procedures on insulin action and B-cell function in type 2 diabetes. *Diabetes Care* 32:514–520, 2009

Franz MJ: The art and science of obesity management. *Diabetes Spectrum* 21:138–172, 2008

Freeman J: Keeping off lost weight. *Diabetes Forecast* 58(2):58–61, 2005

Foster GD, Nonas C: *Managing Obesity: A Clinical Guide.* Alexandria, VA: American Diabetes Association, 2003

Hamman RF, Wing RR, Edelstein SE, Lachin JM, et al.: Effect of weight loss with lifestyle intervention on risk of diabetes. *Diabetes Care* 29:2102–2107, 2006

Huzinga MM: Weight-loss pharmacotherapy: a brief review. *Clinical Diabetes* 25:135-144, 2007

Ponder SW, Anderson MA: Teaching families to keep their children SAFE from obesity. *Diabetes Spectrum* 21:50–53, 2008

Raynor HA, Jeffery RW, Ruggiero AM, Clark JM, et al.: Weight loss strategies associated with BMI in overweight adults with type 2 diabetes at entry into the Look AHEAD trial. *Diabetes Care* 31:1299-1305, 2008

Rizzotto J-A: Meal planning in groups. *Diabetes Spectrum* 18:132–134, 2005

Roberts S: Carb counting: a flexible way to plan meals. *Diabetes Forecast* 60(5):25–27, 2007

Roth MA: Web-based weight management program in an integrated health care setting: a randomized controlled trial. *Obesity* 14:266–272, 2006

Svetkey LP, Stevens VJ, Brantley PJ, et al.: Comparison of strategies for maintaining weight loss. *JAMA* 299:1129–1148, 2008

Ulen CG, Huzinga MM, Beech B, Elasy TA: Weight regain prevention. *Clinical Diabetes* 26:100–114, 2008

◐ Nutrients and Calories in Food Groups

Food Group	Nutrient(s)	Effect on Blood Glucose*	Calories per Bite
Starch	**Carbohydrate** Protein	Large	Low
Fruit	**Carbohydrate**	Large	Low
Milk	**Carbohydrate** Protein Fat	Large	Low (higher if 2% or whole milk)
Vegetable	**Carbohydrate** Protein	Small	Low
Meat	**Protein** Fat	—	High (lower if very low fat)
Fat	**Fat**	—	High

* Within 2 hours of eating.

#18   Eating for a Healthy Heart

▶ ▶ ▶ ▶ ▶

STATEMENT OF PURPOSE

This session is intended to provide information about fats, fiber, and sodium and their impact on the risks for cardiovascular complications. Sources and effects of the different types of dietary fat and fiber are included.

PREREQUISITES

It is recommended that each participant have attended session #5, *Planning Meals* (p. 69), or have achieved those objectives. This session also builds on information about the food label in session #6, *Stocking the Cupboard* (p. 101).

OBJECTIVES

At the end of this session, participants will be able to:

1. define lipids;

2. identify factors that influence blood lipids;

3. state the benefits of managing blood lipids for people with diabetes;

4. explain the effect of dietary cholesterol on blood cholesterol;

5. identify foods high in cholesterol;

6. distinguish between the effects of saturated, unsaturated, and trans fat on blood lipids;

7. identify two sources of each of the three types of dietary fat;

8. explain the two types of dietary fiber and give two examples of foods high in each;

9. state two benefits and two reasons for caution in the use of dietary fiber;

10. state the rationale for limiting sodium in the diet;

11. identify foods high in sodium;

12. identify personal food habits or behaviors that may contribute to increasing risk for cardiovascular complications;

13. identify personal barriers and benefits of reducing risks for the cardiovascular complications.

CONTENT

Preventing long-term complications and incorporating nutritional management into lifestyle.

MATERIALS NEEDED

VISUALS PROVIDED	ADDITIONAL
1. Reasons for Meal Planning 2. Types of Fat in Blood 3. Types of Fat in Food	■ Commercial food product containers or labels

Handouts (one per participant)
1. Sources of Cholesterol and Fat
2. Sources of Fiber
3. High-Sodium Foods
4. Alternative Seasonings

METHOD OF PRESENTATION

Start by introducing yourself and telling what you do. Ask participants to introduce themselves. Explain that the purpose of this session is to provide information about blood fats and the reasons why it is important for people with diabetes to work toward recommended levels.

Present material in a question/discussion format, using the first question as a starting point. Provide appropriate content outlined below in response. Ask if there are additional questions, and respond, repeating the process for the entire session. Use the questions in the Instructor's Notes section to generate discussion if no questions are forthcoming after a period of silence. Keeping track of the content discussed in each session, using the Diabetes Self-Management Record, the Participant Follow-up Record, or another form, helps you to evaluate if all needed content has been discussed.

Guidelines for maintaining normal blood fat levels are consistent with guidelines for healthy eating. Although designed for people with diabetes, this content can be used by anyone to improve blood lipid levels.

CONTENT OUTLINE

CONCEPT	DETAIL	INSTRUCTOR'S NOTES
1. **Review goals for meal planning**	1.1 Managing blood fats or lipids is a major reason for meal planning for many people with diabetes, because of the increased risk for heart attacks and vascular disease.	Ask, "What concerns/questions do you have about eating for a healthy heart?" Review goals for meal planning. Use Visual #1, Reasons for Meal Planning. Ask, "What reason is most important for you?"

CONTENT OUTLINE

CONCEPT	DETAIL	INSTRUCTOR'S NOTES
	1.2 *Lipid* is a medical term used for fat and/or cholesterol.	
	1.3 Your weight and your blood glucose levels affect the fat in your blood. Staying at a desirable weight and in your target blood glucose range helps keep your blood lipids at the right level. Heredity and exercise also affect blood lipid levels.	Refer to Outline #4, *Food and Blood Glucose* (p. 53).
	1.4 People with diabetes are two to four times more likely to have heart and circulation (blood flow) problems. Normal blood lipids and blood pressure can help lower that risk.	Lipid management is aimed at lowering LDL cholesterol and triglycerides and raising HDL cholesterol.
	1.5 Most people can improve their lipids with modest adjustments in saturated fat intake, physical activity, and gradual weight loss (1/2–1 lb per week). A diet high in fruits, vegetables, whole grains, cold-water fish, and nuts may also be beneficial.	Rapid weight loss can increase lipid levels.
2. Tests for blood lipids	2.1 Three kinds of lipids are present in your blood: ■ low-density lipoprotein (LDL) cholesterol ■ high-density lipoprotein (HDL) cholesterol ■ triglycerides. Each of these lipids in your blood can be measured, and your total cholesterol level can be determined.	Ask, "Do you know your LDL, HDL, and triglyceride levels? What are your targets?" Use Visual #2, Types of Fat in Blood.
	2.2 The total cholesterol level is used as a screening tool.	A fasting lipid profile is recommended annually for all people with diabetes. Atherosclerotic disease is generally not seen in people with cholesterol levels lower than 150 mg/dl.

CONTENT OUTLINE

CONCEPT	DETAIL	INSTRUCTOR'S NOTES
	2.3 LDL cholesterol is the lipid that builds up inside your blood vessels and slows or blocks blood flow. It is called the "bad" or "lousy" cholesterol. Recommended LDL level for people with diabetes is less than 100 mg/dl. For persons with heart disease, a lower LDL of <70 mg/dl is recommended.	LDL = total cholesterol – HDL $-$ $\dfrac{\text{triglycerides}}{5}$ Currently, LDL cholesterol and triglycerides are most closely associated with the development of atherosclerosis.
	2.4 Decreasing saturated and trans fat intake may help to lower LDL cholesterol.	Maximal medical nutrition therapy typically reduces LDL by 15–25 mg/dl.
	2.5 HDL cholesterol is the lipid that helps remove cholesterol from the blood. It is called the "good" or "helpful" cholesterol. The higher your HDL level, the lower your risk of heart disease. The recommended HDL level is more than 40 mg/dl for men and 50 for women. Levels above 60 mg/dl are considered protective.	HDL level is modestly affected by diet, but may be increased through exercise, weight reduction (1% kg lost), and smoking cessation (3–6%). Medications increase by 2–3%.
	2.6 Triglycerides in the blood tend to be high when blood glucose is high. High triglycerides also tend to lower HDL cholesterol. The recommended triglyceride level is less than 150 mg/dl.	Triglycerides are used to calculate LDL cholesterol. Point out that some people are particularly sensitive to the effects of carbohydrates, sugar, alcohol, dietary fat, or large meals. These factors can also elevate triglyceride levels even without high blood glucose levels.
3. Cholesterol	3.1 The amount of cholesterol and, primarily, the amount and type of fat in your diet affect the level of cholesterol in your blood.	To some extent, lipid abnormalities associated with diabetes are thought to be part of the disease. Genetics may also influence a person's response to diet.
	3.2 Fat and cholesterol are two types of lipids (fatty substances) found in food.	Use Visual #3, Types of Fat in Food.

CONTENT OUTLINE

CONCEPT	DETAIL	INSTRUCTOR'S NOTES
	3.3 Cholesterol in your food may increase the cholesterol in your blood if eaten in excessive amounts.	
	3.4 Cholesterol is a soft, waxy substance made by all animals, including humans. It is essential for life, but the body makes all it needs.	Cholesterol is made in the liver. It is used to make bile acid, hormones, and vitamin D.
	3.5 Cholesterol is found in all foods that come from animals. Examples are meat, cheese, egg yolk, whole or 2% milk, and ice cream. The American Diabetes Association and The American Dietetic Association recommend limiting cholesterol to less than 200 mg/day.	Ask, "What foods contain cholesterol?" Use Handout #1, Sources of Cholesterol and Fat. Ask, "Which foods high in cholesterol do you eat often?" Note that cholesterol is part of the cell wall of animals and cannot be removed as fat can. Cholesterol is not present in egg whites. Some foods contain much more cholesterol than others, but all animal foods contain cholesterol.
4. Fat	4.1 All fats are high in calories and can contribute to excess weight.	1 gram of fat = 9 calories.
	4.2 Different people need different amounts of fat depending on their weight and lipid goals. Work with a dietitian to learn the best amount for you.	A total of 25–30% of total calories or 50–70 g of fat per day is a reasonable initial target for most people.
	4.3 Fat contributes flavor and texture to foods and gives you a sense of fullness.	Fat transports the fat-soluble vitamins A, D, E, and K and provides linoleic acid, an essential fatty acid.
	4.4 Only some fats in food can directly increase the cholesterol in blood.	
	4.5 Saturated, trans, and unsaturated are the three types of fat in food.	Refer again to Visual #3, Types of Fat in Food.
5. Saturated fat and hydrogenated and trans fatty acids	5.1 Saturated fat and trans/hydrogenated fatty acids increase blood cholesterol levels because your body makes cholesterol from these fats. This fat is solid at room temperature.	Limiting saturated fat to less than 7% of total calories is recommended. Eliminating trans fatty acids is recommended.

CONTENT OUTLINE

CONCEPT	DETAIL	INSTRUCTOR'S NOTES
	5.2 All animal products contain saturated fat. Examples are whole milk, meat, bacon, butter, sour cream, and cheese. Check meat packages for percentage of fat. The higher the percent of fat, the higher the saturated fat content.	Ask, "Which foods containing saturated fat do you eat?" Less expensive cuts of meat contain less marbling and are lower in fat, but more expensive ground meat (e.g., ground round or sirloin) is higher in fat.
	5.3 Some vegetable products are high in saturated fat. Palm and coconut oil are vegetable fats naturally high in saturated fat.	Coconut oil is not an oil, but is solid at room temperature.
	5.4 Vegetable oils that have been processed (hydrogenated) to become solid are trans fats. Trans fats are now listed on food labels and are banned in some places. The recommended intake of trans fats is less than 1% of your diet. Hydrogenated fats are man-made saturated fat and have a negative impact on your blood lipid levels.	Shortening is an example of hydrogenated vegetable oil. Foods listing this first on the label contain higher amounts. Margarine, commercial baked goods, and snack foods may contain trans or hydrogenated fats. Show examples (or labels) of these products. Trans fatty acids are believed to have a more negative impact than saturated fat.
	5.5 A product may contain saturated and hydrogenated fat even though the label truthfully says that it contains no cholesterol. Since 1990, an item labeled "cholesterol free" can contain no more than 2 mg saturated fat per serving.	Illustrate with commercial food products (or labels) that contain saturated fat but no cholesterol but can still have a negative impact on cholesterol synthesis.
	5.6 To reduce saturated and trans/hydrogenated fats in your diet, you can eat fewer or smaller portions of these foods or substitute other products.	Ask, "How could you eat fewer saturated and trans/hydro-genated fats?" Show examples of products or labels such as reduced-fat cheeses, imitation or low-fat sour cream, and baked goods made with liquid oils.
	5.7 Many low- and no-fat products can be found in the grocery store; however, they may be higher in carbohydrate and may be no lower in calories than foods they are meant to replace.	Show examples of products low in fat but high in carbohydrate. Ask, "How might you fit this product into your meal plan?"

CONTENT OUTLINE

CONCEPT	DETAIL	INSTRUCTOR'S NOTES
6. Monounsaturated and polyunsaturated fats	6.1 Unsaturated fat lowers blood cholesterol. These fats are liquid at room temperature. Unsaturated fats are either polyunsaturated or monounsaturated. Check the label to be sure that these do not contain palm or coconut oil. These are often used in semi-solid spreads, microwave popcorn, and pastries.	The more liquid the fat, the more unsaturated it is—tub margarine is more unsaturated than stick margarine; liquid is more unsaturated than tub. Even though palm and coconut oil come from plants, they are saturated fats.
	6.2 Polyunsaturated fats lower both LDL and HDL cholesterol. Some polyunsaturated fat is essential to life.	Linoleic acid, the essential fatty acid, is a polyunsaturated fat.
	6.3 Polyunsaturated fats are found in safflower, sunflower, corn, and soybean oil; margarines made from these liquid oils; mayonnaise; and nuts such as walnuts.	Ask, "What foods do you eat that contain polyunsaturated fats?"
	6.4 Monounsaturated fats are liquid at room temperature but become too thick to pour when cold.	It is recommended that the remainder of the fat content be made up of polyunsaturated and monosaturated fat.
	6.5 Monounsaturated fats are found in high concentrations in olive, peanut, and canola oil; olives and avocados; and almonds, cashews, peanuts, and pistachios.	Ask, "What foods do you eat that contain monounsaturated fat?"
	6.6 Monounsaturated fat lowers LDL cholesterol without lowering HDL cholesterol.	Replacing some carbohydrate with added monounsaturated fat may help to lower blood glucose and triglycerides in some people without worsening lipid levels. Ask, "Are there ways you can substitute monounsaturated for unsaturated fat in your diet?"
	6.7 Omega-3 fats are found in fish oil, flaxseed, and soybean oil. These lower triglycerides and protect the heart.	Ask, "What foods do you eat that contain omega-3 fats?"

CONTENT OUTLINE

CONCEPT	DETAIL	INSTRUCTOR'S NOTES
	6.8 Tuna, salmon, lake trout, mackerel, herring, and sardines are high in omega-3 oil. Use tuna and sardine products that are not packed in oil. Two or more servings per week are recommended.	These are all "fatty" cold water fish.
	6.9 Omega-3 oil is available in capsule form. A prescription is available for people with high triglyceride levels. If you buy over-the-counter products, pay particular attention to the DHA and EPA amounts as this is the active ingredient that helps to prevent inflammation. The sum of these two ingredients is the amount of omega-3 oil you are receiving.	Inflammation damages blood vessels. The precise therapeutic dose has not been determined, but 3 grams per day is the highest recommended dose.
	6.10 Food products are available that may help to lower cholesterol levels, if eaten in therapeutic amounts.	Show examples of products (i.e., margarine). Plant products are added to decrease absorption of the cholesterol and saturated fat.
7. Guidelines for choosing foods lower in fat	7.1 Guidelines for limiting fat: ■ Choose lean meats, fish, and poultry. ■ Use skim or low-fat milk. ■ Limit egg yolks and organ meats. ■ Limit high-fat animal products such as bacon, hot dogs, cheese, and butter. ■ Limit commercially prepared baked and snack foods. ■ Use monounsaturated fat for cooking and replace other oils when making salad dressing or baking.	Ask, "What are some of your ideas for eating less than 200 mg cholesterol and less than 25–30% fat?" Write down responses on the board and add to list. ■ Eat 4–6 oz lean meat per day. ■ Drink skim milk only. ■ Eat no more than three to four egg yolks per week. ■ Use small amounts of mono-unsaturated oil for cooking and as a substitute oil in food preparation. Note that this way of eating is recommended for everyone.
8. Fiber	8.1 Fiber is the undigestible part of plant food. It provides bulk but does not add to blood glucose levels.	Ask, "What foods high in fiber do you eat?"

CONTENT OUTLINE

CONCEPT	DETAIL	INSTRUCTOR'S NOTES
	8.2 There are two types of fiber. The coarse or stringy kind called insoluble fiber helps prevent constipation.	Insoluble fiber speeds up the passage of food through the digestive system.
	8.3 Insoluble fiber is found in whole-grain bread and cereal, wheat bran, fresh fruit, and vegetables.	Ask, "What foods help prevent constipation?" Use Handout #2, Sources of Fiber.
	8.4 The other kind of fiber absorbs water like gelatin and is called soluble fiber.	Soluble fiber slows down the passage of food through the digestive system.
	8.5 Water-soluble fiber is found in okra, oat bran, rice bran, dried beans, dried peas, lentils, and most fresh fruits and vegetables.	Water-soluble fiber has a tendency to lower lipid levels.
	8.6 To eat the recommended amount of fiber, you can include ■ fresh fruits ■ fresh vegetables ■ whole grains ■ bran cereal ■ legumes.	The recommended goal for dietary fiber is 20–35 g/day, or 14 g/1,000 calories per day. Legumes are various dried beans, dried peas, and lentils.
	8.7 One way to add fiber is to use legumes, dried beans, dried peas, and lentils in soups and casseroles.	
	8.8 Some high-fiber foods may cause gas and cramping. Gradually adding fiber into your diet helps control this problem.	Ask, "Have you had any problems with eating fiber?" Drinking adequate fluid is necessary to prevent constipation. Fiber requires enzymes to prevent gas formation. As we age, we are less able to make those enzymes, but they are available over the counter.
	8.9 If the stomach empties slowly (as with autonomic neuropathy), high-fiber diets can make the problem worse.	If participants report feeling full quickly, suggest that they consult their provider before adding high-fiber foods.
	8.10 Some people find that a high-fiber diet helps them feel full and more able to limit calories.	Ask, "What ideas do you have for ways you could increase the fiber in your diet?" Provide information about how to deal

CONTENT OUTLINE

CONCEPT	DETAIL	INSTRUCTOR'S NOTES

		with fiber when counting carbs, either by subtracting half the total mount of fiber, or by subtracting the total fiber from the number of carbohydrates when there are more than 5 grams of fiber.
9. Sodium	9.1 Over half of the people with diabetes also have high blood pressure. High blood pressure increases your risk for heart and blood vessel disease.	Ask, "Do you know your blood pressure target?" The recommended blood pressure for people with diabetes is generally 130/80.
	9.2 Reducing dietary sodium may help to reduce your blood pressure.	Sodium restrictions do not help everyone (they do help 10–20% of the general population and 60% of those with hypertension).
	9.3 The sodium recommendation for people with diabetes, whether or not they have high blood pressure, is 2,300 mg of sodium per day, along with a diet high in fruits, vegetables, and low-fat dairy products.	The recommendation for people with diabetes and symptomatic heart failure is 2,000 mg/day.
	9.4 The body needs no more than 500 mg of sodium per day (the amount in 1/4 tsp of salt). The naturally occurring sodium in food and water easily supplies that amount.	
	9.5 Table salt is high in sodium, but soup, pickles, olives, canned vegetables, lunch meats, snack, and convenience foods also tend to be very high in sodium. Restaurant food, especially fast food, is often high in sodium. Many of these items provide more than 1,000 mg per serving.	Ask "What foods contain sodium?" Show Handout #3, High-Sodium Foods.
	9.6 To reduce sodium in your diet, you can eat fewer or smaller portions of these foods or substitute other foods.	Ask, "How could you lower the sodium in your diet?" Mean effects of moderate sodium restriction is about 5 mmHg for systolic and 2 mmHg for diastolic blood pressure among

CONTENT OUTLINE

CONCEPT	DETAIL	INSTRUCTOR'S NOTES
		hypertensive patients and about 3 and 1 mmHg among normotensive patients.
	9.7 A guideline is to choose foods that are: ■ less than 400 mg per serving ■ less than 800 mg per entree or frozen meal.	Ask, "Where is information about sodium on the food label?" Show product labels; include low-salt foods. If possible, have the class taste some reduced-salt products.
	9.8 Products are now available to help lower sodium intake, such as reduced-sodium soups. Many food products are lower in sodium than they used to be. These can help you meet your goals.	Salt substitutes contain potassium and must be used cautiously. People with renal disease and those treated with potassium-sparing diuretics should avoid substitutes that contain potassium.
	9.9 Many seasonings and spices can add flavor without sodium. Several sodium-free seasoning blends are available. Try small amounts of unfamiliar herbs and spices from bulk food stores. Your ability to taste other flavors and enjoy foods without sodium improves with time.	Use Handout #4, Alternative Seasonings. If possible, offer samples of Mrs. Dash and other salt-free seasonings.
	9.10 Modest weight loss has beneficial effects on blood pressure as does moderate (e.g., 30–45 minutes of brisk walking) physical activity. Smoking cessation and limiting alcohol intake are also recommended.	Diastolic and systolic blood pressure each drop approximately 1 mm/Hg for every kilogram of weight loss.
10. Planning for change	10.1 If your lipid profile or blood pressure is not on target, or if you want to make changes in your diet to help prevent heart disease, there are many food choices available.	Ask, "Are there changes you could make in your eating or exercise habits to help lower your heart disease risk?" Note that exercise is also a key factor in blood lipid control. See Outline #7, *Physical Activity and Exercise* (p. 121). Ask, "What barriers do you anticipate? Are there strategies you can use to overcome those barriers?"

CONTENT OUTLINE

CONCEPT	DETAIL	INSTRUCTOR'S NOTES
	10.2 It's important to begin making changes one step at a time. You could start by: ■ deciding what your long-term blood lipid and blood pressure goals are ■ planning how to work toward that goal ■ choosing one step to take right now.	Ask participants to: ■ set a reasonable blood lipid goal ■ develop a plan on which they are willing and able to work ■ choose one thing they will try before the next session.
	10.3 Working with a registered dietitian can help you choose and reach your goals.	

SKILLS CHECKLIST

None.

EVALUATION PLAN

Knowledge will be evaluated by achievement of learning objectives and by responses to questions during the session. The ability to apply knowledge will be evaluated by the development of personal blood lipid goals, by the development and implementation of a plan to achieve those goals, and through program outcome measures.

DOCUMENTATION PLAN

Record class attendance and achieved objectives as appropriate using the Diabetes Self-Management Record, Participant Follow-up Record, or another form.

SUGGESTED READINGS

American Diabetes Association: Nutrition recommendations and interventions for diabetes. *Diabetes Care* 31:S61–S78, 2008

Franz MJ, Wylie-Rosett J: The 2006 American Diabetes Association Nutrition recommendations and interventions for the prevention and treatment of diabetes. *Diabetes Spectrum* 20:49–52, 2007

Pereira RF, Franz MJ: Prevention and treatment of cardiovascular disease in people with diabetes through lifestyle modification: current evidence-based recommendations. *Diabetes Spectrum* 21:189–193, 2008

Yantis MA, Velander R: Get the skinny on trans-fatty acids. *Nursing* 37(12):26–28, 2007

➲ Reasons for Meal Planning

■ Maintain blood glucose as close to your target range as possible.

■ Maintain cholesterol (blood fats) as close to your target levels as possible.

■ Maintain blood pressure as close to your target level as possible.

■ Prevent, delay, or treat diabetes-related complications.

■ Improve health through food choices.

■ Meet individual nutritional needs.

☜ Types of Fat in Blood

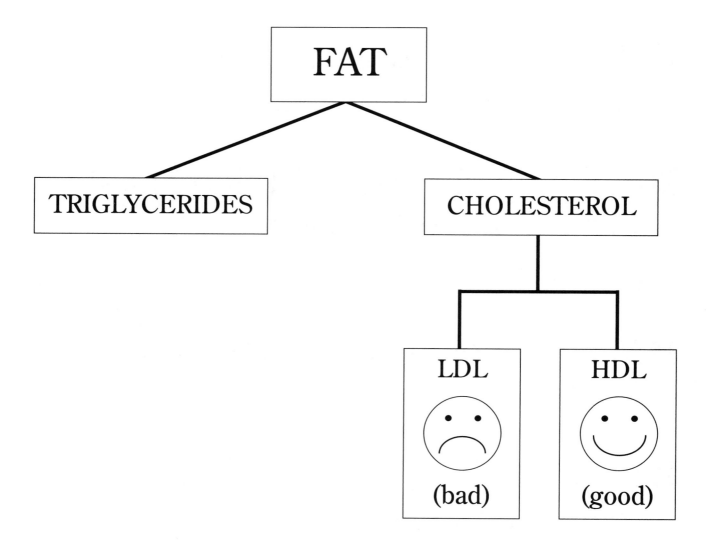

⊜ Types of Fat in Food

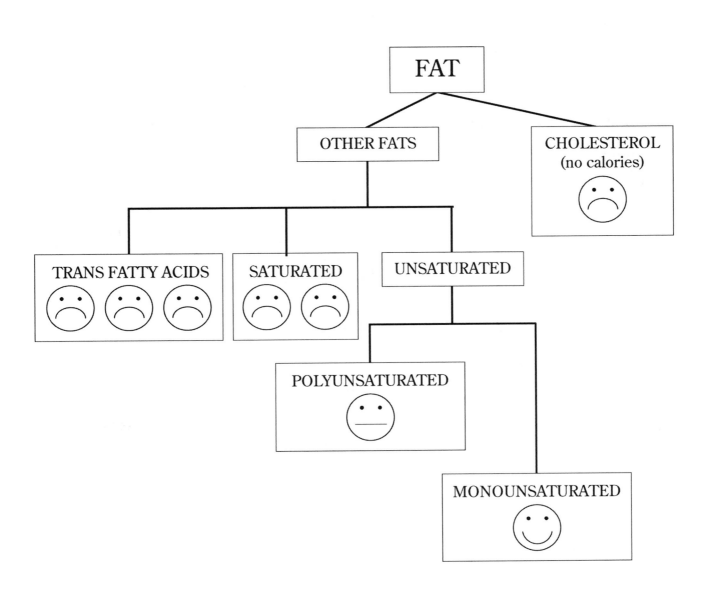

➲ Sources of Cholesterol and Fat

Cholesterol (limit these)	Saturated Trans Fat (limit these)	Unsaturated Fat
Meat	Meat	Safflower oil
Cheese	Cheese	Sunflower oil
Egg yolks	Egg yolks	Corn oil
Whole milk	Whole milk	Soybean oil
Reduced fat (2%) milk	Reduced fat (2%) milk	Sesame oil
Ice cream	Ice cream	Salad dressing
Butter	Butter	Mayonnaise
Organ meats	Cream cheese	Walnuts
	Sour cream	Sesame seeds
	Palm oil	Margerine (in soft tubs)
	Coconut oil	
	Cocoa butter	Olive oil
	Hydrogenated vegetable oil	Canola oil
	Poultry with skin	Peanut oil
	Fatback	Olives
	Chitterlings	Avocados
		Almonds
		Peanuts
		Cashews
		Pecans
		Almonds
		Sesame seeds
		Peanut butter

Polyunsaturated

Monounsaturated (choose more often)

⬲ Sources of Fiber

Soluble Fiber	Insoluble Fiber (to help prevent constipation)
Raw vegetables Fresh fruits Barley Dried peas Brown rice Okra Kidney beans Lentils Pinto beans Black-eyed peas Black beans Whole-grain products: ■ Oat, oat bran, and rice bran cereals ■ Soy pasta ■ Oat bran, rye, and pumpernickel breads ■ Oat and rye crackers	Some raw vegetables Wheat bran products: ■ Cereal (100% bran) ■ Whole grain products ■ Pasta ■ Bread ■ Crackers

⬤ High-Sodium Foods

Baking powder

Baking soda

Bouillon

Brine

Canned and dried soups

Canned meats and vegetables

Dill pickles

Disodium phosphate

Fast foods

Frozen mixed dishes

Macaroni, noodle, rice, and stuffing mixes

Monosodium glutamate (MSG)

Olives

Processed meat (corned beef, ham, frankfurters, lunch meat, and sausage)

Salty snack foods (crackers, chips, and nuts)

Sauerkraut

Seasoned salts (e.g., onion, garlic, and celery)

Sodium _____
(Any word that starts with "sodium" or has the word "sodium" in it)

Soy sauce

Steak, teriyaki, and tartar sauce

Table salt

➲ Alternative Seasonings

Herbs/Spices	Ways to Use Them
Basil	Egg, fish, tomato sauce, and vegetables
Bay leaves	Soups, stews, and boiled beef or pork
Caraway seeds	Roast pork, vegetables of the cabbage family, carrots, onions, and celery
Celery powder	Soups, salads, and deviled eggs
Curry powder	Chicken, lamb, eggs, and rice
Dill	Salads, deviled eggs, chicken, and fish
Fennel	Pork, poultry, and seafood dishes
Garlic	Meats, stews, soups, and salads
Nutmeg	Apple dishes and vegetables
Onion powder	Meat, soups, stews, and casseroles
Oregano	Italian dishes, stews, and soups
Paprika	For color; also aids browning of roasted chicken and turkey
Parsley	Eggs, soups, stews, and vegetables
Pepper, black	Salads, fish, meat, eggs, and vegetables
Pepper, red	Meats, sauces, gravies, eggs, fish, vegetable dishes, and stews (this is a strong spice)
Rosemary	Potatoes, peas, squash, lamb, veal, duck, pork stews, and salmon
Sage	Stuffing, poultry, pork, lamb, and veal
Thyme	Italian dishes, meat, and vegetables

| #19 | Carbohydrate Counting |

▸ ▸ ▸ ▸ ▸

STATEMENT OF PURPOSE

This session is intended to provide information on two methods of carbohydrate counting as a meal-planning approach. Using carbohydrate counting may improve blood glucose levels regardless of whether diabetes medications are also used. It is important for participants to work with a dietitian to develop a meal plan with the amount and distribution of carbohydrate that helps them reach their targets and goals.

PREREQUISITES

This session builds on the basic carbohydrate-counting information in session #5, *Planning Meals* (p. 69). It is recommended that each participant have attended sessions #3, *The Basics of Eating* (p. 37), #4, *Food and Blood Glucose* (p. 53), and #5, *Planning Meals* (p. 69), or have achieved those objectives. This session is intended for individuals who have some experience living with diabetes and who want a more calculated meal plan to meet their goals. It is suggested that participants who have meal-planning booklets and meal plans bring them to class.

OBJECTIVES

At the end of this session, participants will be able to:

1. describe carbohydrate counting;

2. state the rationale for using carbohydrate counting for meal planning;

3. name three food groups high in carbohydrate;

4. describe two methods of carbohydrate counting;

5. identify three sources of information on the carbohydrate content of food;

6. list 12 food items they often eat or drink and the carbohydrate content of each;

7. calculate the amount of carbohydrate in their serving size from a food label;

8. identify personal benefits and barriers of carbohydrate counting and strategies to overcome barriers;

9. define pattern management and carbohydrate/insulin ratios.

CONTENT

Incorporating nutritional management into lifestyle.

MATERIALS NEEDED

VISUALS PROVIDED	ADDITIONAL
1. Carbohydrate Servings	■ Chalkboard and chalk/Board and markers
	■ Food models or pictures of foods
Handouts Provided (one per participant)	■ Commercial food product containers or labels
1. Carbohydrate Foods	■ *Basic Carbohydrate Counting* and *Advanced*
2. Tips for Counting Carbohydrate Servings	*Carbohydrate Counting* (available from the
3. Carbohydrate in My Food	American Diabetes Association, www.diabetes.org,
4. How to Calculate Carbohydrate Grams	or 800-232-6733)
in Your Serving	
5. Practice Worksheet	

METHOD OF PRESENTATION

Start by introducing yourself and telling what you do. Ask participants to introduce themselves. Explain that the purpose of this session is to provide information about the carbohydrate-counting method for meal planning.

Present material in a discussion/question format using the first question as a starting point. Provide appropriate content outlined below in response. Ask if there are additional questions, and respond, repeating the process for the entire session. Use the questions in the Instructor's Notes section to generate discussion if no questions are forthcoming after a period of silence. Keeping track of the content discussed in each session, using the Diabetes Self-Management Record, the Participant Follow-up Record, or another form, helps you to evaluate if all needed content has been discussed.

CONTENT OUTLINE

CONCEPT	DETAIL	INSTRUCTOR'S NOTES
1. What is carbohydrate counting?	1.1 Counting just the carbohydrate in the food you eat is one method for meal planning that works well for many people. With this method, you count only the amount of carbohydrate at each meal and snack.	Ask, "What questions or concerns do you have about carbohydrate counting?"
	1.2 Carbohydrate counting focuses the attention on food choices that most affect blood glucose levels.	This method only addresses blood glucose management— the reason for meal planning unique to diabetes. Other

CONTENT OUTLINE

CONCEPT	DETAIL	INSTRUCTOR'S NOTES
		nutrition issues, such as the levels of fat, protein, vitamins, and minerals, can be addressed after blood glucose levels are stable and at later visits with the patient. This is one way to encourage the practice of an underlying educational principle: changes need to be made in steps. Optimal nutrition may need to wait until blood glucose levels are in the target range.
	1.3 Carbohydrate counting does not always mean reducing the total amount of carbohydrate, but keeping track of the amount in any one meal or snack.	Ask, "What carbohydrate foods do you currently eat?" What carbohydrate foods are important or have meaning for you?"
	1.4 The amount of carbohydrate at each meal or snack may be consistent from day to day or flexible, depending on the type of carbohydrate-counting meal plan used.	
	1.5 This approach can be used as part of blood glucose self-management. You can learn to eat more or fewer carbohydrate foods based on your blood glucose response and personal preferences.	Stress the value of blood glucose monitoring as a method to evaluate the impact of food choices with this approach to meal planning. The American Diabetes Association's target capillary plasma glucose levels are: 70–130 mg/dl preprandial and <180 mg/dl postprandial.
	1.6 Some people calculate their premeal bolus insulin dose based on the amount of carbohydrate they plan to eat at that meal and their premeal blood glucose.	The amount of bolus (rapid-acting or short-acting) insulin needed before a meal is closely related to the amount of carbohydrate eaten at that meal. Offer referral to a dietitian as needed.
	1.7 Carbohydrate-counting meal plans may have the same amount of carbohydrate, but differ in total	Ask, "How much flexibility do you want and need for meal planning?" Point out that

CONTENT OUTLINE

CONCEPT	DETAIL	INSTRUCTOR'S NOTES
	content based on calorie needs, blood glucose targets, food preferences, daily schedule, diabetes medicines, exercise plans, monitoring, and desire for flexibility. Ask a dietitian to help you create a plan that works for you.	carbohydrate counting does not control protein or fat. Two people could have the same number of carbohydrates but have very different amounts of calories, fat, and protein.
2. Why use carbohydrate counting?	2.1 Carbohydrate affects blood glucose more than any other nutrient.	Review the material from Outline #4, *Food and Blood Glucose* (p. 53), as needed.
	2.2 Carbohydrate counting may offer blood glucose management with more ease and flexibility in food choices than other meal-planning methods.	If weight is a concern, decreasing fat or total calories may also be needed.
	2.3 Using carbohydrate counting to distribute carbohydrate throughout the day can improve blood glucose levels regardless of whether you also take diabetes pills or insulin.	If participants do not understand why their blood glucose is high after some meals, carbohydrate counting may help gain insight.
3. Planning to use carbohydrate counting	3.1 To use carbohydrate counting, you need to be familiar with foods that contain carbohydrate and with your carbohydrate needs.	Point out that foods high in carbohydrate are not "bad," they just need to be counted.
	3.2 Food groups high in carbohydrate: ■ starch ■ fruit ■ milk ■ any foods that contain sugar, honey, molasses, or syrup.	Ask, "What foods do you eat that contain carbohydrate?" Look at Handout # 1, Carbohydrate Foods. Review information from Outline # 4, *Food and Blood Glucose* (p. 53), as needed.
	3.3 The vegetable group is low in carbohydrate. Vegetables usually can be ignored unless you have 1 1/2 cups or more at a meal or snack (cooked). Remember starchy vegetables are in the starch/bread group.	Hold up containers or models of several different foods and ask participants to identify whether they are high in carbohydrate. Ask whether each item fits into the starch, fruit, milk, vegetable, or other carbohydrate category.
	3.4 The carbohydrate content of foods in the other carbohydrate group varies.	
	3.5 Carbohydrate needs usually range from 40 to 60% of total calorie needs.	To estimate carbohydrate needs, assume that 50% of the day's

CONTENT OUTLINE

CONCEPT	DETAIL	INSTRUCTOR'S NOTES

calories come from carbohydrate. Divide carbohydrate (CHO) calories by 4 calories per gram. Example:

$$1800 \text{ cal} \times 50\% = 900$$

$$\frac{900 \text{ CHO cal}}{4 \text{ cal/g}} = 225 \text{ g CHO}$$

This is equal to 15 carbohydrate servings or choices.

3.6 There are two methods of carbohydrate-based meal planning:
- basic: counting carbohydrate servings
- advanced: counting carbohydrate grams and using carbohydrate/insulin ratios (adjusting rapid- or short-acting insulin dose to the amount of carbohydrate you plan to eat).

Basic carbohydrate counting involves understanding the relationships among food, medication, activity, and blood glucose levels. Advanced carbohydrate counting includes pattern management and insulin-to-carbohydrate ratios.

4. Basic carbohydrate counting

4.1 The basic carbohydrate-counting method uses the food groups of the food guide pyramid or the exchange system. Each starch, fruit, and milk serving counts as one carbohydrate serving.

The basic carbohydrate-counting method was introduced in Outline #5, *Planning Meals*. Review this material and/or use the *Basic Carbohydrate Counting* booklet as needed. count both carbohydrate servings and carbohydrate grams may be confusing to participants. Review each so they can decide which best fits their needs. Patients with limited math skills or those who want a more simple approach may prefer to count carbohydrate servings.

4.2 For example, one carbohydrate serving is:
- 1 orange = 1 fruit
- 1 slice bread = 1 starch
- 1/2 cup corn = 1 bread
- 1 cup milk = 1 milk.

Review and demonstrate with food models. Understanding food groupings and serving sizes is helpful for learning to use basic carbohydrate counting.

CONTENT OUTLINE

CONCEPT	DETAIL	INSTRUCTOR'S NOTES
	Although these are very different foods, they count the same in terms of carbohydrate and should have a similar effect on your blood glucose.	
	4.3 Each carbohydrate serving is about 15 g of carbohydrate. You can count either servings or grams of carbohydrate	Use Handout #2, Tips for Counting Carbohydrate Servings.
	4.4 Servings of starch, fruit, and milk are used interchangeably to create meals with a similar carbohydrate content. For example, your lunch might have 2 starches, 1 fruit, and 1 milk—this would be 4 carbohydrate servings.	2 starches = 2 carbohydrate servings 1 fruit = 1 carbohydrate serving 1 milk = 1 carbohydrate serving
	4.5 A meal plan for the day might be 3 carbohydrate servings at breakfast, 4 at lunch, and 4 at dinner.	Use Handout #3, Counting Carbohydrate In My Food. Ask participants to list meals that they frequently eat and also meals they would like to eat but typically avoid, and count the carbohydrate servings as a group.
5. Changing foods to carbohydrate servings	5.1 When the food group of an item is unknown: ■ look up the grams of carbohydrate per serving and divide by 15, or ■ count the grams of carbohydrate.	Have carbohydrate content books available. Ask participants to identify favorite foods and look up the carbohydrate amounts.
	5.2 If you have used exchanges in the past, you may already know the number of starch, fruit, and milk exchanges in many foods. For example: ■ 1 cup noodle soup = 1 starch (1 carbohydrate serving) ■ 1 cup ice cream = 2 starches and 4 fats (2 carbohydrate servings).	Meat/protein and fat exchanges do not affect the number of carbohydrate choices, however, they do contain calories. If you are concerned about your weight, pay attention to meat and fat portions.

CONTENT OUTLINE

CONCEPT	DETAIL	INSTRUCTOR'S NOTES

5.3 Several reference books are available to look up the carbohydrate value in foods you don't know.

Instructor's Notes: Demonstrate using food composition references. Use Use Handout #2, Tips for Counting Carbohydrate Servings.

5.4 When the grams of carbohydrate are available, dividing by 15 gives the number of carbohydrate servings. The carbohydrate content is listed on almost all food labels.

Instructor's Notes: Demonstrate using product labels and food composition books to find the grams of carbohydrate in other food items. Show Visual #1, Carbohydrate Servings.

5.5 Round off the number of choices to the nearest half choice. Examples:
■ Big Mac = 45 g
   Carbohydrate = 3 servings

■ 16 Cheese Tidbits = 8 g
   Carbohydrate = 1/2 serving.

$$\frac{45}{15} = 3$$

$$\frac{8}{15} = 0.53$$

5.6 Counting carbohydrate servings is not as precise as counting actual grams of carbohydrate, because the carbohydrate content of one serving can range from 10 to 20 g. This means the carbohydrate content of 3 choices could range from 30 to 60 g.

Instructor's Notes: It is more difficult to calculate insulin doses based on carbohydrate intake with this degree of variability.

5.7 For many people, this method is accurate enough to meet their goals. The smaller numbers may be easier to remember (e.g., 3–4 servings rather than 45–60 g).

Instructor's Notes: This method is most appropriate for:
■ people with type 2 diabetes
■ children
■ adults with type 1 diabetes who are new to carbohydrate counting
■ adults with type 1 diabetes for whom increased precision and complexity is not needed or wanted.

5.8 This approach may be easier for those familiar with the exchange system or who eat few foods in the other carbohydrate category.

Instructor's Notes: Use the *Basic Carbohydrate* booklet to reinforce information about carbohydrate servings. The booklet also discusses meat and meat substitutes, fat, measuring, and label reading, and provides

CONTENT OUTLINE

CONCEPT	DETAIL	INSTRUCTOR'S NOTES
		lists of foods equal to 1 carbohydrate serving.
6. Counting carbohydrate grams	6.1 Counting grams of carbohydrate is another carbohydrate-based method for meal planning.	Use the *Basic Carbohydrate Counting* or *Advanced Carbohydrate Counting* booklets to reinforce information.
	6.2 You can plan a specific number of carbohydrate grams for each meal and snack or vary the carbohydrate content and adjust other aspects of your plan (e.g., your insulin bolus dose).	It is easier initially to eat a consistent amount of carbohydrate to establish target carbohydrate levels and insulin ratios.
	6.3 Grams of carbohydrate, the information needed to use this method, is on every food label.	A reasonable target range when counting carbohydrate grams is ±3 g.
	6.4 A wide variety of meals can be planned to match a given carbohydrate amount.	Any food with a known carbohydrate content can be used and still fit the plan.

6.5 For example, a meal equal to 60–65 carbohydrate grams could be:

- 1 cup 2% milk — 12
  ham sandwich — 32
  1/2 cup applesauce — <u>17</u>
  61

- muffin — 24
  apple cinnamon oatmeal — <u>41</u>
  65

- large baked potato — 30
  1 cup broccoli — 10
  6 oz steak — 0
  2 cups tossed salad — 3
  2 Tbsp ranch dressing — 2
  1/2 cup ice cream — <u>15</u>
  60

Instructor's notes (for 6.5): Nutrient value can vary. Carbohydrate counting helps people reach blood glucose targets. Other information may be needed to address other nutrition goals. Use Handout #4, How to Calculate Carbohydrate Grams in Your Servings.

Use Handout #3, Carbohydrates In My Food. Ask participants to list meals they eat frequently and also meals that they would like to eat but typically avoid, and count the number of carbohydrate as a group.

6.6 Foods high in sugar may easily be included using this method.

Instructor's notes (for 6.6): Use *Advanced Carbohydrate Counting* to reinforce and build on the information in this section. The booklet offers support for using carbohydrate

CONTENT OUTLINE

CONCEPT	DETAIL	INSTRUCTOR'S NOTES
		counting for pattern management.
7. Using carbohydrate/ insulin ratios	7.1 Patterns are trends in your blood glucose over time. Pattern management refers to changes you make in food, medication, or physical activity based on comparing your blood glucose trends with your targets.	Ask, "What adjustments do you currently make in your medication or food to reach your blood glucose targets?" American Diabetes Association's target blood plasma glucose levels are: 70–130 mg/dl preprandial <180 mg/dl postprandial
	7.2 It is easier to see trends when your records have more information than just your blood glucose levels. Other helpful information is: ■ insulin time and dose ■ missed meals/snacks ■ extra or unusual foods ■ new food ■ more or less physical activity than usual ■ hypoglycemia and treatment ■ stress or illness ■ alcohol intake.	Stress the importance of recording or downloading meter results.
	7.3 To start pattern management, you will need to monitor multiple times during the day.	Ask, "What do you learn from pre- and post-prandial readings? How do you use this information?"
	7.4 When looking at your blood glucose records, ask yourself: ■ What patterns do I see? ■ What other information would help? ■ What could be causing or influencing these values? ■ What strategies could I use to address this trend?	Ask participants for examples. Stress the importance of reviewing trends, not just individual numbers. Ask, "How do you deal with the frustration of unexpected numbers?"
8. Calculating carbohydrate/ insulin ratios	8.1 The next step is to figure out your carbohydrate/insulin ratio. In this approach, the premeal bolus insulin dose is based on the amount of carbohydrate you plan to eat at that	Before using carbohydrate/ insulin ratios, it is helpful if blood glucose is close to the target range using a set basal and bolus insulin program and a consistent

CONTENT OUTLINE

CONCEPT	DETAIL	INSTRUCTOR'S NOTES

meal. People who use this method take rapid-acting or short-acting insulin before each meal. Monitoring after the meal helps determine if the dose was adequate for the carbohydrate eaten.

carbohydrate intake for 3–7 days. Rapid-acting insulin may be particularly useful for carbohydrate/insulin ratios.

8.2 Carbohyrate/insulin ratios vary with individual sensitivity; however, most people need 1–3 units of insulin per 15 g of carbohydrate. For people taking 1 unit for every 15 g of carbohydrate, the ratio is 1:15.

Weight (lb)	Insulin units/15 g Carbohydrate
<150	1
150–200	2
>200	3

If the participant has a history of sensitivity to insulin, then start with 1 unit per 30 g of carbohydrate. Demonstrate using participants' meal and insulin plans and provide an opportunity for the group to practice.

8.3 It will be easier if you begin with a baseline meal plan and insulin dose. You can calculate your insulin/ carbohydrate ratio or begin by taking 1 unit of rapid-acting or short-acting insulin for each 15 g of carbohydrate you eat. If your blood glucose level is higher than you want it to be after the meal, increase the dose to 2 units per 15 g carbohydrate, and higher as needed. Use your blood glucose record to look for patterns and make adjustments.

Most participants benefit from a baseline meal plan and insulin dose to establish the ratio. Participants need to develop their plans in collaboration with their health care teams and will be in frequent contact with their team initially. Review Visual #1 if participants will be calculating their own ratio. Use Handout Handout #5, Practice Worksheet.

8.4 Once you know your carbohydrate/ insulin ratio, you can use it to calculate your bolus dose and/or to estimate insulin needs for varying carbohydrate intake.

Stress the importance of post-prandial glucose checks.

8.5 You will need to fine-tune your ratio over time. Remember that a ratio of 1:20 is **less** insulin per gram of carbohydrate than a ratio of 1:15.

CONTENT OUTLINE

CONCEPT	DETAIL	INSTRUCTOR'S NOTES
	8.6 Some foods require more or less insulin per 15 g carbohydrate.	Foods usually requiring more insulin are Chinese and Italian dishes (e.g., pizza). Foods usually requiring less insulin are dishes containing large amounts of whole grains, legumes, and beans, as well as vegetarian dishes. Use *Advanced Carbohydrate Counting* to reinforce and build on this section.
	8.7 You may also have a correction dose to correct pre-meal blood glucose levels. The correction dose is added to or subtracted from the pre-meal dose.	One formula for calculating the correction dose is to divide 1,800 by the total daily insulin dose (both basal and bolus). The result is the insulin sensitivity factor or the approximate change in blood glucose per unit of insulin.
	8.8 A correction dose can be given when blood glucose levels are too high, using your insulin sensitivity factor. Checking glucose levels two hours after a correction dose helps you know if the dose was effective for you.	Provide participants with the opportunity to practice by showing different examples and asking that they calculate their dose.
9. Sources of information on carbohydrate content of food	9.1 Sources of information on the carbohydrate content of foods are: ■ food labels ■ exchange list references ■ food-composition references.	
	9.2 Food labels tell the amount of carbohydrate per serving. Note that it is the total carbohydrate, not just sugar, that matters in carbohydrate counting.	Ask participants to find the carbohydrate content on several food labels.
	9.3 If you use a food label to calculate your ratio and your blood glucose isn't where you'd predict, remember: ■ food labels can be slightly inaccurate ■ subtract fiber from total carbohydrate.	Fiber is unabsorbed carbohydrate and needs to be subtracted from the carbohydrate total on the label.

CONTENT OUTLINE

CONCEPT	DETAIL	INSTRUCTOR'S NOTES
	9.4 Food composition references also tell you the grams of carbohydrate in a food.	Show samples of food composition references. Provide time for participants to look up favorite foods. Continue to use Handout #3.
	9.5 If the serving size on the label is not the same as your serving size, you can calculate the amount of your carbohydrate from the information on the label.	Use Handout #4, How to Calculate Carbohydrate Grams in Your Serving, to demonstrate and practice how to calculate the carbohydrate content of different serving amounts.
10. Other factors influencing blood glucose	10.1 Even when carbohydrate, medication, stress, and exercise levels stay the same, blood glucose levels may vary. Some other factors influencing blood glucose are: ■ fiber ■ fat ■ weight change ■ glycemic index ■ gastroparesis.	Review only the portions of this section that are relevant to your audience. Ask, "What have you noticed that affects your blood glucose levels?"
Fiber	10.2 Fiber cannot be broken down and absorbed by the digestive system. It does not increase blood glucose.	
	10.3 Because fiber does not affect your blood glucose, you need to subtract the fiber from the total carbohydrate. Example: All Bran Total carbohydrate 22 g Fiber 13 g Sugar 5 g $22 - 13 = 9$ g of carbohydrate that affect blood glucose or $22 - 6.5 = 15.5$ g of carbohydrate that affect blood glucose.	This is most important for people using intensive insulin and adjusting their insulin dose based on the carbohydrate content of their meal. Use the example to teach the method used in your setting. Participants who are very sensitive to insulin may need to subtract all of the fiber. Remind participants that they need to monitor post-meal to determine their response.
Fat	10.4 Fat leaves your stomach more slowly and may delay the blood glucose rise after a meal up to 10 hours when eaten in large amounts.	Eating a high-fat bedtime snack may not cause a rise in blood glucose until the following morning and could result in hypoglycemia during the night.

CONTENT OUTLINE

CONCEPT	DETAIL	INSTRUCTOR'S NOTES
Weight	10.5 Your carbohydrate/insulin ratio may change if you gain or lose weight.	
	10.6 The improved glucose levels and flexibility of carbohydrate counting may lead to weight gain. If that is a concern, talk with your dietitian about weight management strategies.	Ask, "Do you think weight gain will be an issue for you? Why or why not? What strategies could you use to avoid weight gain?" Weight gain with improved blood glucose levels is more often an issue among patients who are severly hyperglycemic.
Glycemic index	10.7 Glycemic index (GI) is a measure of how different foods containing the same amount of carbohydrate affect your blood glucose levels. Fat and fiber may lower the GI of a food.	Tables listing the GI of foods are available and may be helpful; however, responses to any one food are variable and individual.
	10.8 Glycemic index varies with the speed of digestion. Carbohydrates that are liquids, thoroughly cooked, or blended are absorbed faster than carbohydrates that are solid, raw, or require thorough chewing.	The type of carbohydrate also makes a difference. For example, the starch in Cornflakes is more quickly digested and has a higher GI than sucrose (glucose + fructose).
	10.9 You can discover your own response to food through postmeal monitoring.	Ask, "Have you noticed different responses to the same amount of carbohydrate?"
	10.10 Your blood glucose response to a given amount of a certain food will be different than the next person's response. Blood glucose monitoring is the only way to discover your response. Your response may also vary from time to time. The only way to discover your response is through monitoring and recording your blood glucose after meals.	Thin people with type 1 diabetes tend to be more sensitive to changes in carbohydrate levels than those with type 2 diabetes who are overweight and/or insulin resistant. Ask, "Have any of you had this experience? How do you handle your frustration with this situation?"
Gastroparesis	10.11 People with nerve damage to the digestive tract from diabetes do not absorb food the same way each time they eat. This means blood glucose levels can vary, even when exactly the same meal is eaten.	Gastroparesis is reviewed in Outline #14, *Long-Term Complications* (p. 283).

CONTENT OUTLINE

CONCEPT	DETAIL	INSTRUCTOR'S NOTES
11. Using carbohydrate counting	11.1 Finding and counting the carbohydrate content of the foods you eat each day takes time and effort; however, your blood glucose levels may improve, and carbohydrate counting provides increased flexibility.	Ask, "What are the benefits to you for using carbohydrate counting? The barriers? Are there strategies you can use to make meal planning less of a chore?" List these on the board and discuss.
	11.2 To use the carbohydrate-counting system: ■ Meet with a dietitian to develop a plan and obtain information about the carbohydrate content of foods. ■ Start with a baseline insulin dose. ■ Weigh or measure the amount of food you plan to eat. ■ Calculate the carbohydrate content for that amount.	
	11.3 Become familiar with the carbohydrate content of the foods you eat: ■ Make a list of 12 foods you eat regularly. ■ Record the number of carbohydrate choices and/or grams of carbohydrate in these foods. ■ Monitor pre- and postmeal blood glucose levels.	Use Handout #5, Carbohydrate in My Food, to do this activity. Review participants' plans and answer questions. This is designed to help participants begin carbohydrate counting more easily and accurately. Use product labels and food-composition books to find the grams of carbohydrate in other food items.
	11.4 Identify a step you can take to use carbohydrate counting.	Close with summary questions and comments.

SKILLS CHECKLIST

Participants will be able to calculate the carbohydrate content of foods they often eat.

EVALUATION PLAN

Knowledge will be evaluated by achievement of learning objectives and by responses to questions during the session. The ability to apply knowledge will be evaluated by the development of personal meal-planning goals, by the development and implementation of a carbohydrate-counting approach to achieve those goals, and through program outcome measures.

DOCUMENTATION PLAN

Record class attendance and achieved objectives as appropriate using the Diabetes Self-Management Record, the Participant Follow-up Record, or another form.

SUGGESTED READINGS

Buethe M: CountCarbs: a 10 step guide to teaching carbohydrate counting. *The Diabetes Educator* 34:67–74, 2008

Kulkarni K: Carbohydrate counting: a practical meal-planning option for people with diabetes. *Clinical Diabetes* 23:120–124, 2005

Papanas N, Mallezos E: Education for dietary freedom in type 1 diabetes? Yes, it's possible. *The Diabetes Educator* 34:54–58, 2008

Roberts S: Carb counting: a flexible way to plan meals. *Diabetes Forecast* 60(5):25–27, 2007

Sheard NF, Clark NG, Brand-Miller JC, Franz MJ, Pi-Sunyet FZ, Mayer-Davis E, Kulkarni K, Geil P: Dietary carbohydrate (amount and type) in the prevention and management of diabetes: ADA Statement. *Diabetes Care* 27:2266-2271, 2004

Carbohydrate Servings

Amount	Food Item	Starch	Fruit	Milk	Other	Carbohydrate Servings
2 oz	1/2 Bagel	2				2
1/2 cup	Orange juice		1			1
1 cup	Milk			1		1
1 cup	Mashed potatoes	2				2
8 oz	Artificially sweetened yogurt			1		1
1 small	Banana		1			2

Combination Foods—Exchange Value Available

Amount	Food Item	Starch	Fruit	Milk	Other	Carbohydrate Servings
1 cup	Potato salad	2				2
1	Ice cream bar	1				1
2 cups	Spaghetti and meatballs	6				6
8 oz	Fat-free vanilla yogurt		1	1 1/2		2 1/2

Combination Foods—Exchange Value Not Available

Amount	Food Item	Starch	Fruit	Milk	Other	Carbohydrate Servings
16	Cheese Tidbits = 8 g carbohydrate					1/2
1	Oreo Big Stuff cookie = 33 g carbohydrate					2
8 oz	Stouffers Vegetable Lasagna = 28 g carbohydrate					2
1	Big Mac = 43 g carbohydrate					3

⬆ Carbohydrate Foods

Food Group	Food
Starch	Bread, rolls, bagels, English muffins, tortillas, pita bread, naan, saltine crackers, and matzoh
	Pasta: noodles, spaghetti, and macaroni
	Rice
	Cereal: dry or cooked
	Legumes: lentils, dried beans (garbanzo, kidney, black, and butter beans), and dried peas (split peas and black-eyed peas)
	Starchy vegetables: potatoes, corn, peas, squash, yams, and taro root
Fruit	Apples, oranges, bananas, and all other fruits—fresh, frozen, canned, or juiced
Milk	All milk
	Yogurt (plain or artificially sweetened)
Vegetable	Carrots, green beans, broccoli, beets, greens, okra, and all other crunchy vegetables (only if 1 1/2 cups or more)
Other	Foods that include any of the above items, such as:
	■ casseroles
	■ soups
	■ stews
	■ pizza
	■ snack foods—chips, pretzels, and french fries
	■ desserts—ice cream, frozen yogurt, cake, cookies, and pie
	■ alcoholic beverages—beer and sweet wine

⊜ Counting Carbohydrate Servings

Meal Time _____:_____

_____ carbohydrate servings OR

_____ grams carbohydrate

_____ meat or meat substitutes

_____ fats

Snack Time _____:_____

_____

_____

Meal Time _____:_____

_____ carbohydrate servings OR

_____ grams carbohydrate

_____ meat or meat substitutes

_____ fats

Snack Time _____:_____

_____

_____

Meal Time _____:_____

_____ carbohydrate servings OR

_____ grams carbohydrate

_____ meat or meat substitutes

_____ fats

Snack Time _____:_____

_____

_____

➡ Tips for Counting Carbohydrate Servings

Grams of carbohydrate	Count as:
0–5 g	Do not count
6–10 g	1/2 carbohydrate serving or 1/2 starch, fruit, or milk serving
11–20 g	1 carbohydrate serving or 1 starch, fruit, or milk serving
21–25 g	1 1/2 carbohydrate servings or 1 1/2 starch, fruit, or milk servings
26–35 g	2 carbohydrate servings or 2 starch, fruit, or milk servings

Know what you are eating. Measure or weigh your foods to help you learn what carbohydrate servings look like. The foods I will measure are:

_____

The food labels I will check are:

_____

Feel good about what you already do. If you decide to make food changes, choose only one or two changes to make. This is what I will do:

_____

_____

Counting carbohydrate in your food allows you more flexibility in food choices and helps keep your blood glucose levels within target range.

➲ How to Calculate Carbohydrate Grams in Your Serving

If you know the serving size for a food product and the grams of carbohydrate in that serving size, you can find the number of grams in a different serving size in two steps:

> 1. **Divide** your serving size by the serving size on the label.
>
> 2. **Multiply** the result by the grams of carbohydrate on the label.

Examples

Label information:

> Serving size = 1/2 cup   Carbohydrate: 22 grams
>
> Your serving = 3/4 cup
>
> 1. **Divide** your serving size by the serving size on the label.

$$\frac{0.75}{0.5} = 1.5$$

> 2. **Multiply** the result by the grams of carbohydrate on the label.
>
> 1.5 x 22 grams = 33 grams

Your serving has 33 grams of carbohydrate.

Sometimes you can estimate the amount without using the formula. In this example, you can see that your serving size is 1 1/2 times as much as the serving size mentioned on the label. You can just add half the carbohydrate (11 grams) to the label amount (22 grams) to get the amount in your serving (33 grams).

continued

HOW TO CALCULATE CARBOHYDRATE GRAMS IN YOUR SERVING *continued*

Label information:

Serving size = 10 oz   Carbohydrate : 15 grams

Your serving = 6 oz

1. **Divide** your serving size by the serving size on the label.

$$\frac{6}{10} = 0.6$$

2. **Multiply** the result by the grams of carbohydrate on the label.

0.6 x 15 grams = 9 grams

Your serving has 9 grams of carbohydrate.

Note:

■ This method works regardless of the serving-size units.

■ This method works whether you eat more or less than the serving size on the label.

⬆ Carbohydrate in My Food

Carbohydrate Grams	Amount	Food Item	Starch	Fruit	Milk	Other	Carbohydrate Servings

⬭ Practice Worksheet

How to Figure Your Carbohydrate-to-Insulin Ratio Using the Carbohydrate Gram Method

1. Record the grams (g) carbohydrate that you consistently eat at each meal based on your blood glucose and food records.

   Breakfast _____ g   Lunch _____ g   Supper _____ g

2. Record the insulin meal doses that consistenly meet target blood glucose. (u = units of insulin)

   Breakfast _____ u   Lunch _____ u   Supper _____ u

3. Determine the carbohydrate g per u insulin for each meal by dividing the total g carbohydrate for each meal by the number of u R.

   Breakfast = B   Lunch = L   Supper = S

   $$\frac{\text{_____ g carbohydrate}}{\text{_____ u insulin}} = \text{_____ g/u}$$

   $$B \frac{\text{\_\_\_\_\_ g}}{\text{\_\_\_\_\_ u}} = \text{\_\_\_\_\_ g/u}$$

   $$L \frac{\text{\_\_\_\_\_ g}}{\text{\_\_\_\_\_ u}} = \text{\_\_\_\_\_ g/u}$$

   $$S \frac{\text{\_\_\_\_\_ g}}{\text{\_\_\_\_\_ u}} = \text{\_\_\_\_\_ g/u}$$

PRACTICE WORKSHEET *continued*

4. If your answers to step 3 vary from each other by no more than 1 g carbohydrate, add the 3 answers together and divide by 3 to get the average grams carbohydrate per unit of insulin.

   B _____

   L _____

   + S _____

   _____ total divided by 3 = _____ g/unit

5. If your answers to step 3 vary from each other by no more than 1 g carbohydrate and you and your health-care team agree that your basal insulin doses are well adjusted, then use your answers to step 3 are your carbohydrate-to-insulin ratios for each meal.

   My carbohydrate-to-insulin ratios are
   B _____ g/u   L _____ g/u   S _____ g/u

6. To make insulin adjustments for more or less carbohydrate eaten, add up the total carbohydrate and divide by the appropriate carbohydrate-to-insulin ratio.

   Total carbohydrate _____ g ÷ g/u (ratio) _____ = _____ u insulin

How to Figure Your Carbohydrate-to-Insulin Ratio Using the Carbohydrate Servings Method

1. Record the insulin meal doses that consistently meet target blood glucose based on your blood glucose and food records.

   Breakfast _____ u   Lunch _____ u   Supper _____ u

2. Record the number of carbohydrate choices that you consistently eat at each meal.

   Breakfast _____   Lunch _____   Supper _____
      carbohydrate   carbohydrate   carbohydrate
      servings   servings   servings

3. Determine the units of insulin per carbohydrate choice for each meal by dividing the number of units by the number of carbohydrate choices.

$$\frac{\text{units}}{\begin{array}{c}\text{carbohydrate}\\ \text{servings}\end{array}} = \underline{\quad} \text{ units per carbohydrate serving}$$

$$\text{B } \frac{\underline{\quad} \text{ units}}{\underline{\quad} \text{ servings}} = \underline{\quad} \text{ units per carbohydrate serving}$$

$$\text{L } \frac{\underline{\quad} \text{ units}}{\underline{\quad} \text{ servings}} = \underline{\quad} \text{ units per carbohydrate serving}$$

$$\text{S } \frac{\underline{\quad} \text{ units}}{\underline{\quad} \text{ servings}} = \underline{\quad} \text{ units per carbohydrate serving}$$

My carbohydrate/insulin ratio is _____ units per carbohydrate serving.

4. If your answers to step 3 are different for one or more meals, use more than one ratio.

    My carbohydrate/insulin ratios are
    B _____ u/carbohydrate serving

    L _____ u/carbohydrate serving

    S _____ u/carbohydrate serving

5. To make insulin adjustments for more or fewer carbohydrate servings, add up the total number of carbohydrate servings and multiply by your ratio (u/carbohydrate serving).

    Total number of carbohydrate servings _____
    x _____ u/carbohydrate serving
    = _____ u R

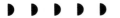

| #20 | **Sexual Health and Diabetes** |

STATEMENT OF PURPOSE

This session is intended to provide information about sexual health and sexual function and how they can be affected by diabetes.

PREREQUISITES

It is recommended that participants have basic knowledge about diabetes and its complications, either from personal experience or from attending previous sessions.

OBJECTIVES

At the end of this session, participants will be able to:

1. express greater insight about their own sexuality;

2. state ways to initiate discussion about sexual concerns with people who are important to them and with members of the health care team;

3. identify effective methods of contraception (if applicable);

4. describe sexual functioning for either men or women that can be affected by diabetes;

5. understand their own emotional response to sexual health issues;

6. state therapies available for sexual dysfunction.

CONTENT

Preventing, detecting, and treating chronic complications. Developing personal strategies to address psychosocial issues and concerns.

MATERIALS NEEDED

VISUALS PROVIDED	ADDITIONAL
1. Sexual Response Cycle—Physical Changes 2. Changes in Sexual Function with Aging 3. Normal Menstrual Cycle 4. Contraceptive Methods	■ Chalkboard and chalk/Board and markers ■ Samples of products available used in treating sexual dysfunction

5. Penile Prostheses—Semirigid
6. Penile Prostheses—Inflatable

METHOD OF PRESENTATION

Start by introducing yourself and telling what you do. Ask participants to introduce themselves. Explain that the purpose of this session is to present information about diabetes and sexual health for both men and women throughout their lifespan.

Present material in a question/discussion format, using the first question as a starting point. Provide appropriate content outlined below in response. Ask if there are additional questions, and respond, repeating the process for the entire session. Use the questions in the Instructor's Notes section to generate discussion if no questions are forthcoming after a period of silence. Keeping track of the content discussed in each session, using the Diabetes Self-Management Record, the Participant Follow-up Record, or another form, helps you to evaluate if all needed content has been discussed.

This outline is only a guide. It does not need to be presented in its entirety, but should be tailored to meet the needs of each group. Participants may feel most comfortable in groups of either all men or all women, with only pertinent content presented. The content can also be provided on an individual basis. As an instructor, you need to be knowledgeable and feel comfortable talking about sexual health issues before leading this session.

CONTENT OUTLINE

CONCEPT	DETAIL	INSTRUCTOR'S NOTES
1. Meaning of human sexuality	1.1 Sexuality is an important dimension of our lives.	Ask, "What do you think of when you hear the word sexuality?" Write responses on the board and incorporate into the discussion throughout. Ask, "What questions or concerns do you have about sexual health and diabetes?"
	1.2 It is present from birth to death.	
	1.3 It involves integrating ideas and emotions with actions.	
	1.4 It involves the giving and receiving of sensual pleasure.	
	1.5 It is involved in all human relationships and is part of having effective, satisfying interpersonal relationships	

CONTENT OUTLINE

CONCEPT	DETAIL	INSTRUCTOR'S NOTES
	with others, including being able to give and receive.	
2. Components of sexual health	2.1 Sexual health involves an awareness and appreciation of your feelings and attitudes about your sexuality.	Include the response on the board as part of the discussion.
	2.2 Male and female roles in relationships, the family, and society play a part as well.	
	2.3 Sexual function fulfills two basic purposes: reproduction and recreation (the giving and receiving of physical and psychological pleasure).	Point out differences between sexuality/sexual role and sexual functioning. The capacity for engaging in satisfying relationships need not be altered because of diabetes.
	2.4 There are four phases of sexual response: ■ excitement ■ plateau ■ orgasm ■ resolution.	Review the four phases of sexual response. Use Visual #1, Sexual Response Cycle—Physical Changes.
	2.5 Sexual function changes as a normal part of the aging process.	Use Visual #2, Changes in Sexual Function with Aging.
3. Impact of diabetes on sexual health	3.1 You need to decide who to tell you have diabetes and how and when to tell them.	Ask, "What have you heard about how diabetes can affect sexual health?" Discuss why it is important to tell certain people, how and when this can be best accomplished, and any fears about how it will affect relationships.
	3.2 It may be hard to tell others that you have diabetes because you may fear losing a friendship or close relationship. If someone ends a relationship for this reason, it may help to know that the person probably didn't have your best interests in mind.	It may be helpful for partners to attend an education program or diabetes support group together.
	3.3 Diabetes can affect sexual roles. For example, if men or women are physically unable to work or to prepare	Ask, "Do you feel that diabetes has affected your role at work or in your family?"

CONTENT OUTLINE

CONCEPT	DETAIL	INSTRUCTOR'S NOTES
	certain foods the family enjoys, they may feel like they are no longer fulfilling their obligations as husbands or wives.	
	3.4 Diabetes can also influence decisions about having children for both men and women. Concerns include: Will my children inherit diabetes? What are the risks involved in pregnancy for a person with diabetes?	Risk if one parent has: ■ type 1: 1–6% ■ type 2: 10–15% ■ MODY (maturity-onset diabetes of the young): 50% See Outline #21, *Pregnancy and Diabetes* (p. 447).
	3.5 Diabetes can also affect sexual functioning in both men and women.	
4. Sexual health issues for women— Menstruation	4.1 Some women experience delayed onset of menses or irregular menstrual cycles. This is often relieved by lowering blood glucose levels.	Ask, "What questions or concerns do you have about menstruation?"
	4.2 Some women experience elevated blood glucose levels before and during their menstrual period that can lead to ketosis and/or diabetic ketoacidosis. This can be treated with a planned increase in insulin dose or a planned decrease in carbohydrate intake.	An increase in estrogen and progesterone levels before menses can cause some insulin resistance. Use Visual #3, Normal Menstrual Cycle. Food cravings associated with the menstrual cycle may also affect blood glucose levels.
	4.3 Some women experience a decrease in blood glucose levels during menstruation, when estrogen and progesterone levels decrease. A smaller insulin dosage may be needed during this time.	Suggest that women seek advice from their provider if this is a problem.
Planning for pregnancy	4.4 Fertility is not **generally** affected by diabetes.	Ask, "What questions or concerns do you have about pregrancy?"
	4.5 More women with diabetes are having healthy babies now than ever before; however, women with high blood glucose levels are at risk for premature births, high-	

CONTENT OUTLINE

CONCEPT	DETAIL	INSTRUCTOR'S NOTES
	birth-weight babies, infants with birth defects, and infant deaths.	
	4.6 For the best possible pregnancy outcome, women should achieve near-normal blood glucose levels before conception and during pregnancy by paying close attention to diet, medicines, exercise, and monitoring.	Regulation of blood glucose before and during pregnancy is a critical factor in promoting a successful pregnancy. An A1C of < 7% is recommended.
	4.7 Along with your partner, talk with your provider about the many factors that will need to be considered with a pregnancy: ■ increased care demands ■ increased financial costs ■ presence and severity of complications ■ burden of care ■ worry about outcome of pregnancy.	Preconception care and counseling are important first steps in pregnancy for women with diabetes. See Outline #21, *Pregnancy and Diabetes* (p. 447).
Contraception	4.8 All of the current methods of birth control are available for people with diabetes. No one method is recommended.	Ask, "What questions or concerns do you have about contraception?"
	4.9 Choose the method that will work best for you. An unplanned pregnancy generally does not allow for the needed blood glucose management before conception.	Use Visual #4, Contraceptive Methods. Discuss each method, how it works, side effects, and effectiveness.
Menopause	4.10 Changes in estrogen and other hormone levels can cause widely varying blood glucose levels.	The current recommendation for hormone replacement therapy (HRT) is the lowest possible dose for the shortest time to manage symptoms.
	4.11 Mood swings are common with the changes in hormone levels.	
	4.12 A decrease in estrogen can also cause hot flashes, fast heartbeat, and flushed skin. It is important not to treat these hot flashes as an insulin reaction.	Ask, "How do you tell the difference between a hot flash and a reaction?"

CONTENT OUTLINE

CONCEPT	DETAIL	INSTRUCTOR'S NOTES
	4.13 Taking estrogen may reduce these symptoms but may increase your risk for other health problems. Talk with your provider about the risks and benefits of hormone replacement therapy for you. Estrogen acts against insulin, so changes in your treatment plan may be needed if you take HRT.	Menopause increases the risk for heart disease, and calcium is depleted from the bones. The risk of vaginal infections increases with changes in vaginal tissue secretions. Encourage women to have frequent visits with both a gynecologist and diabetes provider during menopause.
Vaginitis	4.14 Vaginitis, especially caused by yeast infections, is more common among women with diabetes.	Recurring vaginal infections can decrease interest in sexual intercourse. Ask, "What questions or concerns do you have about infections?"
	4.15 This occurs because high blood glucose levels provide an excellent medium for growth of these organisms. These infections are not related to sexual activity, age, or personal hygiene.	
	4.16 Treat promptly at first sign of symptoms: itching, foul-smelling discharge, or pain.	
	4.17 Antifungal preparations are the treatment of choice for yeast infections and are available without a prescription. If the infection is not gone after a week, contact your provider.	Infections that are not responsive may need a more potent prescriptive preparation or may be trichomonas or bacterial vaginosis. These generally respond to metroniadazole.
5. Sexual dysfunction in women with diabetes	5.1 Not as much is known about sexual dysfunction in women with diabetes. It seems to develop slowly.	Ask, "What questions or concerns do you have about sexual function?"
	5.2 Damage to the autonomic nerves from neuropathy may make a woman unable to experience orgasm, or it may take longer for	

CONTENT OUTLINE

CONCEPT	DETAIL	INSTRUCTOR'S NOTES
	a woman to reach high levels of arousal and require more intense stimulation.	
	5.3 Painful intercourse is related to vaginitis or a lack of lubrication. Inadequate lubrication is often a problem in women with decreased estrogen production after menopause. Preparations to relieve vaginal dryness are available without a prescription.	Preparation with vitamin E may be helpful.
	5.4 Because women need to feel desire, feeling stressed, tired, depressed, or undesirable can affect how women respond sexually.	Ask, "How do you keep the romance and desire in your relationship?"
6. Treatment of sexual dysfunction in women	6.1 Evaluation is the first step of treatment. Tell your health care professional the nature of your concerns and when you first noticed the problem. A pelvic exam may be needed as part of the evaluation.	
	6.2 Keeping blood glucose levels in the target range can help. Often, high or low blood glucose levels may detract from overall well-being and sexual functioning.	
	6.3 Specific types of treatment may include: ■ medications for vaginitis ■ use of water-soluble lubricating gels ■ use of estrogen-based lubricating gels ■ postmenopausal hormone replacement therapy.	
7. Sexual health issues for men— puberty	7.1 Some men experience delayed onset of puberty and sexual maturation.	Ask, "What questions or concerns do you have about sexual function?"
Parenthood	7.2 Fertility is generally not affected by diabetes, except in retrograde ejaculation.	Retrograde ejaculation occurs rarely.

CONTENT OUTLINE

CONCEPT	DETAIL	INSTRUCTOR'S NOTES
	7.3 Retrograde ejaculation is the flow of liquid and sperm back into the bladder, rather than forward out of the penis. Orgasm is experienced, but less fluid is released in a forward direction. This does not affect sexual enjoyment, but may affect fertility because few sperm are deposited during intercourse.	Neuropathy may affect the valve that normally closes off the bladder during ejaculation.
	7.4 Treatment for infertility caused by retrograde ejaculation includes harvesting sperm from urine.	
	7.5 Several methods of birth control are available for people with diabetes. No one method is recommended.	Use Visual #4, Contraceptive Methods. Discuss each method, how it works, side effects, and effectiveness.
	7.6 Hypoglycemia may occur during sexual activity.	One carbohydrate exchange before sexual activity is usually adequate to prevent a reaction.
8. Sexual dysfunction in men with diabetes	8.1 Erectile dysfunction (ED) occurs in at least half of all men who have diabetes. It is often caused by damage to autonomic nerves from neuropathy. Changes in blood vessels are also common.	"Erectile dysfunction" is the preferred term because of negative connotations associated with the term "impotence." Prevalence rates range from 27–75%. Erectile dysfuction is the first sign of diabetes in about 12%.
	8.2 Erectile dysfunction can also be caused by: ■ drugs, including some blood pressure and depression medicines ■ decreased testosterone levels ■ alcohol ■ hardening of arteries in the pelvis ■ psychological factors ■ smoking.	Inability to achieve/sustain an erection more than 50% of the time is considered ED. Many drugs can affect sexual functioning. Men taking any of these drugs should bring this to the attention of the health care team for evaluation.
9. Treatment of sexual dysfunction	9.1 Tell your health care professionals about your concerns and when you first noticed a problem. You may be referred to a urologist for further evaluation.	Encourage participants to discuss sexual problems—problems cannot be treated if health care professionals are unaware of them.

CONTENT OUTLINE

CONCEPT	DETAIL	INSTRUCTOR'S NOTES

9.2 A blood sample may be taken for male hormone measurement, and a nocturnal penile tumescence study may be done (this involves the placement of a device around your penis while you sleep to measure the number of erections that occur with deep sleep). This test is not painful.

The presence of three to six erections during two to three nights of sleep generally indicates that the impotence is not organic.

9.3 High or low or fluctuating blood glucose levels may affect sexual functioning and overall well-being. Keeping blood glucose levels in the target range is often the first step in treatment.

The risk of ED is 1.7 times higher if the A1C is greater than 9% compared with an A1C of 7.5.

9.4 Inspite of recent publicity about erectile dysfunction and its treatment, no one therapy is effective for everyone. Some current treatment options include:
- avoidance of alcohol
- change in drug therapy
- psychological counseling
- hormonal treatment

Hormonal treatment is effective in 3–4% of men.

- drug therapies

New medications for the treatment of sexual dysfunction for men and women are under development.

- devices to assist with erection

These devices are effective in 90% of patients.

- surgery.

Surgery has high success rates.

9.5 Sildenafil (Viagra), vardenafil (Levitra), and tadalafil (Cialis): oral medications that will cause or improve reactions. About 50–65% of all failures with these medications are related to not following the directions (e.g., not waiting, no stimulation, taking after high-fat meals, etc).

These medications are less effective among men with diabetes than the general population.

CONTENT OUTLINE

CONCEPT	DETAIL	INSTRUCTOR'S NOTES
	■ Caverject and Edex: prostaglandin injections	These medications are effective for 70–83% of men. They are injected near the based of the penis. Using an injection device makes the process easier.
	■ Muse: prostaglandin urethral suppository.	
	9.6 Devices to assist with erection are available.	
	■ Erection and rigidity are achieved by creating a vacuum around the penis. Once the penis is engorged with blood, an entrapment band is placed around the penis to maintain rigidity.	This is the most common type of device used. Units include the Osbon ErecAid, VED, Elite ImpoAid, and Vacurect. These have effectiveness rates of 50–80%.
	■ Entrapment bands are worn around the penis to increase rigidity for the man who can achieve but not maintain an erection.	The unit is called Restore. All of these devices are contraindicated in men using anticoagulants, with bleeding disorders, or with a history of priapism.
	■ Penile orthoses (to support the penis) or external penile prostheses substitute for a dysfunctional penis.	The unit is called Rejoyn support sleeve.
	9.7 Surgical intervention includes placement of a prosthesis into the penis. The two types of prostheses are semirigid and inflatable. All are implanted into both sides of the penis, just above the urethra.	Stress the need for a thorough evaluation by a urologist and counseling for both partners.
	■ **Semirigid.** This method involves two semirigid rods inserted beside each other into the penis. The man then has a constantly erect penis that can be bent down.	Use Visual #5, Penile Prostheses—Semirigid.
	■ **Inflatable.** Two cylinders are placed inside the penis. A fluid reservoir is implanted in the groin The man can inflate the chambers to have an erection and collapse	Inflatable prostheses are more complicated and expensive, but allow for more familiar functioning. These are effective for 90–95% of men. Use Visual

CONTENT OUTLINE

CONCEPT	DETAIL	INSTRUCTOR'S NOTES
	the chambers when an erection is no longer wanted.	#6, Penile Prostheses— Inflatable.
10. Treatment resources for men and women	10.1 Difficulties with sexual functioning can lead to many behaviors, such as: ■ anxiety ■ sexual avoidance ■ poor communication ■ anger ■ feelings of hopelessness or rejection ■ loss of self-esteem ■ searching for explanation (myths) ■ partner dissatisfaction.	Suggestive comments and acting out may also occur among people who are experiencing sexual dysfunction.
	10.2 Sexual dysfunction contributes to depression and decreases quality of life.	
	10.3 One of the keys to success in treatment is being able to have good communication with your partner.	
	10.4 A health professional, counselor, or sexual therapist in whom you have confidence, and to whom you can relate, will be invaluable.	Counseling is often recommended as treatment for sexual dysfunction and may also be beneficial for patients with physiologically based problems.
	10.5 Other avenues of treatment are available, such as support groups, couples retreats (often sponsored by church groups), and sexual counselors.	There are national support and information sources. Have a list of community resources available. Note: Sex therapists and marriage counselors do not have standard education requirements— participants need to be careful to find a reputable therapist.
	10.6 There is help available, and the first step is to talk with a health care professional about your concern. Don't wait to be asked.	The Impotence Hot Line is 312-725-7722. Additional information can be found at http://www.webmd.com/ erectile-dysfunction/default.htm.

SKILLS CHECKLIST

None.

EVALUATION PLAN

Knowledge will be evaluated by achievement of learning objectives and by responses to questions during the session. The ability to apply knowledge will be evaluated through program outcome measures.

DOCUMENTATION PLAN

Record class attendance and achieved objectives as appropriate using the Diabetes Self-Management Record, the Participant Follow-up Record, or another form.

SUGGESTED READINGS

Brown JS, Luft J: Urinary incontinence. *Diabetes Self-Management* 22(3):48–50, 2005

D'Arrigo: Diabetes in the bedroom. *Diabetes Forecast* 59(9):55–57, 2006

Enzlin P, Rosen R, Wiegel M, Brown J, et al.: Sexual dysfunction is women with type 1 diabetes. *Diabetes Care* 32:780–785, 2009

Ezzell A, Baum N: When Viagra doesn't work. *Diabetes Self-Management* 25(2):29–32, 2008

Ezzell A, Baum N: Treatment of erectile dysfunction in diabetic men. *Practical Diabetology* 36(4):18–21, 2007

Hatzimouratidis K, Hatichristou D: Erectile dysfunction and diabetes mellitus. *Insulin* 4:114–122, 2009

Jackson SL, Scholes D, Boyko EJ, Abraham L, Fihn SD: Urinary incontinence and diabetes in postmenopausal women. *Diabetes Care* 28:1730–1738, 2005

Owens MD: Diabetes and women's health issues. *Diabetes Spectrum* 16:146–173, 2003

Penckofer S, Ferrans CE, Velson-Redrich, Savoy S: The psychological impact of living with diabetes: women's day-to-day experiences. *The Diabetes Educator* 33:680–690, 2007

Rice D, Jack L, Jr: Use of an assessment tool to enhance diabetes educators' ability to identify erectile dysfunction. *The Diabetes Educator* 32:373–380, 2006

Roszler J: Diabetes and sexual health. *Practical Diabetology* 28(2):26–30, 2009

Roszler J, Rice D: *Sex and Diabetes.* Alexandria, VA: American Diabetes Association, 2008

Ruder K: Woman and diabetes. *Diabetes Forecast* 60(11):38–42, 2007

Salonia A, Lanzi R, Scavini M, Pontillo M, et al.: Sexual function and endocrine profile in fertile women with type 1 diabetes. *Diabetes Care* 29:312–316, 2006

Weeks B, Picorelli CT: How new drugs help treat erectile dysfunction. *Nursing* 36(1):18–19, 2006

Weeks B, Picorelli CT: Treating erectile dysfunction without first-line drugs. *Nursing* 36(3):26–27, 2006

❂ Sexual Response Cycle—Physical Changes

Phase	Woman	Man
Excitement	■ Vaginal lubrication ■ Expansion and lengthening of the inner 1/3 of the vagina ■ Increase in size of clitoris ■ Erection of nipples	■ Erection of penis ■ Smoothing out of skin ridges of scrotum ■ Rising of testes toward the pelvis ■ Erection of nipples (in some men)
Plateau	■ Blood vessels filled with more blood than usual in the outer 1/3 of the vagina ■ Opening of vagina narrows, "gripping" action occurs ■ Rash may appear on chest or elsewhere	■ Blood vessels filled with more blood than usual cause further increase in size of testes ■ Deepening in color of penis ■ Small amounts of fluid may appear from urethra at end of penis ■ Rash may appear on chest or elsewhere

continued

SEXUAL RESPONSE CYCLE—PHYSICAL CHANGES *continued*

Phase	Woman	Man
Orgasm	■ Rhythmic contractions of uterus, outer 1/3 of the vagina, and rectal sphincter ■ Total-body response ■ May have more than one orgasm before resolution	■ Rhythmic contractions of testes and penis cause movement of fluid into the urethra and then suddenly out of the penis (ejaculation) ■ Total-body response ■ Has only one orgasm, requires period of resolution before another erection and orgasm are possible
Resolution	■ Orgasm disappears as muscle contractions move blood away from genital area ■ Uterus, vagina, and clitoris return to normal position and size	■ Blood leaves penis, which becomes limp ■ Testes and scrotum return to normal position and size

Adapted from Masters WH, Johnson VE. *Human Sexual Response.* Boston, MA: Little, Brown and Co., 1966

➲ Changes in Sexual Function with Aging

	Younger Women	Older Women
Breasts	■ Nipple erection ■ Increase in size, areolar engorgement, flush	■ Same ■ Intensity of reactions may diminish
Sex flush	■ Vasocongestive skin response to tension	■ Diminishes
Clitoris	■ High degree of responsivity	■ Same
Major labia	■ Flatten, separate, and elevate with increased sexual tension	■ Response diminishes
Minor labia	■ Vasocongestive thickening; color change from cardinal red to burgundy before orgasm	■ Color change and thickening diminish
Bartholin's glands	■ Small amount of mucoid secretion during plateau	■ Response diminishes
Vagina	■ Walls thickened; vaginal lubrication within 10–30 seconds of stimulation ■ During resolution, slow collapse of expanded portion of vagina	■ Walls thin; vagina shortens; expansibility decreases; lubrication may take >1–3 minutes
Uterus	■ Expulsive contractions (3–5 with orgasm)	■ Decrease in number

continued

CHANGES IN SEXUAL FUNCTION WITH AGING *continued*

	Younger Men	**Older Men**
Breasts	■ Nipple erection	■ Diminishes
Penis	■ Erection develops within 3–5 seconds of stimulation, full erection early in cycle	■ Erection takes 2–3 times longer after 50 years of age; full erection not attained until just before orgasm
	■ Ejaculatory control varies	■ Maintain erection longer without ejaculation
	■ May attain and partially lose full erection several times	■ When erection partially lost, difficulty in returning to full erection
	■ Forceful ejaculation; expulsive contractions during orgasm	■ Force diminishes; sensual experience may be reduced
	■ Refractory phase variable	■ Prolonged refractory period after orgasm; rapid penile detumescence
Ejaculation	■ Two-stage, well-differentiated process	■ Single-stage expulsion of seminal fluid
	■ Awareness of fluid emission and pressure	■ May experience seepage rather than expulsion; fewer, less visible sperm
Testes	■ Testicular elevation in late excitement or early plateau; increase in size	■ Diminished response
	■ Testicular descent during resolution	■ Rapid descent

Adapted from Masters WH, Johnson VE. *Human Sexual Response*. Boston, MA: Little, Brown and Co., 1966

Normal Menstrual Cycle

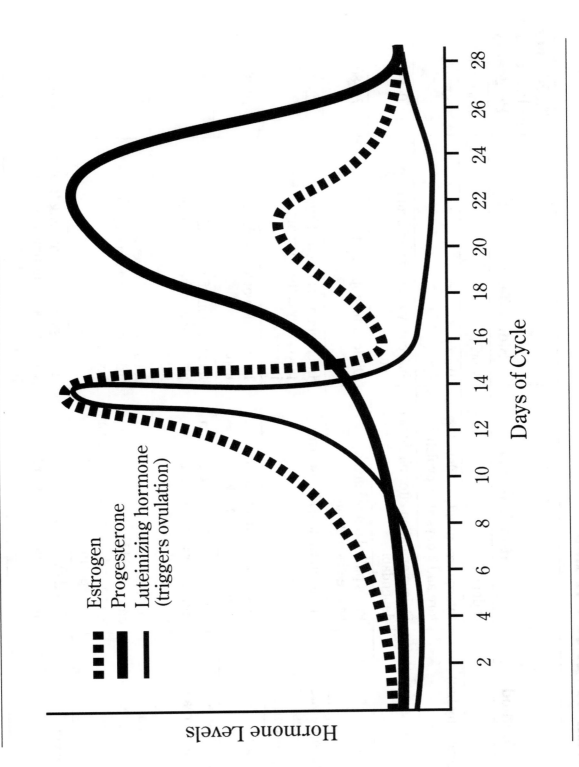

Estrogen

Progesterone

Luteinizing hormone
(triggers ovulation)

Hormone Levels

Days of Cycle

2   4   6   8   10   12   14   16   18   20   22   24   26   28

➔ Contraceptive Methods

Method	How It Works	Side Effects	Effectiveness in Preventing Pregnancy
None	It doesn't	Worry	20% (luck!)
Biological (rhythm)	Intercourse avoided 3 days before and 3 days after ovulation	Worry	60–80%
Breast-feeding	Delays ovulation after birth; not dependable	Insecurity about when ovulation returns	0–84%
Withdrawal	Penis pulled out of vagina before ejaculation	Difficult to stop and do	75–80%
Contraceptive vaginal creams, jellies, foams, and suppositories	Placed in vagina, kills sperm	Interruption of lovemaking to place; may cause burning or itching	72–90%
Diaphragm*	Fits over mouth of uterus to block sperm entry	Interruption of lovemaking to place	70–85%
Diaphragm plus spermicidal cream or jelly	Fits over cervix to block sperm entry; spermicidal barrier to sperm and kills sperm	Interruption of lovemaking to place; may cause burning or itching	85–97%
Cervical cap plus spermicidal cream or jelly	Fits over cervix to block sperm entry; held in place by suction; spermicidal barrier to sperm and kills sperm	Interruption of lovemaking to place; may cause burning or itching	60–90%
Male condom*	Placed over penis, prevents sperm from entering vagina	Interruption of lovemaking to place; some decrease in sensation; some people allergic to latex	85–90%

*A diaphragm or condom should be used with spermicidal cream or jelly. Make sure your cream or jelly is not one just for lubrication. Be sure the expiration date of the product has not passed.

© 2009 American Diabetes Association

CONTRACEPTIVE METHODS *continued*

Method	How It Works	Side Effects	Effectiveness in Preventing Pregnancy
Female condom	Inserted into vagina; blocks entry of sperm	Interruption of lovemaking to place; some reduction of sensation; awkward to insert correctly	74–79%
Condom plus spermicidal cream or jelly	Barrier to sperm and kills sperm	Interruption of lovemaking to place; some decrease in sensation; some people allergic to latex	95–97%
Vaginal ring	Placed in the vagina every 28 days; left in place for 21 days; provides low dose combination hormones	Estrogen may decrease effectiveness of insulin although doses of estrogen low; headache, breast tenderness	95–99%
Intrauterine device (IUD)	Placed in uterus by doctor, prevents planting of egg	Heavier menstrual periods and cramping; possible infection	95–98%
Birth control pill or patch (combined estrogen and progestin, and progestin only [mini-pill] available)	Blocks ovulation, thickens mucus of uterine lining to block sperm	Estrogen may decrease effectiveness of insulin; increased vascular disease; mood changes; weight gain	95–99%
Long-acting progestin (available by injection every 2 or 3 months, or subdermal implants [NorPlant])	Blocks ovulation, thickens mucus of uterine lining to block sperm	Has not been tested with women who have diabetes; irregular and longer menstrual periods and spotting; decreased libido	Nearly 100%
Sterilization (vasectomy for men; tubal ligation for women)	Blocks passage of sperm or egg	Requires surgery; usually permanent (hard to reverse surgically)	Nearly 100%

*A diaphragm or condom should be used with spermicidal cream or jelly. Make sure your cream or jelly is not one just for lubrication. Be sure the expiration date of the product has not passed.

© 2009 American Diabetes Association

➤ Penile Prostheses—Semirigid

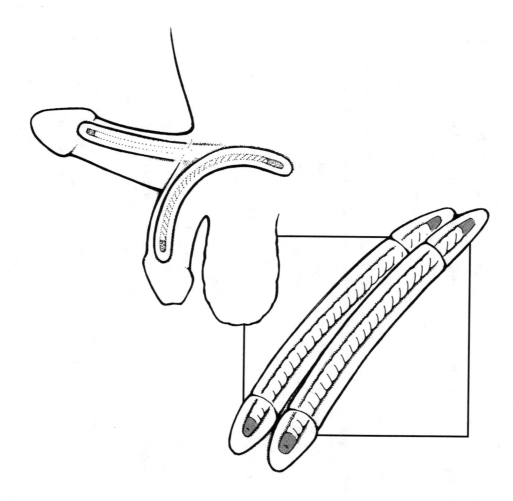

⬌ Penile Prostheses—Inflatable

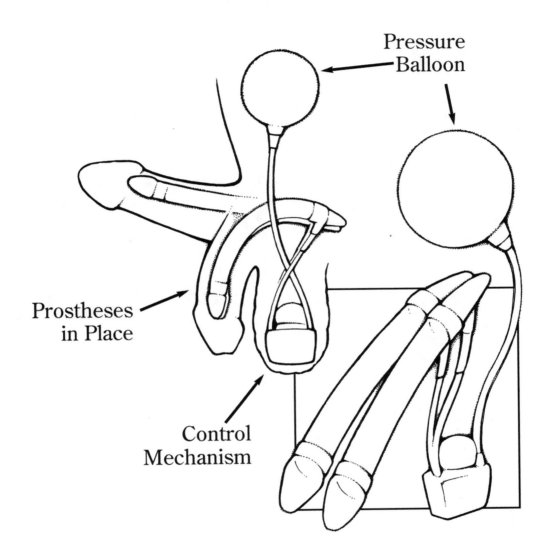

Pressure
Balloon

Prostheses
in Place

Control
Mechanism

| #21 | **Pregnancy and Diabetes** |

STATEMENT OF PURPOSE

This session is intended to provide information about preconception care for women with existing diabetes, care of diabetes during pregnancy, gestational diabetes, and the effect diabetes has on pregnancy and its outcomes.

PREREQUISITES

It is recommended that participants have a basic understanding of both diabetes and pregnancy.

OBJECTIVES

At the end of this session, participants will be able to:

For Preconception Counseling:

1. identify the need for normal blood glucose levels before pregnancy;

2. identify that blood glucose levels have an effect on the outcome of pregnancy;

3. identify one risk of pregnancy for the woman with diabetes;

4. identify personal concerns about pregnancy and diabetes;

5. list tests for diabetes complications that need to be done before pregnancy.

For Gestational Diabetes:

6. define gestational diabetes;

7. state the purpose of a meal plan during pregnancy;

8. identify the effect that blood glucose levels have on birth weight;

9. identify the personal value of monitoring blood glucose levels;

10. describe the treatment for hypoglycemia during pregnancy;

11. identify two emergency situations in which a provider should be notified;

12. identify personal barriers for self-management and strategies to address those barriers;

13. define areas of special care that her baby might receive;

14. identify post-partum care needs specifically for women with gestational diabetes.

For Preexisting Diabetes and Pregnancy:

15. identify that blood glucose control has an effect on the outcome of pregnancy;

16. state the personal value of intensification of insulin therapy during pregnancy;

17. identify personal benefits of monitoring blood glucose levels;

18. identify the effects insulin, different types of food, and exercise have on blood glucose levels;

19. describe the correct treatment for hypoglycemia during pregnancy;

20. identify two emergency situations in which a doctor should be notified;

21. identify personal barriers for self-management and strategies to address those barriers;

22. define one specialized test that the pregnant woman with diabetes may undergo;

23. define areas of special care that her baby might receive.

24. identify post-partum care needs specifically for women with diabetes.

CONTENT

Pregnancy; Preconception Care.

MATERIALS NEEDED

VISUALS PROVIDED

1. Insulin Action Times
2. Where Weight Goes During Pregnancy
3. Insulin Needs During Pregnancy

Handouts (one per participant):
1. Menstrual Chart
2. Treatment of Low Blood Glucose During Pregnancy

ADDITIONAL

- Samples of prenatal vitamins
- Samples of glucose products
- Insulin pump and tubing
- Information about childbirth options, high-risk clinics or medical centers, local hospital policies and tours, childbirth classes, La Leche League, child care classes, and smoking cessation programs

METHOD OF PRESENTATION

Start by introducing yourself and telling what you do. Ask participants to introduce themselves and their partners, if present. If most of the participants are pregnant, ask that they tell their due dates, if they have other children, and any other information they wish. Explain the purposes of this session and that although some of the information may be frightening, it is important to know so that they can be alert for early signs of problems, seek help promptly when needed, and understand the purpose of recommended therapy.

Present material in a question/discussion format, using the first question as a starting point. Provide appropriate content outlined below in response. Ask if there are additional questions, and respond, repeating the process for the entire session. Use the questions in the Instructor's Notes section to generate discussion if no questions are forthcoming after a period of silence. Keeping track of the content discussed in each session, using the Diabetes Self-Management Record, the Participant Follow-up Record, or another form, helps you to evaluate if all needed content has been discussed.

This topic is divided into three main sections: Preconception Counseling, Gestational Diabetes, and Preexisting Diabetes and Pregnancy. Present only the sections appropriate for the participants. It is probably most reasonable to present preconception information and pregnancy information in separate sessions. Preconception information should be provided to all women of child-bearing age who have diabetes.

CONTENT OUTLINE

CONCEPT	DETAIL	INSTRUCTOR'S NOTES
PRECONCEPTION COUNSELING		
1. Overview	1.1 Pregnancy is often an exciting time of joy and anticipation.	Ask, "What feelings do you have about becoming or being pregnant? What questions or concerns do you have?"
	1.2 It may also be a time when you are more concerned about your health.	
	1.3 In the past, some women with diabetes experienced unsuccessful pregnancies.	Ask, "What questions do you have about diabetes?" Review the basic pathophysiology of diabetes.
	1.4 Today, the chances are better than ever that a woman with diabetes will have a healthy baby.	
	1.5 Keeping blood glucose levels near the target range before and during pregnancy helps to ensure a positive outcome.	Ask, "What are your current target blood glucose values?" Recommended levels for non-pregnant adults with diabetes before meals: 70–130 mg/dl; after meals: <180 mg/dl. Recommended capillary blood glucose levels for women with GDM are: before meals <95 mg/dl; 1 hour post meals <140; 2 hours post meal <120 mg/dl.
	1.6 A careful balance of your meal plan, activity, and insulin needs to be	Recommended capillary blood glucose levels for pregnant

CONTENT OUTLINE

CONCEPT	DETAIL	INSTRUCTOR'S NOTES
	achieved and maintained before and during pregnancy. Blood glucose monitoring and frequent medical care are also an important part of preparing for pregnancy.	women with diabetes are: before meals: 60–99 mg/dl; peak after meals are: <129 mg/dl. Recommended target values may vary. Provide information appropriate for your participants.
2. Need for care	2.1 It is true that having diabetes increases the risk of problems for you and your baby.	Ask, "What have you heard about the effects of diabetes on pregnancy?"
	2.2 During pregnancy, some of the glucose in the mother's bloodstream goes to the baby so that it can grow and develop.	The glucose provides nourishment to the baby.
	2.3 However, blood glucose levels that are too high are harmful. They can lead to birth defects and other problems.	If most women in the group are already pregnant, present information about preconception care with sensitivity to their situation. If all women are pregnant, do not present this information.
	2.4 Because the baby's organs are formed during the first 6 weeks of pregnancy, the risk for birth defects is greatest if blood glucose levels are too high during that time. (This may be before you know you're pregnant.)	Incidence is 6–10% for women with diabetes, compared to 2% in the general population; however, with near-normal glucose control in the first trimester, incidence decreases to that of the general population.
	2.5 You can reduce the risks by having an A1C level as close to normal as possible and blood glucose levels consistently in your target range before you become pregnant.	Ask, "What is your target A1C level? Why is this number important to you?" Note that individual targets may vary.
	2.6 You will need to continue to use contraception until your blood glucose levels are in the preconception target range (A1C <7%).	
3. Caring for your diabetes	3.1 It is a good idea to begin working before pregnancy with the health care team who will provide your prenatal care. The team includes an obstetrician, pediatrician, nurse	Ask, "Do you have a care team to help you manage your diabetes?" Define team members' roles. Encourage women to seek care at a high-risk

CONTENT OUTLINE

CONCEPT	DETAIL	INSTRUCTOR'S NOTES
	educator, dietitian, and perhaps a social worker.	clinic or tertiary care center.
	3.2 If you take oral agents, you will stop taking them and begin taking insulin. Talk with your provider about all medications, vitamins, and herbal products you take.	Oral agents may be harmful to the developing fetus. ACE inhibitors and ARBs will be replaced. Other drugs may be stopped or changed as well.
	3.3 Your insulin needs may increase, and you may take more than one type of insulin to keep your blood glucose levels more consistent throughout the day.	Use Visual #1, Insulin Action Times.
	3.4 Most insulin programs will include two to four insulin injections a day before and during pregnancy. Some women use an insulin pump.	Show an insulin pump, if available.
	3.5 Your meals, activity, and insulin program need to be carefully balanced.	
	3.6 You will work with the dietitian to develop a meal plan that fits your life and includes the foods you and your family like and enjoy.	
	3.7 If you have a regular exercise program, you can continue it. You will need to check your blood glucose more often when you exercise. You may need an exercise snack with a more intensive insulin program.	Ask, "Do you exercise now? Do you plan to continue once you become pregnant?"
	3.8 If you plan to start an exercise program, choose something less strenuous, such as walking or swimming, that you can continue throughout your pregnancy.	Ask, "Are you planning to start to exercise when you become pregnant?"
	3.9 You will need to check and record your blood glucose at least four times a day to be sure that the balance is working.	Review recommended times and how to use the information provided. Ask, "How do you use the information you get from monitoring now?"

CONTENT OUTLINE

CONCEPT	DETAIL	INSTRUCTOR'S NOTES
	3.10 Because your blood glucose targets are lower, you are more likely to experience hypoglycemic reactions.	Ask, "How do you know when your blood glucose is too low? How do you treat it?" Review treatment.
	3.11 You need to carry a quick-acting source of sugar with you at all times, such as glucose tablets or gels.	Show sample products. Stress the value of wearing diabetes identification.
	3.12 There is a lot to do to get ready for pregnancy and a healthy baby. It will help to anticipate barriers and plan strategies to address these barriers. Using strategies that have worked for you in the past is often an effective approach.	Ask, "What barriers do you anticipate in managing your diabetes more intensively during this time? What strategies can you think of to help overcome these barriers?" Write barriers and strategies on the board and discuss.
4. Health considerations	4.1 Cigarette smoking and alcohol are harmful to your unborn child. If you smoke, now is a good time to stop. Alcohol should be avoided during pregnancy.	Provide information about smoking cessation programs in your area.
	4.2 Pregnancy can negatively affect some of the long-term complications of diabetes. You need a thorough medical and diabetes checkup before you become pregnant.	Blood pressure, including orthostatic measures, and heart, vascular, thyroid, and kidney function need to be evaluated. It is also important to test for signs of autonomic and peripheral neuropathy.
	4.3 Retinopathy can become worse during pregnancy. You need to see an eye specialist for a dilated eye exam before pregnancy and receive treatment for any retinal damage.	Define *retinopathy* and *eye specialist*. Laser therapy can be done safely during pregnancy.
	4.4 After this exam, you, your partner, and your health care team should discuss any risks of pregnancy.	
	4.5 A prenatal vitamin is needed.	Sufficient vitamins, iron, calcium, and supplemental folic acid are needed. Show samples.
5. Other considerations	5.1 There is very little chance your baby will be born with diabetes. If you	Men with type 1 diabetes have a 6% chance of having a child with

CONTENT OUTLINE

CONCEPT	DETAIL	INSTRUCTOR'S NOTES
	have type 1 diabetes, there is a 1–2% chance your child will ever get diabetes. If you have type 2 diabetes, there is a 10–15% chance your child will get diabetes as an adult and up to a 33% chance for glucose intolerance.	diabetes. The risks are higher if both parents have diabetes. Risks for both types decrease the older parents are at the time of diagnosis.
	5.2 There is no best age to be pregnant. Women who have their children between 20 and 40 years of age have fewer health risks.	A pelvic exam and pap smear are needed before pregnancy. It may be harder to become pregnant as you get older.
	5.3 A pregnancy is very demanding when you have diabetes. It takes knowledge, time, effort, and money for the extra health care costs. You may need to take time off from work or have help caring for other children or with housework.	Point out that this can be a stressful time. Encourage participants to talk with their partners and other supporters about the demands of pregnancy Ask, "What do you think will help you to handle the demands of pregnancy and caring for diabetes?"
6. Becoming pregnant	6.1 Once your A1C and your blood glucose levels are in your target range, you can safely become pregnant.	Encourage participants to talk with their providers before becoming pregnant.
	6.2 You can become pregnant 1–2 h after you ovulate. Ovulation occurs 12–16 days before your period starts.	
	6.3 Your basal temperature goes up slightly just before you ovulate. Your basal temperature is your temperature first thing in the morning, before you get out of bed.	
	6.4 Keeping track of your basal temperature and menstrual cycle or using home prediction kits will help you know when you ovulate.	Distribute and review Handout #1, Menstrual Chart. Participants may want to use the commercial ovulation predictor test kits.
	6.5 Diabetes does not affect fertility for women. You may get pregnant right away, or it can take 6–12 months. If it takes longer, talk with your health care team.	Remind participants that they need to maintain target blood glucose levels during this time. PCOS does affect fertility.

CONTENT OUTLINE

CONCEPT	DETAIL	INSTRUCTOR'S NOTES
7. Conclusion	7.1 Pregnancy can be stressful but it can also be a happy time and a time to look forward to good things ahead.	Ask, "Have you noticed a change in your moods? What are your concerns about your pregnancy or becoming pregnant? What are you looking forward to?"
	7.2 Planning your pregnancy helps to ensure the best outcome for you and your baby.	
GESTATIONAL DIABETES		
8. Why does it occur?	8.1 This type of diabetes appears for the first time during pregnancy. It occurs in approximately 4% (range 1–14%) of all pregnant women.	Ask, "What questions or concerns do you have about gestational diabetes?" Review the pathophysiology of diabetes, normal metabolism, and the role of insulin. Refer to Outline #1, *What is diabetes* (p. 3)?"
	8.2 Women who are older, have had babies weighing 9 lb or more, have a family history of diabetes, are from certain ethnic groups, or are overweight are at an increased risk.	Oher risks of PCOS, being over 25, and women who are multiparous.
	8.3 Gestational diabetes may occur because hormones produced by the placenta in all pregnant women may make insulin less effective (insulin resistance).	Review the purpose of the placenta. Review insulin resistance. In late pregnancy, insulin sensitivity falls by 50%.
	8.4 These hormones increase as pregnancy progresses. More insulin is needed to maintain normal glucose levels. If the pancreas is unable to produce enough insulin, gestational diabetes occurs.	Use Visual #3, Insulin Needs During Pregnancy.
	8.5 Gestational diabetes is usually found in the 5th to 6th month (24–28 weeks) of pregnancy. A special screening blood test is done at that time.	Ask, "How did you find out you had diabetes?" Review the value and results of the glucose challenge tests used during pregnancy in your setting.

CONTENT OUTLINE

CONCEPT	DETAIL	INSTRUCTOR'S NOTES
9. Caring for gestational diabetes	9.1 The purpose of the treatment is to keep the blood glucose near the target range. The target capillary blood glucose levels for pregnancy are as follows: fasting, <95 mg/dl; 1 hour after a meal, <140 mg/dl; and 2 hours after a meal, <120 mg/dl.	The actual recommended target blood glucose values may vary. Provide information appropriate for your setting and the participant's situation. Plasma blood glucose targets are: fasting, <105 mg/dl; 1 hour post meal, <155 mg/dl; and 2 hours post meal, 130 mg/dl.
	9.2 The first treatment is a meal plan. This is not a diet to lose weight, but a plan to spread your food out over the day so that your blood glucose levels are more even. You will work with a dietitian to develop your personal meal plan that will include the foods your family likes and enjoys. Carbohydrates will generally be restricted, but not to less than 40% of calories per day.	Provide participants with the name of a dietitian. Explain the rationale for frequent, small meals. For obese women (BMI >30), a moderate calorie restriction of 30% of the estimated caloric need may reduce hyperglycemia and triglyceride levels with no ketonuria.
	9.3 Exercise helps to lower blood glucose levels by decreasing insulin resistance. Recommended exercises are those that use the upper-body muscles. Talk to your provider about the safety of upper-body exercise.	When the lower body is kept from an excessive weight-bearing load, the load can be increased safely without fear of fetal distress.
	9.4 Check and record your blood glucose levels. Use this information to see how food, activity, and insulin (if taken) affect your blood glucose. Bring this record with you to each of your appointments.	Refer to Outline #10, *Monitoring Your Diabetes* (p. 211). Ask, "What have you noticed about how food affects your blood glucose? Exercise? Insulin?" Checking ketones may be recommended for women using caloric restricted meal plans.
	9.5 Insulin injections may be needed to maintain blood glucose levels in the target range.	Refer to Outline #9, *All About Insulin and Other Therapies* (p. 165). Oral hypoglycemic agents are generally contraindicated during pregnancy. Ask, "What questions or concerns do you have about using insulin?"
	9.6 You will be asked to visit your obstetrician more often than women	

CONTENT OUTLINE

CONCEPT	DETAIL	INSTRUCTOR'S NOTES

without gestational diabetes. It is very important that you do so. You may be referred to a specialist in diabetes or high-risk pregnancies.

9.7 There is a lot to do to care for diabetes when you are pregnant. It will help to anticipate barriers and plan strategies to address these barriers. Using strategies that have worked for you in the past is often an effective approach.

Ask, "What barriers do you anticipate in managing diabetes during your pregnancy? What strategies can you think of to help overcome these barriers?" Write barriers and strategies on the board.

9.8 Caring for diabetes is very demanding when you are pregnant. It takes knowledge, time, effort, and support. It may feel unfair to have diabetes during what should be a very happy time in your life and you may find youself feeling angry, guilty, or depressed. Although these feelings are common, seeking the support of a good listener often helps. If these feelings become overwhelming or are interfering with your ability to care for yourself, talk with your health care team about getting the support you need.

Point out that this can be a stressful time. Encourage participants to talk with their partners and other supporters about their fears and feelings? Ask, "What are your thoughts and feelings about developing diabetes? What would help you to cope with these feelings?"

10. Risks related to gestational diabetes

10.1 Gestational diabetes does increase the risks of certain problems for the mother and baby. The risks are greatest in the last trimester and if the blood glucose levels are too high.

Explain what is meant by "trimester?" Birth defects generally occur early in pregnancy and are not thought to be related to gestational diabetes that develops later in pregnancy.

10.2 Although it is frightening to hear about these possible problems, it is important to understand why glucose management is so important during pregnancy.

A pregnant woman who has experienced any of these problems in the past should be referred to a perinatologist or high-risk pregnancy clinic.

10.3 Some of the problems are:
■ large babies at birth (more than 9 lb)

Birth weight is closely related to the mother's blood glucose level in the last trimester. The baby's pancreas becomes functional at

CONTENT OUTLINE

CONCEPT	DETAIL	INSTRUCTOR'S NOTES

11–13 weeks. If the mother is hyperglycemic, the baby also becomes hyperglycemic and produces excessive amounts of insulin, which is a growth factor for fetal tissue. Large babies can cause difficult deliveries.

- low blood glucose (hypoglycemia) and breathing problems for the baby after birth

- jaundice or yellowish skin in the baby 2–3 days after birth

Hypoglycemia occurs because the baby has been producing insulin in response to the mother's elevated blood glucose levels. After birth, the baby's glucose drops.

- preeclampsia (a combination of high blood pressure, protein in the urine, and swelling in the mother's hands, face, and feet)

Ask, "What is your blood pressure target?" Remind participants to tell their provider of any excessive edema.

- hydramnios (too much amniotic fluid around the baby), which may cause the uterus to stretch and may lead to early delivery

Hydramnios occurs in 25% of diabetic pregnancies. Bed rest and glucose control is recommended.

- urinary tract infections

Ask, "What are symptoms of a urinary tract infection?" Remind participants to inform their providers of any symptoms.

- stillbirth or neonatal death.

10.4 After pregnancy, the symptoms of diabetes usually disappear. Only 2% still have diabetes after delivery. You need to have your blood glucose checked after delivery to be sure you no longer have diabetes.

Define type 2 diabetes. Explain the importance of a 2-hour glucose tolerance test 6 weeks post-partum or after stopping nursing. Encourage women who have a history of gestational diabetes to seek preconception care.

10.5 Type 2 diabetes may return later in your life. The chances for developing diabetes in the 5–10 years after delivery are about 50%; however, rates are lower among women with a lower BMI.

Review the symptoms and diagnostic criteria for type 2 diabetes and the results of the Diabetes Prevention Program. Stress the need to lose weight after delivery as one way to prevent subsequent type 2 diabetes. Maintaining a regular exercise program also helps prevent type 2.

CONTENT OUTLINE

CONCEPT	DETAIL	INSTRUCTOR'S NOTES
	10.6 If you no longer have diabetes, you will need to be screened for diabetes at least every 3 years. If you plan to become pregnant again, ask for a screening glucose test before becoming pregnant. Once you become pregnant again, ask to have your blood glucose checked early in the pregnancy.	Women with impaired fasting glucose or impaired glucose tolerance in the postpartum period should be screened annually. If there are women in the class who had diabetes before becoming pregnant, continue with Concept 11. If not, go on to Concept 14.
	10.7 If you continue to have diabetes after delivery, you need to be sure that you seek care and maintain blood glucose levels as close to normal as possible before becoming pregnant again.	Children of women with GDM are prone to obesity and type 2 diabetes. Adopting a healthy lifestyle can help to prevent future problems for the entire family.

PREEXISTING DIABETES AND PREGNANCY

CONCEPT	DETAIL	INSTRUCTOR'S NOTES
11. Changes during pregnancy	11.1 Women with diabetes are affected by all of the normal changes that occur during a pregnancy. Some of these changes can make blood glucose management more difficult.	Ask, "What questions or concerns do you have about diabetes and your pregnancy?"
	11.2 The amount of glucose lost into the urine increases.	Define *glycosuria*. Stress that blood glucose monitoring is essential during pregnancy.
	11.3 All women produce ketones more easily during pregnancy. Thus, ketosis and diabetic ketoacidosis (DKA) can occur more rapidly.	Ask, "Do you check for ketones?" Remind participants that ketones result when body fats are broken down for energy. In type 1 diabetes, this usually happens because there is not enough insulin to use the glucose in the bloodstream for energy. Ketones cross the placental barrier and may affect fetal cognitive development.
	11.4 The placenta produces hormones that counteract insulin action. These hormones increase as pregnancy progresses. This leads to an increase in insulin needs during pregnancy.	The hormones "act against" or "block" insulin. Show Visual #3, Insulin Needs During Pregnancy. You'll need more insulin as the weeks go by. Insulin sensitivity decreases by 50% late in pregnancy.

CONTENT OUTLINE

CONCEPT	DETAIL	INSTRUCTOR'S NOTES
	11.5 When you have an infection such as a cold, the need for insulin increases and the risk for DKA increases.	If you have an infection, check your urine for ketones. Provide guidelines for when to contact a health professional.
12. Diabetes-related risks in pregnancy	12.1 Diabetes increases the risk for certain problems in the mother and baby:	A pregnant woman who has experienced any of these problems in the past should be referred to a perinatologist or high-risk pregnancy clinic.
	■ preeclampsia (a combination of high blood pressure, protein in the urine, and swelling in the hands, face, and feet)	Ask, "What is your blood pressure target?" Remind participants to tell their doctor about any excessive edema. Bed rest and hospitalization are usual treatments.
	■ urinary tract infections	Ask, "What are symptoms of a urinary tract infection?" Remind participants to inform providers of any symptoms.
	■ hydramnios (too much amniotic fluid around the baby), which may cause the uterus to stretch and may lead to early delivery	Hydramnios occurs more often in diabetic pregnancies. Bed rest and glucose control is recommended.
	■ large babies at birth (more than 9 lb)	Birth weight is closely related to the mother's blood glucose level in the last trimester. If the mother is hyperglycemic, the baby also becomes hyperglycemic and produces excessive amounts of insulin, which is a growth factor for fetal tissue. The baby's pancreas becomes functional at 13 weeks. Large babies can cause difficult deliveries.
	■ low blood glucose and breathing problems for the baby	Hypoglycemia occurs because the baby has been producing insulin in response to the mother's elevated blood glucose levels.
	■ physical defects of the baby	The incidence is 6–10% for women with diabetes who have elevated

CONTENT OUTLINE

CONCEPT	DETAIL	INSTRUCTOR'S NOTES

		blood glucose levels, compared with 2% in the general population.
	■ stillbirth or neonatal death.	
	12.2 While it is frightening to hear about these possible problems, it is important to know why blood glucose management is so important. Keeping your blood glucose in the target range can help prevent these problems.	Ask, "What are your usual target blood glucose levels? What are your target blood glucose values during your pregnancy?" Point out that these will likely be lower than their usual targets.
13. Caring for diabetes during pregnancy	13.1 The purpose of the treatment is to keep blood glucose in the target range. The target blood glucose levels for pregnancy are: 60–99 mg/dl before meals; 100–129 mg/dl peak post meal; and mean daily blood glucose = 110 mg/dl (A1C <6%).	Ask, "What questions or concerns do you have about the care you need during pregnancy?" The actual recommended target blood glucose values may vary. Provide information appropriate for your setting and the participants' situations.
	13.2 Your prenatal care will probably be provided by a team of health professionals. The team includes an obstetrician, endocrinologist/ diabetologist, nurse educator, dietitian, and perhaps a social worker.	Define team members' roles.
	13.3 You need to visit your doctor every other week during the first and second trimesters, and then every week until delivery.	Provide information according to the participant's situation.
	13.4 Check and record your blood glucose levels frequently. Use this information to see how the food you eat, your activity, and your insulin affect your blood glucose levels. Bring your record with you to each of your appointments. Some women use continuous glucose monitoring (CGM) during pregnancy.	Post-meal blood glucose levels are generally at their peak 1 hour after the meal. Pre- and post-prandial monitoring, along with bedtime and an occasional 2–4 a.m. reading is optimal. A1C levels are checked monthly until target levels are reached and then every 2–3 months.
	13.5 Do not take any medicine (including OTC medicines, vitamins, and herbal medicines) until you talk with your health care	Remind participants of the risks of alcohol and smoking. Provide information about smoking cessation programs in your area.

CONTENT OUTLINE

CONCEPT	DETAIL	INSTRUCTOR'S NOTES
	team. This is for your safety and that of your baby.	
	13.6 You may already be taking insulin, using a meal plan, exercising, and checking your blood glucose levels. Your treatment plan will probably change during your pregnancy.	Monitoring ketone levels on arising may also be recommended.
14. More about managing your blood glucose— meal plan	14.1 Your meal plan will change during pregnancy. Eating the meals and snacks as recommended throughout the day and at bedtime will help to keep your blood glucose levels in the target range and prevent hypoglycemia. You will work with a dietitian to develop a meal plan that includes the foods you and your family like and enjoy.	Ask, "What questions or concerns do you have about self-care during pregnancy? Do you currently use a meal plan or count carbohydrates?" Refer participants to a dietitian for a personal meal plan. A decrease in carbohydrate may be recommended.
	14.2 Do **NOT** go on a weight-reduction diet during pregnancy. More calories are needed to meet the energy needs of the growing baby.	Starvation ketosis can occur and may be dangerous to the developing baby.
	14.3 You can expect to gain about 25–35 pounds. Talk with your health care team about your recommended weight gain.	Use Visual #2, Where Weight Goes During Pregnancy.
	14.4 Prenatal vitamins with folic acid are recommended.	Show samples of prenatal vitamins. If you feel nauseated in the morning, try taking your vitamin at dinner.
Exercise	14.5 Exercise burns calories, decreases blood glucose levels, and increases feelings of well-being.	Ask, "What are the barriers of exercise for you? What are the benefits?"
	14.6 If you have a regular exercise program, such as aerobics or swimming, check with your health care team about continuing.	Bicycling is generally not recommended late in pregnancy because of the risk for falls.
	14.7 Walking is a safe activity if started early in pregnancy; otherwise, upper-body exercise is recommended during pregnancy. Check with your doctor before starting	Ask, "What exercise would you consider doing while you are pregnant?"

CONTENT OUTLINE

CONCEPT	DETAIL	INSTRUCTOR'S NOTES
	any exercise, including walking. In general, 30 minutes per day is recommended.	
	14.8 Monitor your blood glucose levels more often when you exercise. If exercise-induced hypoglycemia occurs often, your meal plan or insulin dose will need to be adjusted, or an exercise snack included.	
	14.9 Your insulin dose will change often, especially during the last half of pregnancy.	Use Visual #3, Insulin Needs During Pregnancy.
Insulin	14.10 Most women take two or more injections of insulin per day. This helps to keep the blood glucose levels in the target range.	Refer to Visual #1, Insulin Action Times. Oral medications are not recommended during pregnancy. Refer to Outline #9, *All About Insulin* (p. 165).
	14.11 The technique for injecting insulin doesn't change. Site rotation is still important. There is no reason to stop using abdominal sites, unless you have trouble pinching up your skin.	
	14.12 You can learn to adjust your insulin dose based on your blood glucose levels and carbohydrate intake.	
	14.13 Some women prefer to use an insulin pump.	Show an insulin pump, if available. See Outline #22, *Insulin Pump Therapy* (p. 479).
15. Hyperglycemia	15.1 High blood glucose may lead to or go along with ketoacidosis.	Ask, "What is high blood glucose during pregnancy?"
	15.2 Signs and symptoms of hyperglycemia are: ■ elevated blood glucose ■ ketones ■ more urine output than usual ■ increased thirst ■ dry skin and mouth	Ask, "What are symptoms you notice when your blood glucose is high?" Stress the importance of ketone testing if blood glucose levels are elevated (>200 mg/dl).

CONTENT OUTLINE

CONCEPT	DETAIL	INSTRUCTOR'S NOTES

■ decreased appetite, nausea, and vomiting
■ fatigue, drowsiness, or no energy
■ fever.

15.3 Hyperglycemia usually develops slowly, over several hours or days.

15.4 Call your doctor right away if you have these symptoms. Do **NOT** skip your insulin dose.

Instructor's Notes: If not nauseated, drink extra sugar-free liquids.

16. Hypoglycemia

16.1 Hypoglycemia in pregnancy is defined as blood glucose levels below 60 mg/dl. It may occur more often during pregnancy, because of the intensification of therapy.

Instructor's Notes: Ask, "What is hypoglycemia during pregnancy?" A blood glucose level of 60 mg/dl is low. Hypoglycemia is not harmful to the baby, but can be to the mother if untreated.

16.2 Signs and symptoms of hypoglycemia are:
■ low blood glucose (<60 mg/dl)
■ sweating
■ weakness, trembling, and fast heartbeat
■ hunger
■ anxiety
■ nausea
■ inability to think straight
■ irritability or grouchiness
■ headache
■ confusion, coma, or convulsions.

Instructor's Notes: Ask, "What symptoms do you have when you have a low blood glucose reaction? How do you treat it?"

16.3 Hypoglycemia occurs suddenly and without warning. You need to carry something with you to treat it at all times.

Instructor's Notes: Show examples of glucose products. Stress the need for diabetes identification.

16.4 The preferred treatment during pregnancy is glucose (3–5 glucose tablets or 1 cup skim milk).

Instructor's Notes: Distribute and review Handout #2, Treatment of Low Blood Glucose During Pregnancy. Stress the need to retest and retreat if needed.

16.5 Treat hypoglycemia promptly. Always carry something with you to treat low blood glucose reactions when you are away from home.

Instructor's Notes: Glucagon injection technique should be taught to families of patients prone to severe hypoglycemia, who have asymptomatic hypoglycemia, or are

CONTENT OUTLINE

CONCEPT	DETAIL	INSTRUCTOR'S NOTES

		using intensive insulin therapy. Refer to Outline #11, *Managing Blood Glucose* (p. 231).
17. Team care	17.1 At each visit to your obstetrician, your weight, blood pressure, general health, and growth of the baby will be evaluated.	Ask, "Do you have any questions or concerns about the care you will receive?" A urine culture is needed if significant pyuria is present.
	17.2 Your urine will be checked each time for glucose, ketones, protein, and bacteria.	
	17.3 At each visit to your diabetologist, your meal plan, insulin needs, and blood glucose levels will be evaluated. Your A1C level will be measured every 4–12 weeks. Be sure to bring your blood glucose monitoring records and meter.	
	17.4 You may meet with a dietitian to learn more about your meal plan or with a nurse to learn more about diabetes during pregnancy.	
	17.5 All team members are available to answer any questions you might have. Between visits, write down any questions or concerns you have so that you remember to ask them.	
	17.6 You may be referred to a medical center in your area for specialized care.	Have information available on centers in your area.
	17.7 If you take insulin, you may be hospitalized at any time, if needed, to better manage your blood glucose.	Pregnant women with diabetes may need to be hospitalized for blood glucose management to ensure the birth of a healthy baby.
	17.8 Contact your doctor right away if you notice: ■ more than trace ketones in your urine ■ two glucose levels >200 mg/dl ■ decreased movement of your baby	Provide specific guidelines for your setting as appropriate.

CONTENT OUTLINE

CONCEPT	DETAIL	INSTRUCTOR'S NOTES

- any infection or illness (fever, nausea, or vomiting)
- lower abdominal (stomach) cramps
- vaginal bleeding
- sharp back pain or abdominal pain
- burning or pain when passing urine
- dizziness, fainting, blurred vision, or spots before your eyes
- rapid weight gain
- swelling of your hands, face, or feet
- hypoglycemia that someone else had to treat, or so severe that you passed out
- severe nausea or vomiting with hyperglycemia and ketonuria.

18. Special tests and procedures

18.1 Special tests may be done during your pregnancy. The results of these tests are used to monitor your health and your baby's development.

Point out that this is done as part of very close monitoring and is for their safety. Although these sound frightening, they help ensure the welfare of the baby.

18.2 An ultrasound test is used to determine the size, growth, and position of the baby and placenta. It may be done several times during your pregnancy.
- This test is safe for your baby and causes no discomfort. It uses sound waves, not radiation.

This is often first done around 8 weeks to date the pregnancy. The timing for each of these tests may vary. Present information that is relevant for your setting and the participants.

- A full bladder is needed to push the uterus into position so the baby can be visualized better. You will be asked to drink water before the test.

The American Pregnancy Association offers information about each of these tests (www.americanpregnancy.org).

- You will lie on your back as the ultrasound instrument is passed over your abdomen. Pulses of light appear on a screen and form a picture of the baby and placenta. Ask for a copy of the picture.

CONTENT OUTLINE

CONCEPT	DETAIL	INSTRUCTOR'S NOTES

■ The test lasts for 15–60 minutes.
■ A more comprehensive ultrasound is done at 18–22 weeks.
■ A fetal echogram in midpregnancy (20–22 weeks) is used to screen for congenital heart defects.
■ Ultrasounds may be done at any time during pregnancy to check on the size and health of your baby.

18.3 Your urine will be checked to measure the protein/creatinine ratio about every trimester. This is an indication of your kidney function. If needed, a 24-hour urine test will be done as a follow up. You will be asked to save all your urine for 24 hours so it can be tested for protein and creatinine. A blood sample will be drawn when you bring in the urine.

Remind patients of the importance of saving all urine on ice during the test. 24-hour testing is most often done if pre-eclampsia is of concern.

18.4 Starting at 28 weeks, a nonstress test (NST) will be done once. Starting at 32 weeks an NST will be done twice a week. An external fetal monitor is used to record your baby's movements and the changes in the fetal heart rate. This test indicates how the baby is adjusting to his or her environment.

This is the primary test of fetal well-being. If there are complications, this test will be done twice a week starting at 28 weeks. This test can indicate if the baby is not receiving enough oxygen or other signs of fetal distress.

18.5 The quad test (or alpha-fetoprotein [AFP] profile) is a blood test done at 16–18 weeks' gestation. This is a screening test to give information about whether your baby is in a high-risk category for defects of the brain and spinal cord (neural tube defects) or genetic syndromes. A high or low level indicates only that further tests are needed. This test is offered to all women, but babies of women with diabetes are at higher risk.

The triple test (or AFP profile) measures:
■ alpha-fetoprotein (believed to be low in a Down's syndrome pregnancy because the fetus is immature; it is high in a fetus with neural tube defects)
■ unconjugated estriol (believed to be low in a Down's syndrome pregnancy because of isolated defects in the endocrine fetoplacental system—immature placenta)
■ human chorionic gonadotropin (believed to be higher in a

CONTENT OUTLINE

CONCEPT	DETAIL	INSTRUCTOR'S NOTES

Down's syndrome pregnancy because normally this chemical declines appreciably between 10 and 20 weeks' gestation; if placenta is immature, this decline would not occur on schedule)
- inhibin A is a protein produced by the placenta and the ovaries. The likelihood of identifying Down syndrome is higher through the evaluation of the levels.

18.6 Starting at 28–32 weeks, you may be asked to monitor and record your baby's movements (kick counting). You will choose an hour each day to lie on your left side and count and record movements you feel.

A baby is usually very active, including kicks, stretches, and rollovers.

18.7 Starting at 28–32 weeks, biophysical profiles may be done if additional information is needed after an NST. This consists of an additional NST combined with an ultrasound viewing of the baby. The obstetrician will directly observe fetal movements, amount of amniotic fluid, fetal breathing motions, heart rate, muscle tones, and condition of the fetus.

19. Labor and delivery

19.1 Your baby will be delivered as close to your due date as is safe. Normal gestation is 40 weeks. The decision about when to deliver the baby is based on how you and your baby are doing.

Ask, "What questions or concerns do you have about your labor and delivery?" Some of the factors considered are insulin needs, blood pressure, kidney functioning, results of the biophysical profiles, daily fetal movement counts, NSTs, and results of the amniocentesis.

19.2 Your baby can be born vaginally, even if you had a low-transverse cesarean section in the past.

A low-transverse cesarean section is also called a "bikini cut."

CONTENT OUTLINE

CONCEPT	DETAIL	INSTRUCTOR'S NOTES
	19.3 If early delivery is needed and the baby is to be delivered vaginally, labor will be induced by medication. A cesarean delivery may be needed in some cases.	The indicators for a cesarean delivery are the same as for women without diabetes.
	19.4 During labor, you will receive any needed insulin intravenously, and your blood glucose levels will be monitored every 1–2 hours.	
	19.5 Most hospitals encourage your partner to be present for either a vaginal or cesarean delivery.	Have a list of area hospitals and their policies available.
	19.6 There are classes in your area on childbirth, including the Lamaze method and cesarean delivery.	Have a list of classes in your area available.
	19.7 Tours of the delivery and nursery area are available at many hospitals.	
20. Care after delivery	20.1 After delivery, your insulin needs drop dramatically.	Ask, "What questions or concerns do you have about your care after delivery?" Refer to Visual #3, Insulin Needs During Pregnancy.
	20.2 Your blood glucose will be monitored very closely.	
	20.3 If you continue taking insulin, your insulin needs will go back to your prepregnancy level in 2–6 weeks.	
21. Care of your baby	21.1 A pediatrician may be present during delivery to care for your newborn.	Ask, "What questions or concerns do you have about your baby's health and care?"
	21.2 Your baby may need to stay in an intensive care nursery so that any problems can be dealt with quickly.	
	21.3 Blood will be obtained through a small prick in your baby's heel to test for blood glucose levels.	Hypoglycemia is often a problem for babies who have mothers with diabetes.
	21.4 Your baby may have an intravenous (IV) line to provide fluids and glucose. The IV line will be placed in a	

CONTENT OUTLINE

CONCEPT	DETAIL	INSTRUCTOR'S NOTES

blood vessel in the baby's scalp, hand, foot, or umbilical cord.

21.5 Your baby may be placed in a crib with radiant heaters to keep him or her warm. Respiration and heart rate may be monitored by special machines.

21.6 The babies are kept without clothing under the warmer so that they can be observed more easily.

21.7 You can visit, hold, and feed your baby in the special care nursery. The doctors and nurses are available to care for your baby and answer any questions you may have.

Review standard practices in your setting.

21.8 Your baby will be transferred to the regular nursery as soon as less intensive care is needed. Some babies require intensive care for only a few hours, or not at all.

22. Postpartum care

22.1 While you are in the hospital, you will develop a plan for glucose monitoring patterns, activity levels, and insulin dosages for home.

Ask, "What questions or concerns do you have about your care after delivery?" The risk for hypoglycemia increases in the first few weeks postpartum.

22.2 The dietitian can help you adjust your diet for breastfeeding or weight loss.

22.3 Coping with a newborn and the demands of diabetes can be overwhelming. It can be hard to balance your health needs with those of your new baby. Some women become depressed. If you feel overwhelmed or depressed, talk with your health care team. There is help available.

Review the signs and symptoms of postpartum depression.

22.4 The doctors and nurses are available to answer any questions about post-delivery care, including sexual activity and contraception.

CONTENT OUTLINE

CONCEPT	DETAIL	INSTRUCTOR'S NOTES
	22.5 Many hospital or community groups offer child care classes.	Have a list of resources available.
	22.6 Before discharge, you will find out when you need to return for a visit. At that time, your weight, blood pressure, blood glucose levels, and any incision will be examined.	
23. Breast-feeding	23.1 Mothers with diabetes are able and encouraged to breast-feed their babies if they want to do so.	Ask, "What are some advantages of breast-feeding for you? What barriers do you anticipate?"
	23.2 About 300 calories per day should be added to the prepregnancy diet to cover the extra needs of milk production. A decrease in your nighttime insulin dose may be needed to prevent hypoglycemia.	Point out the need to work with a dietitian after delivery.
	23.3 Breast-feeding may be postponed for a short time until the mother and baby are more fully recovered. Breast pumps are available to use until the baby is able to nurse. You will be able to hold and feed your baby using a bottle of milk you have expressed.	Because of the initial low blood glucose level, some infants may not suck well at first. Also, if they are getting IV fluids and glucose, they may not be hungry.
	23.4 Support groups, such as the La Leche League, are available in many communities.	Have a list of resources available.
24. Summary	24.1 Diabetes increases the risks associated with pregnancy and requires more work on the part of the expectant parents.	
	24.2 Keeping blood glucose levels in the target range increases the chances for a healthy mother and baby.	Risk for birth defects is the same for women with well-controlled diabetes as for women without diabetes.
	24.3 There is a lot to do to care for diabetes when you are pregnant. It will help to anticipate barriers and plan strategies to address	Ask, "What barriers do you anticipate in managing diabetes more during your pregnancy? What strategies can you think of

CONTENT OUTLINE

CONCEPT	DETAIL	INSTRUCTOR'S NOTES
	these barriers. Using strategies that have worked for you in the past is often an effective approach.	to help overcome these barriers?" Write barriers and strategies on the board and discuss.
	24.4 Caring for diabetes is very demanding when you are pregnant. It takes knowledge, time, effort, and support. It may feel unfair to have diabetes during what should be a very happy time in your life and you may find yourself feeling angry, guilty, or depressed. Although these feelings are common, seeking the support of a good listener often helps. If these feelings become overwhelming or are interfering with your ability to care for yourself, talk with your health care team about getting the support you need.	Point out that this can be a stressful time. Encourage participants to talk with their partners and other supportive people about their fears and feelings. Ask, "What are your thoughts and feelings about this pregnancy and caring for your diabetes? What would help you to cope with these feelings?"

SKILLS CHECKLIST

None.

EVALUATION PLAN

Knowledge will be evaluated by achievement of learning objectives and by responses to questions during the session. The ability to apply knowledge will be evaluated through program outcome measures.

DOCUMENTATION PLAN

Record class attendance and achieved objectives as appropriate using the Diabetes Self-Management Record, the Participant Follow-up Record, or another form.

SUGGESTED READINGS

American Diabetes Association: Proceedings of the fifth international workshop-conference on gestational diabetes mellitus. *Diabetes Care* 30 (Suppl 2):S105–S261, 2007

Bradley C: Managing diabetes while breast-feeding. *Diabetes Self-Management* 23(6):84–89, 2006

Brian SR, Nickless N, Thung SF, Inzucchi SE: Gestational diabetes update. *Practical Diabetology* 26(1):10–18, 2007

Case J, Willoughby D, Haley-Zitlin V, Maybee P: Preventing type 2 diabetes after gestational diabetes. *The Diabetes Educator* 32:877–881, 2006

Chu, SY, Callaghan WM, Kim SY, et al.: Maternal obesity and risk of gestational diabetes mellitus. *Diabetes Care* 30:1070–1076, 2007

Clausen TD, Methiesen ER, Hansen T, et al.: High prevalence of type 2 diabetes and pre-diabetes in adult offspring of women with gestational diabetes mellitus or type 1 diabetes. *Diabetes Care* 21:340–346, 2008

Evert AB, Vande Hei K: Gestational diabetes education and diabetes prevention strategies. *Diabetes Spectrum* 19:135–139, 2006

Gonzalez-Quintero VH, Istwan NB, Rhea DJ, et al.: The impact of glycemic control on neonatal outcome in singleton pregnancies complicated by diabetes. *Diabetes Care* 30:467–470, 2007

Guerin A, Nisebaum R, Ray JG: Use of maternal GHB concentration to estimate the risk of congenital anomalies in the offspring of women with prepregnancy diabetes. *Diabetes Care* 30:1920–1925, 2007

Jovanovic L: Diabetes and pregnancy. *Diabetes Spectrum* 20:82–107, 2007

Kim C, Berger DK, Chmany S: Recurrence of gestational diabetes mellitus: a systematic review. *Diabetes Care* 30:1314–1319, 2007

Kim C, Herman WH, Vijan S: Efficacy and cost of postpartum screening strategies for diabetes among women with histories of gestational diabetes mellitus. *Diabetes Care* 30:1102–1106, 2007

Kim C, McEwen LN, Kerr EA, Piette JD, Chames MC, Ferrara A, Herman WH: Preventive counseling among women with histories of gestational diabetes mellitus. *Diabetes Care* 30:2489–2493, 2007

Kitzmiller JL: *Managing Preexisting Diabetes and Pregnancy.* Alexandria, VA: American Diabetes Association, 2008

Kitzmiller JL, Block JM, Brown FM, Catalano PM, et al.: Consensus statement: managing preexisting diabetes for pregnancy. *Diabetes Care* 31:1060–1080, 2008

Lee AJ, Hiscock RJ, Wein P, Walker SP, Permezel M: Gestational diabetes mellitus: clinical predictors and long-term risk of developing type 2 diabetes. *Diabetes Care* 30:878–883, 2007

Luerssen M, Bernasko J, Winsch A: Lows and your pregnancy. *Diabetes Forecast* 58(4):61–64, 2005

Michel B, Charron-Prochownik D: Diabetes nurse educators and preconception counseling. *The Diabetes Educator* 32108–32116, 2006

Nicholson W, Bolen S, Witkop CT: Neale D, et al.: Benefits and risks of oral diabetes agents compared with insulin in women with gestational diabetes: a systematic review. Obstetrics and *Gynecology* 113:193–205

Perkins JM, Dunn JP, Jagasia S: Perspectives in gestational diabetes mellitus: a review of screening, diagnosis and treatment. *Clinical Diabetes* 25:57–62, 2007

Setji TL, Brown AJ, Feinglos MN: Gestational diabetes mellitus. *Clinical Diabetes* 3:17–23, 2005

Temple RC, Aldridge VJ, Murphy HR: Prepregnancy care and pregnancy outcomes in women with type 1 diabetes. *Diabetes Care* 29:1744–1749, 2006

Insulin Action Times

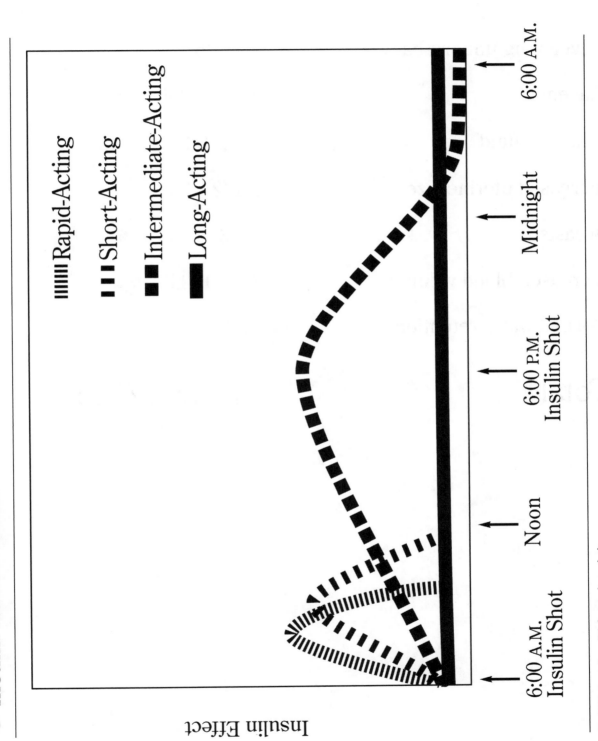

Insulin Effect

Rapid-Acting
Short-Acting
Intermediate-Acting
Long-Acting

6:00 A.M.
Insulin Shot

Noon

6:00 P.M.
Insulin Shot

Midnight

6:00 A.M.

➲ Where Weight Goes During Pregnancy

Developing unborn baby	=	7 – 8 lb
Placenta	=	1 1/2 – 2 lb
Amniotic fluid	=	2 – 2 1/2 lb
Increased uterine size	=	2 1/2 – 3 lb
Breasts	=	2 – 3 lb
Increased blood volume	=	3 – 3 1/2 lb
Normal water retention	=	3 – 3 1/2 lb

Total   = 21 – 25 1/2 lb

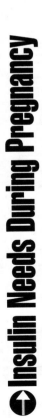

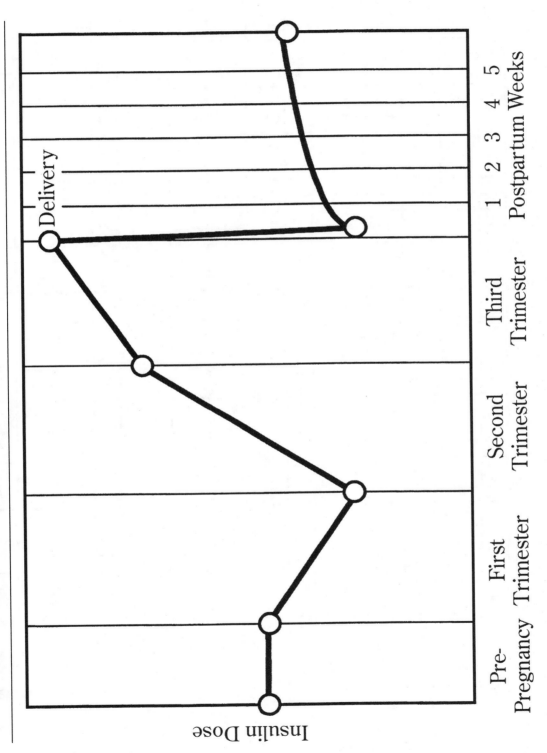

Insulin Needs During Pregnancy

Insulin Dose

Pre-Pregnancy | First Trimester | Second Trimester | Third Trimester | Delivery | 1 2 3 4 5 Postpartum Weeks

Menstrual Chart

Put an X in each box for each day of your period. This will help you determine when your next period will occur. By knowing this, you can count 12–16 days ahead to determine your time of ovulation.

Month:

Days of cycle	1	2	3	4	5	6	7	8	9	10	11	12	13	14	15	16	17	18	19	20	21	22	23	24	25	26	27	28	29	30	31	32	33	34	35	36	37	38	39	40
Date																																								
Period																																								
Temperature																																								

Month:

Days of cycle	1	2	3	4	5	6	7	8	9	10	11	12	13	14	15	16	17	18	19	20	21	22	23	24	25	26	27	28	29	30	31	32	33	34	35	36	37	38	39	40
Date																																								
Period																																								
Temperature																																								

Month:

Days of cycle	1	2	3	4	5	6	7	8	9	10	11	12	13	14	15	16	17	18	19	20	21	22	23	24	25	26	27	28	29	30	31	32	33	34	35	36	37	38	39	40
Date																																								
Period																																								
Temperature																																								

◗ Treatment of Low Blood Glucose During Pregnancy

Low blood glucose (hypoglycemia) can happen to anyone with diabetes who uses insulin—even if diabetes has only occurred during pregnancy. Hypoglycemia is also called an insulin reaction or low blood glucose. A low blood glucose reaction is easily treated. If it is not treated, a reaction usually will become more serious, and you may pass out.

The symptoms and signs of a reaction are caused by the body's response to a low level of glucose in the blood. This is most likely to happen:

- at the time insulin has its peak effect
- during exercise, or up to 24 hours after hard exercise
- if too much insulin has been taken
- if a meal or snack is late or has been missed
- if you are more active than usual
- between 2:00 and 4:00 a.m., when your body is most sensitive to insulin

How Can You Tell If You Are Having A Low Blood Glucose Reaction?

You can learn to notice the early signs and symptoms of a low blood glucose reaction. Some signs are:

- sudden mood changes
- nervousness
- anxiousness
- heart beating rapidly or forcefully
- excess hunger
- sweating
- irritability
- nausea (symptoms of morning sickness will worsen)

If a reaction is more severe, you may notice other symptoms:

- blurred vision
- nightmares
- tingling or numbness around your mouth or your tongue
- headaches
- impaired thinking
- slurred speech

Not everyone has the same symptoms. Sometimes you may have no symptoms at all. When your blood glucose is low, you may feel signs other than those listed here.

continued

TREATMENT OF LOW BLOOD GLUCOSE DURING PREGNANCY *continued*

Whatever your symptoms are, you will usually have the same ones each time you have a reaction. Remember that you may not notice these signs yourself. Instead, others may notice sudden mood changes or confusion.

How Do You Treat A Mild Low Blood Glucose Reaction?

The treatment for a low blood glucose reaction during pregnancy is slightly different than for a person with diabetes who is not pregnant. Glucose tablets or skim or low-fat milk is used instead of juice or another sugar. If you think that you are having a reaction:

1. Check your blood glucose level. If you are not able to do this, yet you feel you are having a reaction, begin with step 2.
2. Treat the reaction if your blood glucose level is less than 60 mg/dl. Take 3–4 glucose tablets or drink 8 oz of fat-free (skim) or low-fat (1%) milk.
3. Wait 15 minutes, then check your blood glucose level again. If it is still less than 60 mg/dl, treat the reaction again.
4. Wait 15 minutes, then check your blood glucose level again.
5. If your blood glucose level is still less than 60 mg/dl, drink 8 oz of fat-free (skim) or low-fat (1%) milk, and eat 15 g carbohydrate (1 serving).
6. After your blood glucose level is above 60 mg/dl, check it again in 1 hour to be sure it has stayed above 60 mg/dl.
7. You may need to eat 30 g (2 servings) carbohydrate AFTER your blood glucose level has risen above 60 mg/dl, especially at night or after exercise.
8. Write down the steps you took to treat the reaction. Think about and write down what may have caused it to happen. This will help you learn how to avoid low blood glucose reactions in the future.

You may show no signs of low blood glucose until it is so bad that you pass out. If this happens, you will need to rely on a relative or friend to treat you with the drug glucagon. Ask your health care provider for information about glucagon.

If no glucagon is available and you are not conscious, **your family should call an ambulance or paramedic immediately!**

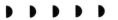

| #22 | Insulin Pump Therapy |

STATEMENT OF PURPOSE

This session is intended to provide information about what continuous subcutaneous insulin infusion therapy is, what can be expected from it, and how to operate and care for a pump.

PREREQUISITES

It is recommended that participants have an understanding of diabetes, insulin therapy, intensive insulin therapy, carbohydrate counting, and self-care and have a desire to explore insulin pump therapy as a treatment option.

OBJECTIVES

At the end of this session, participants will be able to:

1. define insulin pump therapy (continuous subcutaneous insulin infusion);

2. state the purpose of pump therapy;

3. state three personal advantages and barriers for pump therapy versus conventional and intensive therapy and strategies to overcome barriers;

4. define basal rate and bolus and correction dose;

5. state that the infusion site and tubing should be changed every 48–72 hours;

6. define both high and low blood glucose and the corrective action to take for each;

7. state two ways in which activities of daily living can be modified to accommodate wearing a pump;

8. identify personal feelings about using pump therapy;

9. demonstrate how to prepare the syringe or cartridge and tubing for use in the pump;

10. demonstrate how to adjust the basal rate and bolus dose;

11. demonstrate how to insert the needle into the subcutaneous tissue;

12. demonstrate how to disconnect and reconnect the syringe or cartridge and tubing;

13. state three symptoms of infection at the infusion site and corrective actions to take;

14. state three steps to take if the pump is not working correctly;

15. verbalize confidence in own ability to perform each of the skills learned and successfully live with pump therapy.

CONTENT

Using medications safely and for maximum therapeutic effectiveness.

MATERIALS NEEDED

VISUALS PROVIDED	ADDITIONAL
1. Normal Blood Glucose and Insulin Levels	■ Instruction booklet prepared by pump manufacturer
2. Insulin Action Times	■ Insulin pump (type patient will use)
Handouts (one per participant)	■ Reservoir, cartridge, or syringe (appropriate for pump)
1. Insulin Program for Infusion Pump	■ Tubing with different types of needles
2. Blood Glucose Profile	■ Battery or batteries (appropriate for pump)
3. Treatment of Low Blood Glucose	■ Occlusive dressing (if needed)
4. How to Use Glucagon	■ Alcohol wipes
	■ Insulin (appropriate for pump)
	■ Glucagon kit
	■ Samples of glucose products
	■ DVD or videotape produced by pump manufacturer
	■ Continuous glucose monitor

METHOD OF PRESENTATION

Start by introducing yourself and telling what you do. Ask participants to introduce themselves. Explain the purpose for this session.

Present the material in a question/discussion format, using the first question as a starting point. Provide appropriate content outlined below in response. Ask if there are additional questions, and respond, repeating the process for the entire session. Use the questions in the Instructor's Notes section to generate discussion if no questions are forthcoming after a period of silence. Keeping track of the content discussed in each session, using the Diabetes Self-Management Record, the Participant Follow-up Record, or another form, helps you to evaluate if all needed content has been discussed.

One of the most important determinants of successful pump therapy is the ability of the individual to adapt to its use. It is therefore important to provide time for the participants to discuss their concerns and feelings. The instructor can facilitate this by asking questions, listening reflectively, and assisting participants with problem solving. It is also helpful if someone who is using a pump can attend and discuss some personal experiences with the participants. One way to begin is to ask participants to identify why they chose pump therapy, their fears and concerns, and the benefits they believe they will receive.

This outline can be used for individual teaching or in a classroom setting. It contains information needed before selecting pump therapy (Concepts 1–5), the necessary information to live with a pump (Concepts 6–13), and the skills to successfully operate a pump (Concepts 14–22). Present only the concepts appropriate for the audience. Because operating a pump is somewhat complex, this material will need to be reviewed with the individual more than once. Provide copies of the manufacturer's DVDs for home use; this gives participants additional information and opportunities to practice. It is important that the participants have an adequate opportunity to practice each skill and receive feedback from the instructor within a short time after is is presented.

CONTENT OUTLINE

CONCEPT	DETAIL	INSTRUCTOR'S NOTES
CHOOSING PUMP THERAPY		
1. Review definition and action of insulin	1.1 Insulin is a hormone, a protein substance, produced in the pancreas.	Ask, "What questions or concerns do you have about pump therapy?"
	1.2 Insulin is secreted continuously in people who do not have diabetes.	Use Visual #1, Normal Blood Glucose and Insulin Levels.
	1.3 In diabetes, there is not enough insulin action.	
2. Purpose of intensive insulin therapy	2.1 Intensive therapy usually consists of combining types of insulin, taking multiple injections, and using carb:insulin ratios.	Ask, "What have your experiences been with intensive insulin therapy?" This information is provided in Outline #9, *All About Insulin* (p. 165).
	2.2 The goal is to maintain near-normal glucose levels.	
	2.3 Insulin pumps also provide intensive therapy without multiple shots and types of insulins.	
3. Definition of pump therapy	3.1 Pump therapy uses a battery-operated device called an insulin infusion pump.	Show participants an actual pump and tubing.
	3.2 The pump gives very small, repeated pulses of short-acting insulin under the skin (basal rate).	Pumps are manufactured by several companies: ■ Animas Corporation 877-937-7867 www.animascorp.com ■ Disetronic Medical Systems 800-591-3455 www.disetronic-usa.com

CONTENT OUTLINE

CONCEPT	DETAIL	INSTRUCTOR'S NOTES

■ Inulet OmniPod Systems
800-280-7801
www.myomnipod.com

■ Medtronic MiniMed, Inc.
800-646-4633
www.minimed.com

■ Nipro
888-651-7867
www.niprodiabetes.com

	DETAIL	INSTRUCTOR'S NOTES
	3.3 This occurs so often that the pump provides an almost continuous flow of insulin.	
	3.4 Larger amounts of insulin are given before meals (bolus dose) by programming the pump.	
	3.5 The pump is worn outside the body, usually attached to a belt or another article of clothing or attached to the skin.	
	3.6 Rapid- and short-acting insulins are approved for pumps.	
	3.7 You need to insert a needle only every 48–72 hours.	
4. Goal of pump therapy	4.1 The goal of pump therapy is to better manage blood glucose levels.	Ask, "What do you think are advantages of pump therapy for you? Why did you choose pump therapy?" Clarify any misconceptions.
	4.2 Most individuals have improved or more even blood glucose levels. They feel better and feel their quality of life improves.	According to long-term follow-up of the DCCT trial participants, more even blood glucose levels reduces the risk for complications.
	4.3 Because of improved blood glucose levels, the risk for the long-term complications of diabetes is decreased.	
	4.4 Pump therapy affords greater flexibility for timing and content of meals and daily scheduling.	Use of carbohydrate counting further increases flexibility. Ask, "Do you currently count

CONTENT OUTLINE

CONCEPT	DETAIL	INSTRUCTOR'S NOTES
		carbs? What has your experience been with carb counting?"
	4.5 Pump therapy can make managing sick days or other acute complications easier.	
	4.6 Fractional doses are easier and more accurate to administer.	
	4.7 Pump therapy can help to manage the "dawn phenomenon."	The dawn phenomenon is fasting hyperglycemia.
	4.8 A "correction dose" makes it easier to respond to blood glucose levels that are out of your target range.	
5. Things to consider when choosing pump therapy	5.1 If delivery of insulin is interrupted, ketoacidosis develops very quickly (within 4–5 hours).	Ask, "What are the disadvantages of pump therapy for you?" Draw out participants' feelings about these problems and ideas for handling.
	5.2 There is a potential increase in hypoglycemia as glucose levels improve. On the other hand, severe recurrent hypoglycemia and post-exercise hypoglycemia may occur less often.	Checking blood glucose levels before giving a bolus dose will help prevent this.
	5.3 The cost of therapy, monitoring, and frequent medical care may be greater.	Participants need to determine insurance coverage before choosing this therapy.
	5.4 Pump therapy gives the person with diabetes greater responsibility for his or her daily care.	Ask, "How do you feel about making so many decisions each day about your diabetes care?"
	5.5 The pump may be visible to others and can be a constant reminder of diabetes.	Ask, "Are you comfortable explaining diabetes to others?"
	5.6 It takes more time to care for a pump.	
	5.7 There is a potential for infusion site discomfort and infections.	
	5.8 You need to be willing to monitor and record blood glucose levels four to eight times a day and check for ketones when needed.	Ask, "How often do you monitor now? What barriers do you encounter to monitoring? How do you deal with these barriers?"

CONTENT OUTLINE

CONCEPT	DETAIL	INSTRUCTOR'S NOTES

5.9 Pump therapy is not for everyone, and it will not cure diabetes.

Ask, "Do you have concerns about pump therapy? Do you think that a pump is a good choice for you? Why? Why not?" Participants should not feel bad or like failures if they discontinue or choose not to start pump therapy.

MECHANICS OF PUMP THERAPY

6. Basal rate

6.1 Basal rate is the amount of insulin that is infused throughout the day and night.

Use Visual #1, Normal Blood Glucose and Insulin Levels, to illustrate the need for continuous infusion.

6.2 It is designed to meet your insulin needs between meals (fasting state) and at night.

A variety of methods are used to determine individual basal rates.

6.3 If basal insulin needs vary over 24 hours, different basal rates can be programmed into the pump.

Pumps offer multiple basal rates and temporary basal rates for special situations.

6.4 Blood glucose levels during fasting periods (e.g., midnight to 6:00 a.m.) are used to determine the basal rate. The basal rate replaces your intermediate- or long-acting insulin doses.

Distribute Handout #1, Insulin Program for Infusion Pump.

7. Bolus dose

7.1 A bolus dose of insulin is delivered by the pump. It is given to keep postmeal blood glucose on target.

Use Visual #1, Normal Blood Glucose and Insulin Levels, to illustrate the need for insulin at mealtimes.

7.2 This is similar to getting an injection of rapid- or short-acting insulin.

Bolus doses can also be used to correct a high blood glucose level. Use Visual #2, Insulin Action Times, to illustrate.

7.3 It is given before each meal and usually before each snack. When your mealtime changes, the time of the bolus dose changes, too. You can vary your mealtime without becoming hypoglycemic.

Bolus doses are generally based on insulin:carbohydrate ratios. A starting ratio is often 1 unit of insulin per 10 grams of carb (1:10). The ratio is adjusted based on response through post-meal monitoring.

7.4 Your dose is determined on the basis of your glucose level at the time the

Some pumps can be programmed to provide an extended or

CONTENT OUTLINE

CONCEPT	DETAIL	INSTRUCTOR'S NOTES
	bolus is to be given and on carbohydrate intake. The correction dose is added to or subtracted from the bolus dose. Some insulin pumps can be programmed to calculate bolus and corrections doses.	"square wave" bolus over a longer time period. One formula for calculating the correction dose is to divide 1,800 by the total daily insulin dose (both basal and bolus). The result is the expected change in glucose per unit of insulin. This is the insulin sensitivity factor.
	7.5 A correction dose can be given when blood glucose levels are too high, using your insulin sensitivity factor. Checking glucose levels two hours after bolus or correction doses, helps you know if the doses were effective for you.	Provide participants with the opportunity to practice by showing different examples and asking that they calculate their dose. Refer to Outline #19, *Carbohydrate Counting* (p. 399) for more information about calculating ratios.
8. Equipment needed to operate pump	8.1 Review the equipment needed: ■ pump ■ battery ■ pump reservoir, cartridge, or syringe to hold insulin ■ tubing ■ rapid or short-acting insulin ■ occlusive dressing (if not included with tubing) ■ controller dense, if needed.	Pass around each item. Demonstrate the type of pump the patient will be using. Use a battery suitable for that pump. This device is different from syringes used for insulin injections. "Op-site" is a common brand name.
9. Wearing a pump	9.1 The pump can be hooked on a belt, carried in a pocket, attached to other clothing, or attached to the skin.	Ask, "What questions or concerns do you have about wearing a pump?" Demonstrate how a pump can be worn comfortably. If the pump is worn hooked onto a belt, be careful that it stays connected when you adjust clothing or go to the bathroom.

CONTENT OUTLINE

CONCEPT	DETAIL	INSTRUCTOR'S NOTES
	9.2 Modifications in clothing may need to be made to accommodate the pump.	Demonstrate modifications. Have a person who wears a pump share successful ideas.
	9.3 Other people may be curious about the pump and ask questions.	Discuss possible statements or questions and have individuals tell how they might respond. Ask, "How comfortable do you feel responding to questions about your diabetes? About a pump? What kind of support do you want/need from your family and friends to use the pump?"
	9.4 Some pumps can be worn in the water. If your pump is not waterproof, remove it for bathing or swimming. The tubing can be worn or removed.	Demonstrate the procedure for bathing or swimming with and without the tubing in place.
	9.5 Generally, a pump can be worn during exercise. During strenuous exercise, a pump is more likely to be damaged.	If the pump is removed for exercise, a bolus dose is generally not necessary before removing it.
	9.6 A pump can be worn during sexual activity or removed, according to personal preference.	
	9.7 During sleep, the pump can be placed beside you, under a pillow, or attached to your pajamas. Be sure there is enough tubing to allow for movement without disconnecting the pump.	Electric blankets may be too warm and overheat the insulin in the tubing, decreasing its potency.
	9.8 When you are traveling, carry enough syringes, tubing, and insulin for the trip, plus extras.	It should not be necessary to change doses when changing time zones.
	9.9 When you are ill and unable to eat, continue the basal rate and do not give bolus doses, unless blood glucose rises.	Stress the need to establish a plan before illness occurs. Ask, "What barriers do you anticipate with using a pump? What strategies can you identify to overcome those barriers?"
10. Review of monitoring	10.1 Blood glucose monitoring gives you the information you need to make decisions.	Ask, "How do you use the information you get from monitoring now?"

CONTENT OUTLINE

CONCEPT	DETAIL	INSTRUCTOR'S NOTES
	10.2 Check your blood glucose before meals and at bedtime, at a minimum. Checking after meals and at 3 a.m. on occasion gives you an overall picture of your control.	Monitoring provides information for daily decision-making. Blood glucose levels are often used to determine bolus and correction doses.
	10.3 Other times to check include whenever you are feeling as if your blood glucose is low or high, or if you feel nauseated.	Ask, "Do you currently have difficulty checking your blood glucose levels? Do you anticipate barriers while using a pump?"
	10.4 Keeping records of blood glucose levels helps you to: ■ learn the effect of factors such as food, activity, and stress on your blood glucose level ■ make effective decisions ■ serve as the basis to model and remodel the treatment program ■ provide information to your health care team.	Some patients use monthly blood glucose profiles. These involve checking blood glucose levels before and 2 hours after eating, at bedtime, midnight, 3 a.m., and 6 a.m. See Handout #2, Blood Glucose Profile, as an example.
	10.5 It is important to check ketones routinely and whenever blood glucose is greater than 300 mg/dl.	Trace ketones on arising may indicate nocturnal hypoglycemia.
	10.6 Many people who use insulin pumps also use continuous glucose monitors (CGM).	Ask, "Have you used CGM? What questions or concerns do you have about CGM?"
11. Hypoglycemia and hyper-glycemia	11.1 Review the signs and symptoms of hypoglycemia.	Ask, "What symptoms do you usually have?"
	11.2 Hypoglycemia should be treated according to a standard plan. You need to carry something with you to treat it at all times. Talk to your health care team about removing the pump if hypoglycemia is severe.	Ask, "How do you prevent and manage low blood glucose levels now?" Show examples of glucose products. Distribute Handout #3, Treatment of Low Blood Glucose. Stress the need for diabetes identification.
	11.3 A family member or friend needs to know how to give glucagon.	Distribute Handout #4, How to Use Glucagon. Demonstrate use.
	11.4 Review the signs and symptoms of hyperglycemia.	Ask, "What are the symptoms of high blood glucose?"

CONTENT OUTLINE

CONCEPT	DETAIL	INSTRUCTOR'S NOTES
	11.5 If you are hyperglycemic for two readings for no apparent reason, change the tubing and site.	Insulin may aggregate and clog the needle or catheter. For people with type 1 diabetes, blood glucose levels typically rise about 45 mg/dl for every hour without insulin.
	11.6 Hyperglycemia should be treated according to a standard plan. Urine should also be checked for ketones.	
	11.7 If moderate to large ketones are present, assume a lack of insulin. If blood glucose is normal or low and ketones are still present, carbohydrates with appropriate insulin coverage is indicated.	Corrective actions include taking an insulin injection, determining if the pump is malfunctioning, and changing the infusion set and site. Provide guidelines for contacting the health care team.
12. Living with a pump	12.1 Care of the pump is time-consuming and may mean changes in daily routine.	Invite someone who wears a pump to talk to the group. Ask, "What do you need to do to plan time to care for the pump and do the necessary monitoring?"
	12.2 The pump will be a constant reminder of diabetes and may prompt questions from others.	Ask, "What are your thoughts and feelings about diabetes and using pump therapy?"
	12.3 People who use pumps are very much in charge of their diabetes and their lives. The pump does not control them.	Review the advantages of pump therapy that the participants identified.
	12.4 Meal planning, exercising, and blood and urine monitoring are part of an effective pump therapy plan.	
PUMP OPERATION **13. Preparing the pump for use**	13.1 Insert the battery into the correct position.	Demonstrate, then observe patient inserting battery and confirming its status.

CONTENT OUTLINE

CONCEPT	DETAIL	INSTRUCTOR'S NOTES
	13.2 Prepare the syringe or insulin cartridge with the correct insulin using the aseptic technique.	Use the same technique as drawing up for injection. You need enough insulin to fill the syringe or cartridge, flush the tubing, and last at least 24 hours.
	13.3 Prime the tubing with a minimal amount of wasted insulin, and free all air bubbles.	Demonstrate, then observe the patient preparing the syringe or cartridge and tubing correctly. Review the rationale for removal all of the air bubbles.
	13.4 Insert the syringe or cartridge into the correct position in the pump. It is **essential** that these be inserted correctly to ensure infusion.	Demonstrate, then observe the patient inserting the syringe or cartridge correctly.
14. Operating the pump	14.1 Set the prescribed basal rate by following the pump programming instructions.	Demonstrate, then observe the patient adjusting the basal rate. Demonstrate the procedure for confirming the basal rate.
	14.2 Review the rationale and timing of a bolus dose.	Say, "Tell me in your own words when and why you need bolus doses of insulin."
	14.3 Deliver a bolus dose according to the pump instructions.	Demonstrate, then observe the patient delivering a bolus dose correctly.
	14.4 Check to determine if the bolus dose was given correctly.	Demonstrate the procedure for confirming the bolus dose.
15. Preparation of the site	15.1 Locate the appropriate site for needle insertion.	Assess the site for lipodystrophy or scars.
	15.2 Appropriate sites can include the abdomen, arms, thighs, and lateral buttocks.	Choice of site depends on personal preference and wearing style.
	15.3 Wash your hands.	Give the rationale for clean technique.
	15.4 Prepare the skin.	Demonstrate, then observe the patient preparing the skin correctly.
	15.5 Pinch 3 inches of skin between your fingers and insert the needle	Demonstrate, then observe the patient inserting the needle of

CONTENT OUTLINE

CONCEPT	DETAIL	INSTRUCTOR'S NOTES
	or use the insertion device.	applying the pump. Remove the needle if using a catheter-type infusion set.
	15.6 Place occlusive dressing over the needle or catheter, if needed.	Demonstrate the proper technique for placement of the dressing. Occlusive dressings decrease risk of infection.
16. Disconnecting procedure	16.1 The pump may be safely disconnected for up to 1 hour, depending on blood glucose levels.	A bolus may be needed before disconnecting if pump is to be off for more than 1 hour.
	16.2 Most people use tubing that can be easily disconnected. If not, disconnect tubing.	Demonstrate, then observe individual disconnecting the pump from the tubing correctly.
	16.3 Place a clean cap on the tubing and a sterile needle with the cover on the end of the reservoir, cartridge, or syringe.	You may use the cap from the infusion set and the needle and cover you saved when you opened your supplies.
	16.4 Leave the reservoir, cartridge, or syringe in the pump while disconnected.	If the syringe is taped to the skin, you may inadvertently administer a bolus dose.
17. Reconnecting procedure	17.1 Before reconnecting, uncap the tubing and fill the top of the tubing with insulin.	This will decrease the risk of air bubbles and a gap in insulin infusion.
	17.2 Keep the tubing below the level of the needle site so that insulin will not infuse inadvertently because of gravity.	Tubing is available with a connect/disconnect mechanism, but it tends to be more expensive.
	17.3 Reconnect the tubing.	
18. Syringes and tubing	18.1 Reservoirs, cartridges, or syringes and infusion tubing need to be ordered from the pump company or from a diabetes supply company.	Provide the telephone number of the pump company's customer service department to place orders for new supplies.
	18.2 There are a variety of tubing and needle sets available. Needle options include non-needle, straight, and bent. Tubing is available in different lengths.	Show infusion set options. Point out that they may need to try different types to see which they prefer.

CONTENT OUTLINE

CONCEPT	DETAIL	INSTRUCTOR'S NOTES
	18.3 Keep at least a 1-week supply of reservoirs, cartridges, or syringes and tubing on hand.	In case of an emergency or shipping delay, the patient will still be able to use the pump.
19. Care of the infusion site	19.1 The tubing should be changed every 48–72 hours, unless the manufacturer indicates otherwise.	The risk of needle plugging and infection is greater when the infusion site and tubing are changed less often.
	19.2 Sites should also be rotated when the tubing is changed.	
	19.3 Look for signs and symptoms of irritation, inflammation, and infection.	Assess for signs and symptoms daily.
	19.4 Measures to prevent irritation, inflammation, and infection include: ■ cleanliness and aseptic technique ■ proper placement of the needle.	Irritation is often caused when the needle tip is placed too close to the surface or at the wrong angle. Catheter-type tubing may be less irritating.
	19.5 Corrective measures for signs and symptoms of infection are: ■ change the site and tubing ■ wash the area with soap ■ apply sterile dressing ■ if infection is still present in 24–48 hours, call your health care team.	Prompt care can prevent serious problems.
20. Battery care	20.1 Change the battery according to the procedure for the specific type of pump.	Review the manufacturer's guidelines. Demonstrate the procedure for inserting a fresh battery and observe the patient doing this.
	20.2 Batteries need to be changed at appropriate intervals.	Advise patients to have extra batteries available.
	20.3 Store batteries in a cool place.	
21. Pump maintenance and repair	21.1 You need to know the purpose and sound of each alarm.	Refer to the manufacturer's guidelines. Demonstrate each alarm system.
	21.2 Understand what corrective action to take for each alarm.	Demonstrate correct action and observe patient doing this.

CONTENT OUTLINE

CONCEPT	DETAIL	INSTRUCTOR'S NOTES
	21.3 Monitor your pump often for signs of malfunction.	
	21.4 If your pump malfunctions, check your blood glucose level, then call your provider and the pump manufacturer immediately. Ask your treatment team for an injection therapy plan in case of pump failure.	Remind participants of the appropriate toll-free numbers. Remind participants to keep insulin on hand so that they are prepared.
	21.5 If your pump becomes very wet, assume it has malfunctioned (unless your pump is waterproof).	Check your blood glucose level, then call your physician and the pump manufacturer.
	21.6 A loaner pump may be available from the manufacturer if repairs are needed.	Participants should not try to make repairs.

SKILLS CHECKLIST

Each participant beginning pump therapy will be able to:

1. Gather all equipment needed.

2. Insert the battery into correct position and confirm its status.

3. Fill a syringe or cartridge using aseptic technique.

4. Prime the tubing without introducing air bubbles.

5. Place the syringe or cartridge into the pump, making sure that it is in the correct position and attached securely to the tubing.

6. Set the prescribed basal program and confirm.

7. Deliver the prescribed bolus dose and confirm.

8. Locate appropriate sites for needle insertion.

9. Prepare the skin.

10. Insert the needle and place occlusive dressing over the needle, if needed.

11. Disconnect the tubing from the syringe while maintaining a closed system, if needed.

12. Reconnect the tubing and syringe with no air in the line.

13. Attach the pump to an appropriate article of clothing (e.g., a belt).

EVALUATION PLAN

Knowledge will be evaluated by achievement of learning objectives and by responses to questions during the session. Skills will be evaluated by observing return demonstration of techniques. The ability to apply knowledge will be evaluated by the choice to use or not use pump therapy, by the appropriate implementation of this therapy, and through program outcome measures.

DOCUMENTATION PLAN

Record class attendance and achieved objectives as appropriate using the Diabetes Self-Management Record, the Participant Follow-up Record, or another form.

SUGGESTED READINGS

American Diabetes Association: Resource Guide. Insulin delivery. *Diabetes Forecast* 62(1):49–52, 2009

Bolderman KM: *Putting Your Patients on the Pump*. Alexandria, VA: American Diabetes Association, 2003

Herman WH, Ilag LL, Johnson SL, Martin CL, et al.: A clinical trial of continuous subcutaneous insulin infusion versus multiple daily injections in older adults with type 2 diabetes. *Diabetes Care* 38:1568–1573, 2005

Kilpatrick ES, Rigby AS, Atkin SL: A1C variability and risk of microvascular complications in type 1 diabetes. *Diabetes Care* 31:2198–2202, 2008

Ponder SW, Skyler JS, Kruger DF, Metheson D, Brown BW: Unexplained hyperglycemia in continuous subcutaneous insulin infusion. *The Diabetes Educator* 34:327–333, 2008

Ritholz MD, Smaldone A, Lee H et al.: Perceptions of psychosocial factors and the insulin pump. *Diabetes Care* 30:549–554, 2007

Skyler JS, Ponder S, Kruger DF, Matheson D, Parkin CG: Is there a place for pump therapy in your practice? *Clinical Diabetes* 25:50–56, 2007

◑ Normal Blood Glucose and Insulin Levels

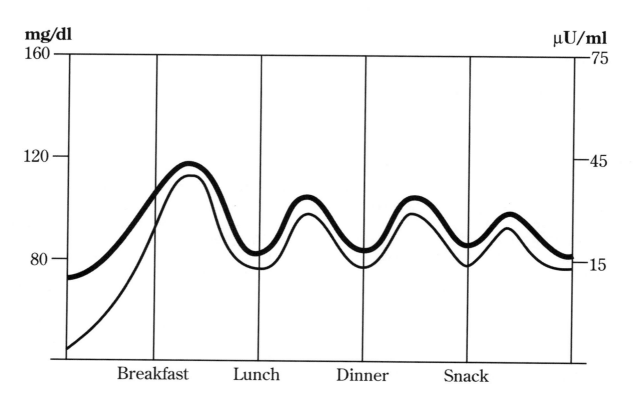

mg/dl

µU/ml

Breakfast   Lunch   Dinner   Snack

▬▬▬ Blood Glucose Level

▬▬ Plasma Insulin Level

⬆ Insulin Action Times

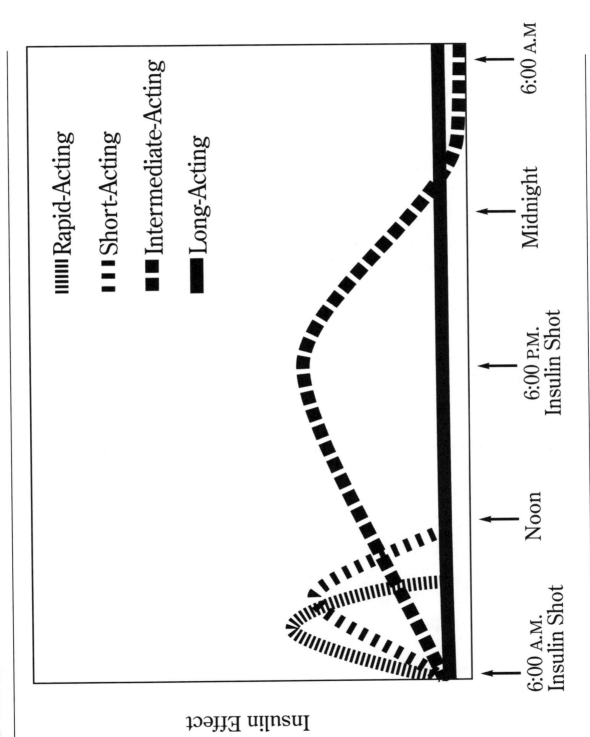

Insulin Effect

Rapid-Acting
Short-Acting
Intermediate-Acting
Long-Acting

6:00 A.M.
Insulin Shot

Noon

6:00 P.M.
Insulin Shot

Midnight

6:00 A.M

⊖ Insulin Program for Infusion Pump

Name _____ Date _____

BASAL INFUSION OF REGULAR INSULIN
Please set your pump to give the following basal doses of insulin.

Infusion Periods (clock time)				
Infusion Rates (units per hour)				
Amount Infused (units per period)				

Total Amount Infused as Basal Dose _____ units per day

continued

INSULIN PROGRAM FOR INFUSION PUMP *continued*

BOLUS INJECTIONS

Please use the scale below to give the premeal bolus dose of insulin, according to your blood glucose level at that time.

Blood Glucose Ranges (mg/dl)	Breakfast	Lunch	Dinner	Bedtime Snack

For each additional 15 grams of carbohydrate, add _____ unit(s) to the designated dose.

For each 15 grams of carbohydrate not eaten, subtract _____ unit(s) from the designated dose.

For exercise, subtract _____ unit(s) from the pre-exercise dose.

For stress, add _____ unit(s) to the designated dose.

➲ Blood Glucose Profile

A blood glucose profile is a "snapshot" of your blood glucose fluctuations throughout the day and can tell you how well your basal and bolus doses are working.

To do a blood glucose profile, check your blood glucose at the following times of the day:

> Before breakfast
> 2 hours after breakfast
> Before lunch
> 2 hours after lunch
> Before dinner
> 2 hours after dinner
> Bedtime
> Midnight
> 3:00 a.m.
> 6:00 a.m.

Do the profile when you are first starting on the pump and before each clinic visit.

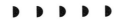 Treatment of Low Blood Glucose

If your blood glucose test is:	The amount of food or drink to take is:
Between 50 and 69 mg/dl	15 g carbohydrate (1 carbohydrate serving **or** 1 cup fat-free [skim] milk)
Less than 50 mg/dl	30 g carbohydrate (2 carbohydrate servings)

You should feel better in 10–15 minutes after you treat yourself. If your blood glucose is still less than 70 mg/dl or you don't feel better 10–15 minutes after the treatment, take 1 more carbohydrate serving. Check your blood glucose an hour after the reaction to make sure that your blood glucose has gone above 70 mg/dl and stayed there.

▶ ▶ ▶ ▶ ▶

EXAMPLES OF TREATMENTS FOR LOW BLOOD GLUCOSE
(All equal about 15 g carbohydrate or 1 fruit serving)

If your blood glucose is between 50 and 69 mg/dl, take the amount listed. If your blood glucose is less than 50 mg/dl, take twice the amount listed.

Foods	Amount
Orange or apple juice	1/2 cup
Grape or cranberry juice	1/3 cup
Non-diet soft drink	1/2 cup
Honey or corn syrup	1 Tbsp
Sugar packets	3
Life Savers	3–8 pieces
Glucose tablets	3–4 tablets

An additional carbohydrate snack may be needed at night or after exercise to keep your blood glucose above 70 mg/dl.

⮑ How to Use Glucagon

Glucagon is an emergency drug that is given as a shot to raise the blood glucose level. It should be given when the person is unable to swallow or is at risk for choking, or in case of a severe insulin reaction or coma.

A prescription is needed to buy glucagon. It comes in two ways: in a kit or in a box to be mixed. If you use the kit, follow the package instructions.

To prepare glucagon for injection if you do not use a kit:

1. Remove the flip-off seals on bottles 1 and 2. Bottle 1 holds a diluting liquid and bottle 2 holds a white powder.

2. Draw the plunger of an insulin syringe (U-100) back to the 50-unit mark.

3. Steady the smaller bottle with the liquid in it (bottle 1) on the table. Push the needle through the stopper.

4. Inject the air from the syringe into the bottle and then turn the bottle upside down.

5. Withdraw as much of the liquid as possible into the syringe.

6. Remove the needle and syringe from bottle 1 and insert this same needle into bottle 2, the bottle with the powder. Inject all of the liquid from the syringe into bottle 2.

7. Remove the needle and syringe. Shake the bottle **gently** until the glucagon powder dissolves and the liquid becomes clear.

8. Withdraw the entire contents of bottle 2 (the mixed glucagon) into the syringe.

9. Inject the glucagon in the same way you would insulin, using the buttock, thigh, or arm.

10. Turn the person onto one side or stomach. (Vomiting is common after glucagon.)

11. As soon as the person is alert and not feeling sick, he or she should eat something, because glucagon acts for only a short period of time. First, give some juice or a non-diet soft drink, and then additional carbohydrate.

12. If the person does not wake up within 15 minutes, the dose may be repeated. Call an ambulance.

13. Always call the doctor after an insulin reaction when coma or seizure occurs.

14. Check the package of glucagon periodically to be sure that it hasn't passed the expiration date. It's a good idea to keep an insulin syringe taped to the box so it will be ready.

Support Materials

Participant Self-Assessment of Diabetes Management

▶ ▶ ▶ ▶ ▶

Name: _____

Date:_____

Date of Birth: ___/___/___ Age: _____ Gender: ❑ F ❑ M

Ethnic Background: ❑ White/Caucasian ❑ Black/African American ❑ Hispanic

❑ Native American ❑ Middle-eastern

What is your language preference: ❑ English Other_____

Address:_____

      Street   City   ST   Zip

Phone: Home (____)_____Work: (____)_____Mobile: (____)_____

1. What type of diabetes do you have? ❑ Type 1 ❑ Type 2 ❑ Pre-diabetes
   ❑ GDM ❑ Don't Know

2. Year/Age of Diabetes Diagnoses:_____/_____
   List relatives with diabetes: _____

3. Do you take diabetes medications? ❑ Y (check all that apply below) ❑ N
   ❑ Diabetes pills ❑ Insulin injections ❑ Other
   ❑ Symlin injections ❑ Combination of pills and injections
   About how often do you miss taking your medication as prescribed? _____

4. Do you have other health problems? ❑ Y ❑ N
   Please list other conditions: _____

5. Do you take other medications? ❑ Y ❑ N
   Please list other medications:_____
   _____

6. What is the last grade of school you have completed? _____

7. Are you currently employed? ❑ Y ❑ N
   What is your occupation? _____

continued

8. Marital Status: ☐ Single   ☐ Married   ☐ Divorced   ☐ Widowed
How many people live in your household? _____

9. How are they related to you? _____

10. From whom do you get support for your diabetes? ☐ Family   ☐ Co-workers
    ☐ Health care providers   ☐ Support group   ☐ No one

11. Do you have a meal plan for diabetes? ☐ Y   ☐ N
    If yes, please describe: _____
    _____

    About how often do you use this meal plan? ☐ Never   ☐ Seldom   ☐ Sometimes
    ☐ Usually ☐ Always
    Do you read and use food labels? ☐ Y   ☐ N
    Do you have any diet restrictions: ☐ Salt ☐ Fat ☐ Fluid ☐ None ☐ Other _____
    Give a sample of your meals for a typical day:
    Time: _____ Breakfast:_____
    Time: _____ Lunch: _____
    Time: _____ Dinner: _____
    Time: _____ Snack:_____
    Time: _____ Snack: _____

12. Do you: do your own food shopping? ☐ Y ☐ N   Cook your own meals? ☐ Y ☐ N
    How often do you eat out? _____

13. Do you drink alcohol? ☐ Y ☐ N   Type: _____
    How many   per day_____   per week_____ occasionally _____
    Do you use tobacco: ☐ cigarette ☐ pipe ☐ cigar ☐ chewing ☐ none
    ☐ quit—how long ago _____

14. Do you exercise regularly? ☐ Y ☐ N   Type: _____
    How Often:_____
    My exercise routine is: ☐ easy ☐ moderately intense ☐ very difficult ☐ intense

15. Do you check your blood sugars? ☐ Y ☐ N
    Blood sugar range: _____ to _____
    How often: ☐ Once a day ☐ 2 or more/day ☐ 1 or more/Week ☐ Occasionally
    When: ☐ Before breakfast ☐ 2 hours after meals ☐ Before bedtime
    What is your target blood sugar range?_____ _____

continued

16. In the last month, how often have you had a low blood sugar reaction:
❏ Never ❏ Once ❏ One or more times/week
What are your symptoms? _____
How do you treat your low blood sugar? _____

17. Can you tell when your blood sugar is too high? ❏ Y ❏ N
What do you do when your sugar is high?_____

18. Check any of the following tests/procedures you have had in the last 12 months:
❏ dilated eye exam ❏ urine test for protein ❏ dental exam ❏ foot exam—self
❏ foot exam—health care professional ❏ blood pressure ❏ weight ❏ cholesterol
❏ HgA1c ❏ flu shot ❏ pneumonia shot

19. In the last 12 months, have you: ❏ used emergency room services ❏ been admitted to a hospital
Was ER visit or hospital admission diabetes related? ❏ Y ❏ N

20. Do you have any of the following: ❏ eye problems ❏ kidney problems ❏ dental problems
❏ numbness/tingling/loss of feeling in your feet ❏ high blood pressure ❏ high cholesterol
❏ sexual problems ❏ depression

21. Have you had previous instruction on how to take care of your diabetes? ❏ Y ❏ N
How long ago:_____

22. In your own words, what is diabetes? _____
_____

23. How do you learn best: ❏ Listening ❏ Reading ❏ Observing ❏ Doing

24. Do you have any difficulty with: ❏ hearing ❏ seeing ❏ reading ❏ speaking
Explain any checked: _____

25. Do you have any special cultural or religious observancespractices or beliefs that influence how
you care for your diabetes? ❏ Y ❏ N Please describe
_____

26. Do you use computers: to ❏ email ❏ look for health and other information

27. Please state whether you agree, are neutral, or disagree with the following statements:
I feel good about my general health: ❏ agree ❏ neutral ❏ disagree
My diabetes interferes with other aspects of my life: ❏ agree ❏ neutral ❏ disagree
My level of stress is high: ❏ agree ❏ neutral ❏ disagree
I have some control over whether I get diabetes complications or not: ❏ agree
❏ neutral ❏ disagree

continued

I struggle with making changes in my life to care for diabetes: ☐ agree ☐ neutral ☐ disagree

28. How do you handle stress? _____
_____

29. What concerns you most about your diabetes? _____
_____

30. What is hardest for you in caring for your diabetes? _____
_____

31. What are your thoughts or feelings about this issue (e.g., frustrated, angry, guilty)?
_____
_____

32. What are you most interested in learning from these diabetes education sessions?
_____

33. **Pregnancy and Fertility:**
   Are you: ☐ Pre-menopausal ☐ Menopausal ☐ Post-Menopausal ☐ N/A
   Are you pregnant? ☐ Y—When are you expecting? _____
                     ☐ N—Are you planning on becoming pregnant? _____
   Have you been pregnant before? ☐ Y ☐ N
   Do you have any children? ☐ Y—Ages: _____ ☐ N
   Are you aware of the impact of diabetes on pregnancy? ☐ Y ☐ N
   Are you using birth control? ☐ Y—please specify _____ ☐ N

Please do not write below this line
EDUCATOR ASSESSMENT SUMMARY:_____
_____
_____
_____
_____
_____

Education Needs/Education Plan: ☐ Diabetes disease process ☐ Nutritional Management
☐ Physical Activity ☐ Medication Use ☐ Monitoring ☐ Acute Complications
☐ Psychosocial Adjustment ☐ Chronic Complications ☐ Behavior Change Strategies
☐ Health Promotion

Date: _____ Educator Signature: _____

Date: _____ Educator Signature: _____

Diabetes Self-Management Education Record

▶ ▶ ▶ ▶ ▶

Participant Name: _____ **Referring Provider:**_____

Assess/Evaluation Ratings: 1=needs instruction 2= needs review 3=comprehends key points
4=demonstrates competency NC=not covered N/A=not applicable

Topics/ Learning Objectives	Pre-Session Assess	Instr. Date Initial	Reinforce Date Initial	Post-session Evaluation	Comments
Diabetes disease process and treatment process *Define diabetes and identify own type of diabetes; list 3 options for treating diabetes*					
Incorporating nutritional management into lifestyle *Describe effect of type, amount, and timing of food on blood glucose; list 3 methods for planning meals*					
Incorporating physical activity into lifestyle *State effect of exercise on blood glucose levels*					
Using medications safely *State effect of diabetes medicines on diabetes; name diabetes medication taking, action, and side effects.*					
Monitoring blood glucose, interpreting and using results *Identify recommended blood glucose targets and personal targets*					

continued

Topics/ Learning Objectives	Pre-Session Assess	Instr. Date Initial	Reinforce Date Initial	Post-session Evaluation	Comments
Prevention, detection, and treatment of chronic complications *Define the natural course of diabetes and describe the relationship of blood glucose levels to long-term complications of diabetes.*					
Developing strategies to promote health/change behavior *Define the ABCs of diabetes; identify appropriate screenings, schedule, and personal plan for screenings; set behavioral goals and action plans.*					
Developing strategies to address psychosocial issues *Describe feelings about living with diabetes; identify support needed and support network.*					
Prevention, detection, and treatment of acute complications *List symptoms of hyper- and hypoglycemia; describe how to treat low blood sugar and actions for lowering high blood glucose levels*					

continued

Identified barriers to learning/self management: _____
_____
_____

Instruction method: _____
_____
_____

Education materials/Equipment provided: _____
_____
_____

DSMS support plan: _____
_____
_____
_____

Behavioral goals/Action plan: _____
_____
_____
_____

Participant Follow-up Record

▶ ▶ ▶ ▶ ▶

Participant Name: Date:

Reassessment:

Ratings: 1=needs instruction   2=needs review   3=comprehends key points
                    4=demonstrates competency   N/A=not assessed

Topic	Reassessment Rating	Comment/Re-education
Knowledge of Diabetes Disease Process		
Nutritional Management		
Physical Activity		
Medication Use		
Monitoring and Using results		
Acute Complications		
Chronic Complications		
Psychosocial Adjustment		
Behavior Change Strategies		
Health Promotion Strategies		

Goal Evaluation:

Ratings: 0%=never   25%=occasionally   50%=half the time
                    75%=most of the time   100%=always

Goal	Evaluation Rating	Comment
Healthy Eating		
Being Active		
Using Medications Safely		
Monitoring		
Reducing Risks: Acute Complications		
Reducing Risks: Chronic Complications		
Healthy Coping		

New goals/Action plan: _____

_____

Follow-up/DSMS Plan: _____

_____

Educator Signature: _____

© 2009 American Diabetes Association

Curriculum Review Guide

▶ ▶ ▶ ▶ ▶

Content/Topic: _____

Date of last review: _____

Date of current review: _____

Curriculum Review Rubric

Assessment Activities:

Does your CQI activity have any implication for curriculum revision?	Yes	No
Do your program outcomes suggest any need for curriculum revision?	Yes	No
Are there any recurrent participant complaints/feedback regarding the topic?	Yes	No
Has there been any change in participant demographics?	Yes	No

Evaluation of New Information:

Are there any new research findings or publications about this topic?	Yes	No

Summary of Findings:
For any "yes" above, provide detail:

Proposed Revision:

Date of approval: _____

Date of implementation: _____

Sample Educational Objectives

▶ ▶ ▶ ▶ ▶

The following sample illustrates how one program cross-referenced their educational objectives to the curriculum content of *Life with Diabetes*. This documentation is not a requirement for programs applying for Recognition. For Recognition requirements, please visit www.diabetes.org/recognition/education or call 1-800-DIABETES.

Learning and Skill Objectives	Outline
A. Overview/Understanding of Diabetes	
1. States:	1
a. excess glucose in blood due to too little insulin in relationship to body needs.	
b. lifelong condition requiring treatment.	
c. which type of diabetes they have.	
B. Stress and Psychosocial Adjustment	
1. Identifies self as having diabetes.	2
2. Identifies thoughts, feelings, and areas of concern about diabetes.	
3. Identifies personal meaning of diabetes.	
4. Identifies effects of stress on blood glucose.	12
5. Identifies one strategy for coping with stress/feelings related to diabetes.	
6. Identifies signs and symptoms of depression.	
7. Identifies personal diabetes care goals.	15
C. Family and Social Support	
1. Identifies desired level of support from family/friends.	2
2. Informs others of ways they can be supportive.	

Learning and Skill Objectives	Outline
3. Identifies local sources for diabetes support.	16
D. Nutrition and Meal Planning	
1. States:	3
a. reasons for meal planning.	
b. rationale for eating meals on time.	
c. rationale for reaching/maintaining desirable weight.	3, 17
d. rationale for eating less fat.	3, 18
e. awareness of types of fat and effects of each.	18
f. awareness of need to change diet with activity changes.	3, 7
2. Has a meal plan.	5
3. Is able to:	
a. describe personal meal plan.	5, 19
b. use meal plan to plan meals.	5, 19
c. use meal plan when eating away from home.	
d. identify behaviors that help control weight.	17
e. identify eating behaviors that help reduce risk of heart disease.	18
f. plan a sick-day diet.	11
g. explain how alcohol affects blood glucose.	

Learning and Skill Objectives	Outline
h. use product labels to choose foods that fit meal plan.	6
i. explain the benefits and cautions of a high-fiber diet.	18
j. plan eating/behavior changes that work toward personal goals.	15
4. Referral to a dietitian.	3
E. Exercise and Activity	
1. States that exercise/activity lowers blood glucose.	7
2. Identifies personal exercise plan.	
3. Identifies when not to exercise.	
4. Describes exercise snack, if needed.	11
5. Identifies insulin adjustment for exercise if needed.	
6. Identifies monitoring needed for exercise.	
F. Medication	
■ **ORAL HYPOGLYCEMIC AGENTS**	
1. States:	8
a. name and dose of agent.	
b. when to take.	
c. effect on blood glucose.	
d. side effects.	
e. precautions	
■ **INSULIN**	
1. States:	9
a. type(s) and dose to take.	
b. when to take.	
c. onset, peak, and duration.	
d. effect on blood glucose.	
e. when low blood glucose is most likely to occur.	11
f. insulin adjustment plan.	
g. how to store insulin.	9
2. Prepares and administers own insulin correctly.	

Learning and Skill Objectives	Outline
a. gently rolls insulin to mix.	
b. injects air into bottle.	
c. checks for/removes bubbles.	
d. draws up correct dose.	
e. disposes of syringes/ lancets correctly.	
3. Selects appropriate injection site.	
a. selects suitable sub-Q tissue.	
b. states rotation plan.	
4. If using intensive therapy, states:	9
a. benefits of intensive therapy.	
b. type of insulin that affects specific blood glucose levels.	
c. need for frequent blood glucose testing.	
d. personal insulin plan and blood glucose goals.	
G. Monitoring and Use of Results	
■ **BLOOD GLUCOSE**	
1. Demonstrates ability to test blood glucose.	10
a. uses appropriate site to obtain blood samples.	
b. uses correct testing technique.	
c. accurately tests blood glucose.	
d. cares for meter and stores strips properly.	
2. States:	
a. need for monitoring.	
b. plan for monitoring blood glucose and record keeping at home.	
c. target blood glucose levels pre and post meals.	
d. personal goal or target range.	
e. appropriate decisions to make about glucose regulation based on results.	11
f. where to obtain glucose meters and supplies.	10

Learning and Skill Objectives	Outline
3. Defines A1C.	
a. states normal value.	
b. states personal goal.	
■ **URINE KETONE TESTING**	
1. States purpose of urine ketone testing.	10
2. Tests urine ketones:	
a. if blood glucose >300 mg/dl.	
b. if ill or unable to eat.	
c. as otherwise prescribed.	
3. Interprets test results correctly.	
4. States proper action to take for ketonuria.	
5. Stores strips properly.	
H. Managing Blood Glucose	
■ **GLUCOSE CONTROL RELATIONSHIPS**	
1. Identifies factors that influence blood glucose levels.	11
2. Identifies personal behaviors that influence blood glucose levels.	
a. relationship of food intake to blood glucose.	4, 11
b. relationship of diabetes medications to blood glucose.	8, 9, 11
c. relationship of exercise to blood glucose.	7, 11
3. States benefits of improved glucose control.	11, 14
4. States risks of improved glucose control.	11
5. Identifies treatment methods to improve glucose control.	
■ **HYPOGLYCEMIA**	
1. States:	11
a. meaning and other names.	
b. personal/common symptoms.	
1) occurring while awake.	
2) occurring while asleep.	
c. causes and how to prevent.	

Learning and Skill Objectives	Outline
d. when to contact health professional.	
e. proper action to be taken to treat hypoglycemia.	
2. Family member/roommate is able to give glucagon.	
3. Wears/carries diabetes identification.	
■ **HYPERGLYCEMIA**	
1. States:	11
a. meaning and other names.	
b. personal common symptoms.	
c. causes and how to prevent.	
d. states proper action to take and when to contact provider.	
e. relationship of ketoacidosis to high blood glucose.	
I. Personal Health Habits	
1. States:	13
a. body areas most susceptible to infection.	
b. signs/symptoms of infection and treatment measures.	
c. effects of smoking on circulation.	
d. need for foot care.	
e. plan for personal foot care.	
f. need for skin care.	
g. plan for personal skin care.	
h. need for regular dental care.	
i. benefits of regular medical care.	
J. Long-Term Complications	
1. States:	14
a. awareness of potential long-term complications and target organs.	
1) cardiovascular.	
2) peripheral vascular.	
3) sensory neuropathy.	
4) autonomic neuropathy.	
5) retinopathy.	
6) nephropathy.	

Learning and Skill Objectives	Outline
b. symptoms indicating onset of complications and importance of early diagnosis.	
c. ways to prevent, delay, or detect complications.	
d. common diabetes-related sexual concerns, dysfunctions, and treatment methods.	20
K. Problem-Solving and Behavior Change	
1. Identifies problem-solving strategies.	15
2. Identifies personal long-term diabetes care goals.	
3. Identifies personal short-term diabetes care goals.	
4. Identifies personal behavior-change goals.	
5. Identifies strategies to achieve goals.	
L. Health Care Systems	
1. States importance of plans for regular health monitoring.	13
a. diabetes management.	
b. ophthalmological exams.	
c. dental care.	
d. regular physical exams.	
e. other as indicated.	
2. Identifies personal risk factors for complications/health problems.	14
3. States how to obtain driver's license and insurance, and employment rights.	16
4. States awareness of community resources.	16
5. States name(s) and phone number(s) of health professional(s) to contact.	
a. stop smoking.	
b. weight control program.	
c. social worker.	
d. visiting nurse/home health.	
e. dietitian.	

Learning and Skill Objectives	Outline
f. diabetes support group.	
g. education program.	
h. other.	
M. Pregnancy	
1. Preconception.	
a. states importance of normal blood glucose levels before pregnancy.	9
b. states need for thorough medical exam before pregnancy.	
2. Preexisting diabetes	21
a. identifies importance of frequent care for changing insulin/dietary needs.	
3. Gestational diabetes.	21
a. defines as hyperglycemia related to hormonal changes during pregnancy.	
b. states importance of follow-up care after delivery.	
4. Blood glucose control.	
a. states need to maintain glucose levels in the target range throughout pregnancy.	
b. lists symptoms of hyperglycemia and when to call a physician.	
c. states symptoms of hypoglycemia and how to treat.	
5. Prenatal care.	
a. lists danger signs during pregnancy; when to call a physician.	
b. identifies tests to monitor health of mother and infant.	
N. Pump Therapy	
1. States:	22
a. correct name of pump used.	
b. correct type of insulin used.	
c. advantages/disadvantages of pump therapy.	

Learning and Skill Objectives	Outline

d. definition of *basal* and *bolus*; how they relate to normal body physiology.
 	
   e. that bolus insulin is given intermittently throughout the day based on:
      1) meals.
      2) blood glucose levels at time bolus is given.
      3) glucose values out of target range other than at meal times.
   f. how pump will affect lifestyle.
   g. proper equipment to be used.
   h. how often to change equipment.
   i. signs/symptoms/treatment of irritation/inflammation/infection.
   j. what to do with the pump for the following activities: sleeping, sexual activities, bathing, swimming, sports, traveling.
   k. awareness of alarms and how to handle.
   l. hotline phone number for appropriate company.
   m. how to obtain pump supplies.
   n. various ways the pump can be worn.
   o. usual battery life.	

Learning and Skill Objectives	Outline

2. Demonstrates ability to:
   a. administer bolus dose three times.
   b. change basal rate three times.
   c. change battery.
   d. fill pump syringe/cartridge with insulin; place in pump.
   e. attach tubing; check for secure connection.
   f. prime tubing with insulin.
   g. select and prepare suitable infusion site.
   h. correctly insert infusion needle and secure.
   i. check pump for correct/current basal rate program.
   j. program bolus dose based on blood glucose reading.
   k. activate pump to deliver bolus dose.
   l. terminate bolus delivery once dose is activated.
3. Able to recognize signs of possible pump malfunction, and steps to address:
   a. change site; administer bolus with syringe.
   b. telephone pump manufacturer for technical help.
   c. monitor ketones for glucose over 300 mg/dl; respond appropriately.
	22

Supplemental Reading

▶ ▶ ▶ ▶ ▶

Supplemental Reading
Patient Education and Empowerment
Anderson RM, Funnell MM, Hernandez CA: Choosing and using theories in diabetes education research. *The Diabetes Educator* 31:513–520, 2005

Anderson RM, Funnell MM: Patient empowerment: reflections on the challenge of fostering the adoption of a new paradigm. *Patient Education and Counseling* 57:153–157, 2005

Anderson RM, Funnell MM: The art and science of diabetes education: a culture out of balance. *The Diabetes Educator* 34:109–117, 2008

Anderson RM, Funnell MM: *The Art of Empowerment: Stories and Strategies for Diabetes Educators*, 2nd edition. Alexandria, VA: American Diabetes Association, 2005

Belton AB: Conversation maps in canada: the first two years. *Diabetes Spectrum* 139–142, 2008

Berikai P, Meyer PM, Kazlauskaite R, Savoy B, Kozih K, Fogelfeld L: Gain in knowledge of diabetes management targets is associated with better glycemic control. *Diabetes Care* 30:1387–1389, 2007

Cochran J, Conn VS: Meta-analysis of quality of life outcomes following diabetes self-management training. *The Diabetes Educator* 34:815–823, 2008

Funnell MM, Anderson RM, Ahroni JH: Empowerment and self-management after weight loss surgery. *Obesity Surgery* 15:417–422, 2005

Funnell MM, Anderson RM, Austin A, Gillespie SJ: AADE Position Statement: Individualization of diabetes self-management education. *The Diabetes Educator* 33:4549, 2007

Funnell MM, Brown TL, Childs BP, Haas LB, Hosey GM, Jensen B, Maryniuk M, Peyrot, M, Piette, JD, Reader D, Siminerio LM, Weinger K, Weiss MA: National Standards for Diabetes Self-management Education. *Diabetes Care* 30:1630–1637, 2007

Funnell MM, Brown TL, Childs BP, Haas LB, Hosey GM, Jensen B, Maryniuk M, Peyrot, M, Piette, JD, Reader D, Siminerio LM, Weinger K, Weiss MA: National Standards for Diabetes Self-management Education. *The Diabetes Educator* 33:599–614, 2007

Funnell MM, Nwankwo R, Gillard ML, Anderson RM, Tang TS: Implementing an empowerment-based diabetes self-management education program. *The Diabetes Educator* 31:53–61, 2005

Marrero DG, Anerson B, Funnell M, Maryniuk M: *1,000 Years of Diabetes Wisdom*. Alexandria, VA: American Diabetes Association, 2008

Mulvaney SA: Improving patient problems solving to reduce barriers to diabetes self-management. *Clinical Diabetes* 27:99–104, 2009

Peragallo-Dittko V: What's urgent? What's important? An open letter to educators in diabetes. *Diabetes Spectrum* 21:154–193, 2008

Peyrot M, Rubin RR: Access to diabetes self-management education. *The Diabetes Educator* 34:90–97, 2008

Piette JD: Interactive behavior change technology to support diabetes self-management. *Diabetes Care* 30:2425–2432, 2007

Robbins JM, Thatcher GE, Webb DA, Valdmanis VG: Nutritionist visits, diabetes classes, and hospitalization rates and charges. *Diabetes Care* 31:655–660, 2008

Seley J, Weinger K: State of the science on diabetes management: strategies for nursing. *American Journal of Nursing* 70:4–73, 2007

Seley JJ: The state of the science on nursing best practices for diabetes management. *The Diabetes Educator* 33:616–627, 2007

Siminerio LM: Conversation maps. *Practical Diabetology* 26(4):39–40, 2007

continued

Siminerio LM: Innovative approaches to diabetes education. *Diabetes Spectrum* 19:76–109, 2006

Smaldone A, Ganda OP, McMurrich S, Hannagan K, Lin S, Caballero AE, Weinger K: Should group education classes be separated by type of diabetes? *Diabetes Care* 29:1636–1638, 2006

Diabetes Self-management Support

Anderson RM: Taking diabetes self-management education to the next level. *Diabetes Spectrum* 20:202–226, 2007

Funnell MM: Providing diabetes self-management support. *Practical Diabetology* 26(1):46–47, 2007

Tang TS, Funnell MM, Anderson RM: Group education strategies for diabetes self-management. *Diabetes Spectrum* 19:99–105, 2006

Tang TS, Gillard ML, Funnell MM, Nwankwo R, Parker E, Spurlock D, Anderson RM: Developing a new generation of ongoing diabetes self-management support interventions: a preliminary report. *The Diabetes Educator* 31:91–97, 2005

Complementary and Alternative Medicine

Balk EM, Tatsioni A, Lichtenstein AH, Lau J, Pittas AG: Effect of chromium supplementation on glucose metabolism and lipids. *Diabetes Care* 30:2154–2163, 2007

Gebel E: Resveratrol: a miracle molecule? *Diabetes Forecast* 62(5):48–51, 2005

Hamilton SJ, Chew GT, Watts GF: Coenzyme Q10 improves endothelial dysfunction in statin-treated type 2 diabetic patients. *Diabetes Care* 32:810–812, 2009

Jones RA: Complementary and alternative medicine use in diabetes. *Practical Diabetology* 26(2):24–26, 2007

Kleefstra N, Houweling ST, Bakker SJL, Verhoeven S, et al.: Chromium treatment has no effect in patients with type 2 diabetes in a western population. *Diabetes Care* 30:1092–1096, 2007

Neithercott T: The A-to-Z of omega-3. *Diabetes Forecast* 62(2)45–47, 2009

Pagan JA, Tanguma J: Health care affordability and complementary and alternative medicine utilization by adults with diabetes. *Diabetes Care* 30:2030–2031, 2007

White Am, Johnston CS: Vinegar ingestion at bedtime moderates waking glucose concentrations in adults with well-controlled type 2 diabetes. *Diabetes Care* 20:2814–2816, 2007

Special Populations: Cultural Concerns

Anderson RM, Funnell MM, Nwankwo R, Gillard ML, Oh M, Fitzgerald JT: Evaluating a problem-based empowerment program for African Americans with Diabetes: results of a randomized controlled trial. *Ethnicity and Disease* 15:671–678, 2005

Al-Arouj M, Bouguerra R, Buse J, Hafez S, Hassanein M, Ibrahim MA, et al.: Recommendations for management of diabetes during Ramaden. *Diabetes Care* 28:2305–2311, 2005

Anderson-Loftin W, Barnett S, Bunn PS, Sullivan P, Hussey J, Tavakoli A: Soul food light: culturally competent diabetes education. *The Diabetes Educator* 31:555–563, 2005

Brown SA, Blozis SA, Kouzekanani K, Garcia AA, Winchell M, Hanis CL: Health beliefs of Mexican Americans with type 2 diabetes. *The Diabetes Educator* 30:300–308, 2007

Brown SA, Blozis SA, Kouzekanani K, Garcia AA, Winchell M, Hanis CL: Dosage effects of diabetes self-management education for Mexican Americans. *Diabetes Care* 28:527–532, 2005

Caban A, Walker EA, Sanchez S, Mera MS: "It feels like home when you eat rice and beans:" perspectives of urban Latinos living with diabetes. *Diabetes Spectrum* 21:120–127, 2008

Fan T, Koro CE, Fedder Do, Bowlin SJ: Ethnic disparities and trends in glycemic control among adults with type 2 diabetes in the US from 1988 to 2002. *Diabetes Care* 29:1924–1925, 2006

Finucane ML, McMullen CK: Making diabetes self-management culturally relevant for Filipino Americans in Hawaii. *The Diabetes Educator* 34:841–853, 2008

continued

Jack L, Jr., Satterfield D, Rodriguez B, Librud L, Rivera M, Lester A, Burley L, Shane-McWhorter L, Kriska A: AADE Position Statement: Cultural sensitivity and diabetes education: recommendations for diabetes educators. *The Diabetes Educator* 33:41–44, 2007

Look MA, Baumhofer NK, Ng-Osorio J, Furubayashi JK, Kimata C: Diabetes training of community health workers serving Native Hawaiians and Pacific People. *The Diabetes Educator* 34:834–840, 2008

Lorig K, Ritter PL, Villa F. Piette JD: Spanish diabetes self-management with and without automated telephone reinforcement. *Diabetes Care* 31:408–414, 2008

Lujan J, Oswald SK, Ortiz M: Promotora diabetes intervention for Mexican Americans. *The Diabetes Educator* 33:660–670, 2007

McCabe M, Gohdes D, Morgan F, Eakin J, Schmitt C: Training effective interpreters for diabetes care and education. *The Diabetes Educator* 32:714–720, 2006

Rhee MK, Ziemer DC, Caudle J, Kolm P, Phillips LS: Use of a uniform treatment algorithm abolishes racial disparities in glycemic control. *The Diabetes Educator* 34:655–663, 2008

Shin JJ: Insights into type 2 diabetes in Asian-Americans. *Practical Diabetology* 26(1):26–29, 2007

Sixta CS, Ostwald S: Strategies for implementing a promotores-led diabetes self-managment program into a clinic structure. *The Diabetes Educator* 34:285–298, 2008

Sixta CS, Ostwald S: Texas-Mexico border intervention for patients with type 2 diabetes. *The Diabetes Educator* 34:299–309, 2008

Tang TS, Brown MB, Funnell MM, Anderson RM: Social support, quality of life and self-care behaviors among African Americans with type 2 diabetes. *The Diabetes Educator* 34:266–276, 2008

Special Populations: Low Literacy

Gerber BS, Brodsky IG, Lawless KA, Smolin LI, Arozullah AM, Smith EV, Berbaum ML, Hcckerling PS, Eiser AR: Implementation and evaluation of a low-literacy diabetes education computer multimedia application. *Diabetes Care* 28:1574–1580, 2005

Hill-Briggs F, Smith AS: Evaluation of diabetes and cardiovascular disease print patient education materials for use with low-health literate populations. *Diabetes Care* 31:667–671, 2008

Ishkawa H, Takeuchi T, Yano E: Measuring functional, communicative, and critical health literacy among diabetic patients. *Diabetes Care* 31:874–879, 2008

Piette JD: Functional health literacy problems. *Practical Diabetology* 26(2):32–34, 2007

Rothaman RL, Malone R, Bryant B, Wolfe C, Padgett P, DeWait DA, Weinberger M, Pignone M: The spoken knowledge in low literacy in diabetes scale. *The Diabetes Educator* 31:215–224, 2005

Special Populations: Older Adults

Bognef HB, Morales KH, Post EF, Bruce ML: Diabetes, depression, and death. *Diabetes Care* 30:3005-3010, 2008

Kemmis K, Stuber D: Diabetes and osteoporotic fractures. *The Diabetes Educator* 31:187–196, 2005

Munshi M: Diabetes in older adults. *Diabetes Spectrum* 19:218–248, 2006

Munshi M, Grande L, Hayes M Ayres D, et al.: Cognitive dysfunction is associated with poor diabetes control in older adults. *Diabetes Care* 29:1794–1799, 2006

Odegard PS, Setter SM, Neumiller JJ: Pharmacy Updates: considerations for the pharmacological treatment of diabetes in older adults. *Diabetes Spectrum* 202–225, 2007

Ruder K. Aging gracefully. *Diabetes Forecast* 2006; 59(12):45–47.

Ruder K: The aging brain. *Diabetes Forecast* 60(5):22, 2007

Ryan CM, Freed ME, Rood JA, Cobitz AR, Waterhouse BR, Strachan MWJ: Improving metabolic control leads to better working memory in adults with type 2 diabetes. *Diabetes Care* 29:345–351, 2006

Selvin E, Coresh J, Brancati FE: The burden and

continued

treatment of diabetes in elderly individuals in the U.S. *Diabetes Care* 29:2415–2419, 2006

Sinclair AJ, Contry SP, Bayer AJ: Impact of diabetes on physical function in older people. *Diabetes Care* 21:233–235, 2008

Trief PM: Depression in elderly diabetes patients. *Diabetes Spectrum* 20:71–75, 2007

Vaughan N: The ears have it. *Diabetes Self-Management* 27(3):6–14, 2006

Health Care Systems Issues for Diabetes Educators

Barlow S, Crean J, Heizler A, Mulcahy K, Springer J: Diabetes educators: assessment of evolving practice. *The Diabetes Educator* 31:359–372, 2005

Cherrington A, Ayala GX, Amick H, Allison J, Corbie-Smith G, Scarinci I: Implementing the community health worker model within diabetes management. *The Diabetes Educator* 34:824–833, 2008

Davidson MB, Ansari A, Karlan VJ: Effect of a nurse-directed diabetes disease management program on urgent care/emergency room visits and hospitalizations in a minority population. *Diabetes Care* 30:24–227, 2007

Davis AM, Sawyer DR, Vinci LM: The potential of group visits in diabetes care. *Clinical Diabetes* 26:58–62, 2008.

Funnell MM, Anderson RM, Nwankwo R, Gillard ML, Butler PM, Fitzgerald JT: A study of certified diabetes educators: Influences and barriers. *The Diabetes Educator* 32:359–372, 2006

Geil PB: Nutrition practice guideline care improves diabetes outcomes. *Diabetes Spectrum* 17:73–77;83–86, 2004

King A, Wolfe G, Healy S, Lineham T, et al.: Exploring methods to extend the reach of diabetes specialist expertise into primary care clinics. *The Diabetes Educator* 33:525–530, 2006

Krein SL, Funnell MM, Piette JD: Economics of diabetes mellitus. *Nursing Clinics of North America* 41:499–511, 2006

Manchester CS: Diabetes education in the hospital: establishing professional competency. *Diabetes Spectrum* 21:268–271, 2008

Peeples M, Austin MM: Toward describing practice: the AADE National Diabetes Education Practice Survey. *The Diabetes Educator* 33:424–433, 2007

Peterson KA, Radosevich DM, O'Connor PJ, Nyman JA, et al.: Improving diabetes care in practice. *Diabetes Care* 31:2238–2243, 2008

Rogers S: Inpatient care coordination for patients with diabetes. *Diabetes Spectrum* 21:272–75, 2008

Rothman RL, So SA, Shin J, Malone RM, Bryant B, Dewalt DA, et al.: Labor characteristics and program costs of a successful diabetes disease management program. *American Journal of Managed Care* 12:277–283, 2006

Siminerio LM, Piatt G, Emerson S, Ruppert K, et al.:Deploying the chronic care model to implement and sustain diabetes self-management training programs. *The Diabetes Educator* 32:253–261, 2006

Siminerio LM, Piatt G, Zgibor JC: Implementing the chronic care model for improvements in diabetes care and education in a rural primary care practice. *The Diabetes Educator* 31:225–234, 2005

Siminerio LS, Funnell, MM, Peyrot M, Rubin RR: U.S. nurses' perceptions of their role in diabetes care: results of the cross-national Diabetes Attitudes, Wishes and Needs (DAWN) study. *The Diabetes Educator* 33:152–162, 2007

Wylie-Rossett J, Tobin JN, Davis N: Revised 2005 Diabetes Quality Improvement checklist. *The Diabetes Educator* 31:669–675, 2005

Resources for People with Diabetes

▶ ▶ ▶ ▶ ▶

DIABETES ORGANIZATIONS
American Diabetes Association
1701 N. Beauregard Street
Alexandria, Virginia 22311
800-232-3472 (membership information)
800-232-6733 (to order publications)
703-549-1500 (National Center)
www.diabetes.org

For information on local chapters and their activities, consult your local white pages.

For information about diabetes, call
800-DIABETES (342-2383)

The American Dietetic Association
To speak with a dietitian, find a dietitian in your area, or order free information:
120 S. Riverside Plaza, Suite 2000
Chicago, IL 60606-6995
800-877-1600
www.eatright.org

Canadian Diabetes Association
1400-552 University Avenue
Toronto, Ontario, M5G 2R5
800-226-8464
www.diabetes.ca

JOURNALS FOR PEOPLE WITH DIABETES

Diabetes Forecast (monthly magazine)
American Diabetes Association; subscription included with ADA membership
800-806-7801
http://www.diabetes.org

Diabetes Health (monthly newspaper)
415-488-1141
www.diabeteshealth.com

Diabetes Self-Management (bimonthly magazine)
800-234-0923 (Customer Service)
www.diabetesselfmanagement.com

Voice of the Diabetic (magazine)
410-296-7760
www.nfb.org

INFORMATION ABOUT EDUCATIONAL MATERIALS
National Diabetes Education Clearinghouse (NDIC)
1 Diabetes Way
Bethesda, MD 20892
301-654-3327
www.yourdiabetesinfo.org

CHILDREN WITH DIABETES
Children with Diabetes Organization
8216 Princeton-Glendale Rd
West Chester, OH 45069
www.childrenwithdiabetes.com

DIABETES IDENTIFICATION

ID Technology, Inc.
117 Nelson Road
Baltimore, MD 21208
1-877-432-2637
www.id-technology.com

Lifetag, Inc.
5857 North Mesa, Suite 19
El Paso, TX 79912
888-543-3824
www.lifetag.com

continued

Medic Alert Foundation U.S.
2323 Colorado Ave.
Turlock, CA 95382
888-633-4298
www.medicalert.org

Goldware
1667-B, S Khei RD
Khei, HI 96753
800-669-7311

Identifind
(iron-on labels for clothing)
PO Box 567
Canton, NC 28716
828-648-6768
www.identifind.com

INSULIN SUPPLIES

Antares Pharma, Inc.
13755 First Avenue North
Minneapolis, MN 55441

Medicool
20460 Gramercy Place
Torrence, CA 90501
(manufactures and sells insulin cases)
800-433-2469
www.medicool.com

Medi-ject Corporation (manufacturer of a needle-free insulin injector)
800-328-3077
www.mediject.com

Patton Medical
(injection port)
3108 N Lamar Blvd
Austin, TX 78705
877-763-7678
www.i-port.com

INSURANCE COVERAGE

John Hall and Associates
P.O. Box 14868
Shawnee Mission, KS 66285-4868
913-268-7878

RESEARCH STUDIES

Centerwatch
100 N. Washington
Suite 301
Boston, MA 02114
617-948-5100
www.centerwatch.com

PRESCRIPTION ASSISTANCE

Partnership for Prescription Assistance
1-888-477-2669
www.pparx.org

SENIOR CITIZENS

American Association of Retired Persons
National Headquarters
601 E Street, NW
Washington, DC 20049
1-888-687-2277
www.aarp.com

Children of Aging Parents
PO Box 167
Richboro, PA 18954
800-227-7294
www.caps4caregivers.org

National Association of Area Agencies on Aging
1720 Rhode Island Ave, NW, Suite 1200
Washington, DC 20036
202-872-0888
www.n4a.org

continued

National Institute on Aging
Resource Directory for Older People
National Institute on Aging
Building 31, Room 5C27
31 Center Drive
Bethesda, MD 20892
301-496-1752
www.nia.nih.gov

National Association for Home Care
228 7th St, NE
Washington, DC 20003
202-547-7424
www.nahc.org

SPORTS/ATHLETICS
Diabetes Exercise & Sports Association
10216 Taylorsville Rd
Louisville, KY 40299
800-898-4322
www.diabetes-exercise.org

TRAVEL
International Association for Medical Assistance to Travelers
1623 Military Rd, #279
Niagara Falls, NY 14304
716-754-4883
www.iamat.org

Resources for Health Professionals

▶ ▶ ▶ ▶ ▶

EDUCATIONAL MATERIALS AND RESOURCES

Altschul Group Corporation
1560 Sherman Avenue, #100
Evanston, IL 60201
847-328-6700
www.marita.com

Braille Translations
20 Roszel Rd
Princeton, NJ 08540
866-732-3585
http://www.rfbd.org

Centers for Disease Control
4770 Buford Highway, NE
Atlanta, GA 30341
800-223-4636
www.cdc.gov

Centerwatch
100 N. Washington, Suite 301
Boston, MA 02114
617-948-5100
www.centerwatch.com

Children with Diabetes
8216 Princeton-Glendale Rd
West Chester, OR 45069
www.childrenwithdiabetes.com

Health Literacy Project
Providence, RI 02903
401-946-7887
www.RIHLP.org

IDC Publishing
3800 Park Nicollet Blvd.
St. Louis Park, MN 55416
888-637-2675
www.parknicollet.com

Leap Program
P.O. Box 2910
Merrifield, VA 22116
888-ASK-HRSA
www.hrsa.gov/leap

Milner-Fenwick
119 LakeFront Drive
Hunt Valley, MD 21093
800-432-8433
www.milner-fenwick.com

National Diabetes Education Program (NDEP)
1 Diabetes Way
Bethesda, MD 20814
888-693-6337
www.ndep.nih.gov

National Guideline Clearinghouse
www.guideline.gov

National Library of Medicine
8600 Rockville Pike
Bethesda MD, 20894

National Oral Health Information Clearinghouse
1 NOHC Way
Bethesda, MD 20892
301-402-7364
www.nidcr.nih.gov

continued

FOOD MODELS

National Dairy Council
10255 W. Higgins Rd., Suite 900
Rosemont, IL 60018
www.nationaldairycouncil.org

Nasco
P.O. Box 901
901 Janesville Avenue
Ft. Atkinson, WI 53538-0901
800-558-9595
www.enasco.com/nutrition

Wisconsin Dairy Council
175 Patrick Blvd, Suite 201
Brookfield, WI 53045
262-432-0686
www.wisdairy.com

DIABETES ORGANIZATIONS

**American Association of Diabetes
  Educators**
200 W. Monroe St., Suite 800
Chicago, IL 60606
800-338-3633 or 312-644-4411
www.diabeteseducator.org

American Diabetes Association
1701 N. Beauregard Street
Alexandria, VA 22311
800-806-7801 (membership information)
800-232-6733 (to order publications)
www.diabetes.org

American Dietetic Association
120 S. Riverside Plaza, Suite 2000
Chicago, IL 60606-6995
800-877-1600
www.eatright.org

American Heart Association
7272 Greenville Avenue
Dallas, TX 75231
800-242-2721
www.americanheart.org

Canadian Diabetes Association
1400-522 University Ave
Toronto, Ontario, M5G 2R5
Canada
800-226-8464
www.diabetes.ca

International Diabetes Center
5000 West 39th Street
Minneapolis, MN 55416
888-825-6315

Joslin Diabetes Center
One Joslin Place
Boston, MA 02215
617-732-2400
www.joslin.org

PUBLICATIONS FOR HEALTH PROFESSIONALS

*Diabetes, Diabetes Care, Diabetes Spectrum,
Clinical Diabetes*
American Diabetes Association

The Diabetes Educator
American Association of Diabetes Educators

Journal of the American Dietetic Association
The American Dietetic Association

Diabetes Dateline
National Diabetes Information Clearinghouse
www.diabetes.niddk.nih.org

Practical Diabetology
Rapaport Publishing, Inc.
150 W 22nd Street, Suite 800
New York, NY 10011
212-989-0200
www.practical-diabetology.com

Insulin
Exerpta Medica
685 US-202
Bridgewater, NJ 08807
www.insulinjournal.com

Other Titles from the American Diabetes Association

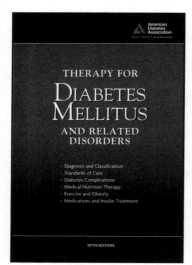

Therapy for Diabetes Mellitus and Related Disorders, 5th Edition

by Harold E. Lebovitz, MD, Editor

For years, Therapy for Diabetes Mellitus and Related Disorders has helped diabetes care professionals deliver proven treatments to their patients. Leading diabetes experts from around the world have contributed to this new revision, offering their insight on new advances in diabetes management and control. Get the latest details on glycemic control, prevention and management of complications, treatment of diabetes in specific populations, information on the newest medications, and much more.

Order no. 5402-04; Price $69.95

Complete Nurse's Guide to Diabetes Care, 2nd Edition

edited by Belinda Childs, ARNP, MN, CDE, BC-ADM, Marjorie Cypress, PhD, MSN, RN, C-ANP, CDE, and Geralyn Spollett, MSN, C-ANP, CDE

Nurses need the latest and most comprehensive diabetes information at hand. This completely revised edition of *Complete Nurse's Guide to Diabetes Care* covers the entire diabetes care continuum for nurses, whether they work in hospitals, clinics, home health care settings, physicians' offices, or nursing schools. This essential resource covers the fundamentals of diabetes care, guidelines for management of acute and chronic complications, risk factors, diabetes in specific populations, and psychological issues.

Order no. 5423-02; Price $59.95

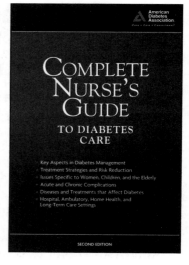

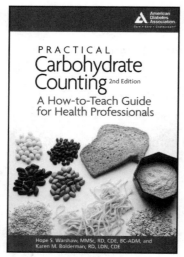

Practical Carbohydrate Counting, 2nd Edition

by Hope S. Warshaw, MMSc, RD, CDE, BC-ADM, and Karen M. Bolderman, RD, LDN, CDE

Written for all clinicians working in diabetes care and education, this second edition of *Practical Carbohydrate Counting* will be your go-to-tool when patients want to improve their glucose control with medical nutrition theraphy. This resource provides clear and practical approaches that will allow you to help your patients achieve glycemic control with Basic or Advanced Carbohydrate Counting.

Order no. 5619-02; Price $22.95

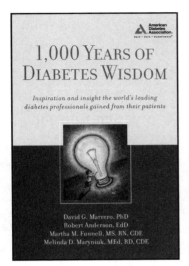

1,000 Years of Diabetes Wisdom

edited by David G. Marrero, PhD; Robert Anderson, EdD; Martha M. Funnell, MS, RD, CDE; and Melinda D. Maryniuk, MEd, RD, CDE
This anthology of more than 50 stories focuses on the other side of treating diabetes—what providers can learn from their patients. With more than 1,000 combined years of patient care experience, the contributors share their knowledge and foresight and the life-altering experiences that both challenge and change the way providers care for their patients.
Order no. 5435-01; Price $19.95

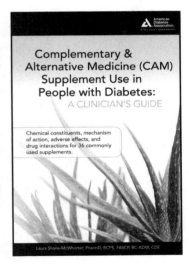

Complementary and Alternative Medicine (CAM) Supplement Use in People with Diabetes

by Laura Shane-McWhorter, PharmD, BCPS, FASP, BC-ADM, CDE
Patients are often interested and excited by the prospects of complementary and alternative medicine supplementation. Keep yourself informed of this growing field, so you-and your patients-can make the safest, most effective decisions when it comes to CAM use.
Order no. 5433-01; Price $39.95

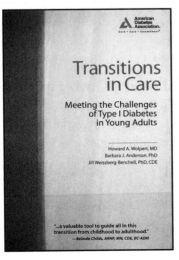

Transitions in Care

by Howard A. Wolpert, MD; Barbara J. Anderson, PhD; and Jill Weissberg-Benchell, PhD, CDE
Transitions in Care serves as a coaching manual for health care providers and parents, and as a guide to self-care and independence for young adults with diabetes. It demystifies a complicated period in a life with type 1 diabetes and makes the passage to adulthood easier for everyone involved.
Order no. 5438-01; Price $24.95

Order this and other American Diabetes Association books and resources for health care professionals at **http://store.diabetes.org** or by calling **1-800-232-6733.**

Provide better outcomes for your patients • Be compensated for more reimbursable services • Grow your practice

Come to the American Diabetes Association for your Education Program Recognition

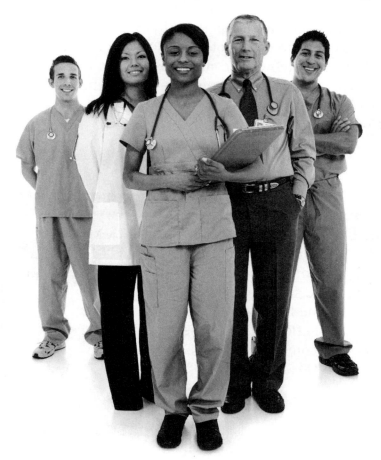

ADA supports your program with our expertise and experience:

ADA's Education Recognition Program provides your staff with tested program guidance and educational tools for optimal operational efficiency—helping your patients successfully learn how to manage their disease and helping you achieve program sustainability.

ADA sets the standards:

As the leader in diabetes treatment and education, ADA annually authors *Clinical Practice Recommendations*—a supplement in *Diabetes Care* that outlines the Standards of Care in Diabetes. ADA also publishes consumer and technical titles written by recognized experts that inform and update you on diabetes care tools and help you achieve the best in patient care and outcomes.

ADA delivers new patients to your practice:

ADA can deliver through the power of a brand rated 15th in the top 100 U.S. nonprofit organizations; through its network of 90 plus nationwide field offices; through its inbound national call center; and through its website. ADA has 450,000 consumer members and 16,500 professional members—nearly a half million people relying on the Association for guidance and advice.

For more information, contact ADA's Education Recognition staff:

**Call 1-888-232-0822
Or visit www.diabetes.org/erp**